GRAVES' DISEASE

PATHOGENESIS AND TREATMENT

ENDOCRINE UPDATES
Shlomo Melmed, M.D., Series Editor

1. E.R. Levin and J.L. Nadler (eds.): Endocrinology of Cardiovascular Function. 1998. ISBN: 0-7923-8217-X
2. J.A. Fagin (ed.): Thyroid Cancer. 1998. ISBN: 0-7923-8326-5
3. J.S. Adams and B.P. Lukert (eds.): Osteoporosis: Genetics, Prevention and Treatment. 1998. ISBN: 0-7923-8366-4.
4. B.-Å. Bengtsson (ed.): Growth Hormone. 1999. ISBN: 0-7923-8478-4
5. C. Wang (ed.): Male Reproductive Function. 1999. ISBN 0-7923-8520-9
6. B. Rapoport and S.M. McLachlan (eds.): Graves' Disease: Pathogenesis and Treatment. 2000. ISBN: 0-7923-7790-7.

GRAVES' DISEASE

PATHOGENESIS AND TREATMENT

edited by

Basil Rapoport, M.B., Ch.B.

and

Sandra M. McLachlan, Ph.D.

Autoimmune Disease Unit
Cedars-Sinai Research Institute
and U.C.L.A. School of Medicine
Los Angeles, California, USA

KLUWER ACADEMIC PUBLISHERS
BOSTON/DORDRECHT/LONDON
2000

Distributors for North, Central and South America:
Kluwer Academic Publishers
101 Philip Drive
Assinippi Park
Norwell, Massachusetts 02061 USA
Telephone (781) 871-6600
Fax (781) 871-6528
E-Mail <kluwer@wkap.com>

Distributors for all other countries:
Kluwer Academic Publishers Group
Distribution Centre
Post Office Box 322
3300 AH Dordrecht, THE NETHERLANDS
Telephone 31 78 6392 392
Fax 31 78 6546 474
E-Mail <orderdept@wkap.nl>

 Electronic Services <http://www.wkap.nl>

Library of Congress Cataloging-in-Publication Data

Graves' disease: pathogenesis and treatment / edited by Basil Rapoport and Sandra M. McLachlan.
    p. ; cm. – (Endocrine updates ; 6)
    Includes bibliographical references and index.
    ISBN 0-7923-7790-7 (alk.paper)
    1.   Graves' disease. I. Rapoport, Basil, 1943- II. McLachlan, Sandra M., 1940- III.. Series.
    [DNLM: 1. Graves' Disease. WK 265 G7753 2000]
    RC657.5 G725 2000
    616.4'43—dc21

                                                     00-024806

Printed on acid-free paper.

Printed in the United States of America

CONTENTS

CONTRIBUTORS

R. A. Ajjan
Division of Clinical Sciences, University of Sheffield, Northern General Hospital, Sheffield , United Kingdom

Osamah Alsanea
Department of Surgery, UCSF/ Mount Zion Medical Center, San Francisco, California, USA

Marcello Bagnasco
Allergy and Clinical Immunology Service, Department of Internal Medicine (DI.M.I.), University of Genoa, Genoa, Italy

Rebecca S. Bahn
Mayo Medical School, Mayo Clinic/Foundation, Rochester, Minnesota, USA

James R. Baker, Jr.
Division of Allergy, Department of Internal Medicine, University of Michigan Medical School, Ann Arbor, Michigan,

Luigi Bartalena
Dipartimento di Endocrinologia, University of Pisa, Pisa, Italy

Lewis E Braverman
Division of Genetics, Brigham and Women's Hospital, Boston, Massachussets, USA

Kenneth D. Burman
Department of Medicine, Washington Hospital Center, Washington, DC, USA

Orlo H. Clark
Department of Surgery, UCSF/ Mount Zion Medical Center, San Francisco, California, USA

Sabine Costagliola
Institut de Recherche en Biologie Humaine et Nucleaire, Universite Libre de Bruxelles, Brussels, Belgium

Terry F. Davies
Division of Endocrinology and Metabolism, Department of Medicine, Mount Sinai School of Medicine, New York, New York, USA

Wolfgang H. Dillmann
Division of Endocrinology and Metabolism, Department of Medicine, University of California, San Diego, San Diego, California USA

Peter H.K. Eng
Division of Genetics, Brigham and Women's Hospital, Boston, Massachussetts, USA

Milton D. Gross
Division of Nuclear Medicine and Department of Internal Medicine, University of Michigan and Department of Veterans Affairs Health Systems, Ann Arbor, Michigan, USA

John E. Freitas
Division of Nuclear Medicine and Department of Internal Medicine, University of Michigan and Department of Radiology, St. Joseph Mercy Hospital, Ann Arbor, Michigan, USA

Michael M. Kaplan
Departments of Medicine and Nuclear Medicine, William Beaumont Hospital, Royal Oak, Michigan, USA

John H Lazarus
Department of Medicine, University of Wales College of Medicine, Heath Park, Cardiff, Wales, United Kingdom

Marian Ludgate
Department of Medicine, University of Wales College of Medicine, Heath Park, Cardiff, Wales, United Kingdom

Claudio Marcocci
Dipartimento di Endocrinologia, University of Pisa, Pisa, Italy

J. Maxwell McKenzie
Department of Medicine, University of Miami School of Medicine, Miami, Florida USA

Donald A. Meier
Department of Nuclear Medicine, William Beaumont Hospital, Royal Oak, Michigan, USA

Paola Montagna
Allergy and Clinical Immunology Service, Department of Internal Medicine (DI.M.I.), University of Genoa, Genoa, Italy

Francesca Paolieri
Allergy and Clinical Immunology Service, Department of Internal Medicine (DI.M.I.), University of Genoa, Genoa, Italy

Giampaola Pesce
Allergy and Clinical Immunology Service, Department of Internal Medicine (DI.M.I.), University of Genoa, Genoa, Italy

David Phillips
MRC Environmental Epidemiology Unit, University of Southampton, Southampton, United Kingdom

Aldo Pinchera
Dipartimento di Endocrinologia, University of Pisa, Pisa, Italy

Matthew D. Ringel
Department of Medicine, Washington Hospital Center, Washington, DC, USA

Claudia Salmaso
Allergy and Clinical Immunology Service, Department of Internal Medicine (DI.M.I.), University of Genoa, Genoa, Italy

B. Shapiro
Division of Nuclear Medicine and Department of Internal Medicine, University of Michigan and Department of Veterans Affairs Health Systems, Ann Arbor, Michigan, USA

James C. Sisson
Division of Nuclear Medicine and Department of Internal Medicine University of Michigan, Ann Arbor, Michigan, USA

Scott A. Rivkees
Department of Pediatrics, Pediatric Endocrinology, Yale University School of Medicine, New Haven, Connecticut, USA

Clark Sawin
Department of Medicine, Boston University School of Medicine, Boston, Massachusetts, USA.

Terry J. Smith
Division of Molecular and Cellular Medicine, Departments of Medicine and Biochemistry and Molecular Biology, Albany Medical College and the Department of Veterans Affairs Medical Center, Albany, NY, USA

Yaron Tomer
Division of Endocrinology and Metabolism, Department of Medicine,
Mount Sinai School of Medicine, New York, New York, USA

Gilbert Vassart
Institut de Recherche en Biologie Humaine et Nucleaire, Universite Libre de
Bruxelles, Brussels, Belgium

Robert Volpé
Department of Medicine, University of Toronto, Toronto, Ontario, Canada

Leonard Wartofsky
Department of Medicine, Washington Hospital Center, Washington, DC, USA

P. F. Watson
Division of Clinical Sciences, University of Sheffield, Northern General Hospital,
Sheffield, United Kingdom

Anthony. P. Weetman
Division of Clinical Sciences, University of Sheffield, Northern General Hospital,
Sheffield, United Kingdom

Peiqing Wu
Division of Allergy, Department of Internal Medicine, University of Michigan
Medical School, Ann Arbor, Michigan, USA

Margita Zakarija
Department of Medicine, University of Miami School of Medicine, Miami, Florida,
USA

PREFACE

Graves' disease is a common disorder afflicting only humans that generates mixed emotions among patients, the clinicians who treat them and the investigators who study its pathogenesis. On the one hand, patients are relieved to be told that Graves' disease is eminently treatable. On the other hand, many are uncomfortable with the prospect of receiving radiation to their thyroids, the need for lifelong post-therapeutic monitoring and the likelihood that another disease, hypothyroidism, will ensue requiring indefinite thyroid hormone replacement. Patients learn that therapy is not synonymous with cure. To the clinician, caring for a patient with uncomplicated Graves' disease is deeply satisfying because of the effectiveness of the therapeutic modalities in reversing thyrotoxicosis. At the same time, the development of severe ophthalmopathy can be a therapeutic nightmare with none of the options being totally satisfactory.

From the perspective of the investigator, Graves' disease is a fascinating disorder with unique features and opportunities for study. The discovery in 1956 that Graves' disease was caused by a humoral factor, later shown to be an antibody to the TSH receptor was a triumph for modern investigative medicine. To our knowledge, spontaneously arising stimulatory autoantibodies to a receptor are unique to Graves' disease. Unlike in many other autoimmune diseases, identification of a single antigenic target, the ability to assay autoantibodies thereto, and the availability of affected tissue with infiltrating lymphocytes provide unparalleled opportunities for investigation. Rapid progress is being made in (i) understanding the molecular interaction between autoantibodies and the TSH receptor, (ii) identifying the genes that contribute to the predisposition to disease, (iii) developing an animal model of Graves' disease and, (iv) identifying the long sought for orbital antigen in ophthalmopathy. Investigations are also progressing rapidly in immunological areas such as apoptosis.

However, a number of major challenges and frustrations remain. For example, (i) generation of recombinant TSH in a form that can be recognized by autoantibodies has been particularly difficult, (ii) the very low precursor frequency of B and T lymphocytes specific for the TSH receptor is a major impedence to characterization of the humoral and T cell-related processes, (iii) the genetic contribution towards developing Graves' disease may be less than previously anticipated and unraveling a relatively weak polygenic background is a daunting undertaking, and (iv) there is still no spontaneous animal model of Graves' disease to rival the utility of the NOD mouse in diabetes mellitus type I. Even in regard to current therapy in standard use for fifty years, much remains to be learned, for example the effect of radioiodine on ophthalmopathy and the immune response to thyroid antigens.

The chapters in this book represent the viewpoints of many prominent clinicians and investigators working in the field. To all, we are grateful for their contributions which cover an unusually comprehensive compendium of subjects relating to the disease. As for the Wright brothers viewing the space shuttle, it would be wonderful to observe the responses of Parry, Graves and von Basedow were they to learn the consequences of their initial clinical insight. Moderately satisfactory treatment has blunted public pressure to 'target' Graves' disease for intensive investigation, perhaps more in the USA than in Europe and in Asia. Nevertheless, the core of dedicated clinicians and investigators that remain focused on this disease feel a special privilege in treating and studying such a remarkable condition. Indeed, lessons learned from Graves' disease may prove valuable for understanding other more fashionable autoimmune diseases. If the progress made from 1956 until the present is repeated in the next 44 years we will be well on the way to the ultimate goal of some form of immunotherapy that will make antithyroid drugs, radioiodine and thyroidectomy obsolete.

Basil Rapoport and Sandra M. McLachlan

GRAVES' DISEASE

PATHOGENESIS AND TREATMENT

1

GRAVES' DISEASE - A HISTORICAL PERSPECTIVE

Robert Volpé and Clark Sawin

INTRODUCTION

While the eponym "Graves' disease" has been generally accepted (at least in the English-speaking world) as the appropriate designation for a condition that we might more properly term "autoimmune hyperthyroidism" or "toxic diffuse goiter", we will continue to employ "Graves' disease" in this chapter, despite the lack of universal agreement regarding this designation and the dispute about the attribution of credit for the original description (see below). We will attempt to provide a historical perspective regarding these matters.

GRAVES' DISEASE IN ANTIQUITY

There is mention of exophthalmos as early as the fifth century BC in writings by Aristotle and Xenophon (1). Abu-l-Fadail Ismail ibn al-Husain al Jurjani, a Persian, completed his system of medicine dedicated to the Shah of Khwarizm, a *Treasure of Medicine,* in 1110 AD (1). In this work, the combination of exophthalmos with goiter is clearly described, although whether this truly represented Graves' disease cannot be determined. Byzantine writers also knew of this combination in the tenth century (2) although once again, one cannot be certain regarding the nature of these cases. Thereafter the field appeared to lay fallow for several hundreds of years, although occasional references by several authors suggest the possibility that they were dealing with Graves' disease .

GRAVES' DISEASE IN THE EIGHTEENTH AND NINETEENTH CENTURIES

In the eighteenth century, and the beginning of the nineteenth century, there were a few reports of patients with exophthalmos and goitre in which the authors did not appear to realize the significance of the connection. Charles de Saint-Yves (1687-1733) mentioned the combination of exophthalmos and goiter as early as 1722 (3) . Guiseppe Flajani (4) (1741-1822) of Ascoli, Italy in 1802 reported on his successful therapy of two patients with exophthalmic goiter, without apparently realizing the significance of the three manifestations, i.e., exophthalmos, goiter, and palpitations, in relation to one another. Flajani's first patient was a young Spanish man living in Rome, age 22, who developed protrusion of the eyes and a "tumor" in the front of the neck, as well as "extraordinary palpitation in the region of the heart". Flajani treated the patient's "tumor" with compresses of vinegar and ammonia, and the tumor resolved within four months. His second case, a young woman with goiter and palpitations, but apparently no eye signs, was treated similarly.

Antonio Testa (5) (1756-1814), Professor of Medicine and Surgery at Ferrara, and Professor of Medicine at Bologna, Italy, made reference in 1800 to the coincidence of prominent eyes and disease of the heart, but this association did not seem to have any significance for him. He was considered to be "a learned theorist, but a mediocre clinician" and by his own writings, was "prone to digressions more curious than useful" (6,7).

While the above observations were tantalizing, credit for the first, truly classical description of exophthalmic goiter should go to Caleb Hillier Parry (1755-1822) a well-known, affluent physician and sheep farmer of Bath, England (8) who treated his first case in 1786. However, the publication of this and subsequent cases was delayed until 1825, three years after Parry's death, when his son finally published these case reports (9). The first patient was a 37 year-old woman who developed palpitations, tachycardia, and goiter a few months after childbirth. "Her eyes protruded from their sockets ... each systole of the heart shook the whole trunk of the body" (this appears to be the first known example of post-partum exophthalmic goiter). His second case, observed in 1802, was precipitated by an acute stress, a type of disease induction that continues to fascinate and interest investigators to this day (10). In 1813, Parry came to realize that there was probably some connection between the malady of the heart and the bronchocele (goiter). He speculated that the condition was probably a type of heart disease, and the goiter developed because the thyroid had to act as a reservoir for the extra blood pumped out by the heart. It should be pointed out, however, that the publication of these reports did not gain much attention at the time (1).

When Robert James Graves (1796-1853) first described three women with goiter and palpitations at the Meath Hospital in Dublin, Ireland, in his lectures during the academic year 1834-1835, he had no idea what was wrong with them, except that they had an odd combination of findings. None of these women had prominent eyes; but, by the time that he published his cases, he had heard of a fourth patient observed by his colleague and friend, William Stokes (1804-1878). This fourth patient did have bulging eyes. Thus the published report by Graves in 1835 (11) described a syndrome of tachycardia and goiter, and now with exophthalmos. Neither Graves nor Stokes knew of the prior publication by Parry, but came independently to the view that these manifestations constituted a syndrome. They thought that it was a form of heart disease, mainly because the most prominent and disturbing complaint was the rapid and powerful heartbeat.

Graves' published series in 1835 raised no more interest than that of Parry's ten years earlier (1). Graves, however, an authoritative figure in Irish medicine (12,13) published a textbook on clinical medicine in 1843 (14), with a second edition in 1848 (15), and this book was read widely in the United Kingdom and Europe. It reprinted in revised form his previously published lectures, including the one on goiter, palpitations and exophthalmos. Most Europeans thought that the textbook of Graves contained his first description of the disease. Stokes (16) in his classic *Diseases of the Heart* published twenty years after Graves' 1835 report recorded a fuller description of the disorder, and framed the cardiac theory more formally than did Graves'.

On the European continent, FP Pauli (17) appears to have published a similar case in 1837. But the most important and accurate European account of this condition was given in 1840 by Carl Adolph von Basedow (18) (1799-1854) of Merseburg, Germany, in a paper entitled "Exophthalmos durch Hypertrophie des Zellgewebes in der Augenhoehle (Exophthalmos caused by hypertrophy of the cellular tissue in the orbit)". His emphasis was certainly on the orbital abnormalities, but he did also mention emaciation, sweating, diarrhea, nervous restlessness, air hunger, and tremor. He also noted a brawny, non-edematous swelling of the legs (localized myxedema). His description of three women and one man with exophthalmos, goiter, and palpitations, gave rise to the phrase "The Merseburg triad". He did not provide a coherent theory regarding causation of the disease.

Basedow did a reasonable search of previous cases, taking note of Parry's and Flajani's cases. Yet he missed Graves' report, leading some Europeans to credit Basedow with the first description of this condition. (The terminology applied to this entity varies regionally to this day, as will be discussed further below.) A physician at St. Bartholomew's Hospital in London, J. Wickham Legge (1843-1921) was later (1882) (19) very critical of Basedow, stating that Basedow's emphasis on the ocular manifestations downplayed the significance of the thyroid and the palpitations. However, Legge was being somewhat unfair in view of the fact that Basedow had introduced the term 'Merseburg triad' to account for all three components.

In France, the first clear description was provided by Jean Martin Charcot (20) (1825-1893) in 1857, reporting on one patient and seven necropsies, and connecting palpitation, goiter, exophthalmos and tremor; he termed it 'cachexia exophthalmica'. Charcot felt that the palpitations were the most important feature, and that, along with the tremor, a neurologic causation seemed to be implicated. He reviewed all the available literature in a reasonable fashion, but, like Basedow, he failed to include the report of Graves' from 1835. He thus initially agreed with the eponymic designation of Basedow's disease for this disorder.

In 1862, an extended discussion of the disease at the French Academy of Medicine over successive meetings took place, in which many theories of etiology and terminology were brought up (1). Armand Trousseau (21) (1801-1867), then the doyen of French medicine, had studied the work of Graves, including his textbook of medicine, and considered Graves' to be a great physician. He strongly disagreed with the eponym Basedow's disease, because Graves' description had preceded that of Basedow's by a decade, and because Trousseau wished to honor Graves', who at this time had been dead for almost ten years. Actually, Trousseau would have preferred no eponym at all, but it was clear that the term exophthalmic goiter was unsatisfactory, because many patients had no obvious exophthalmos, and a few had no obvious goiter. Trousseau argued strongly for the designation, 'Graves' disease', and his authoritative influence prevailed. Curiously, it did so mainly in English-speaking countries.

Basedow's name by then had become entrenched in most of Europe as a designation for this entity, and remains so today (6,7). Occasionally, in Italian circles, the disease is referred to as 'Flajani's disease' (6,7). It should also be added that in 1898, Sir William Osler (22,23) (1849-1919) in the third edition of his textbook of medicine changed his mind from his second edition and gave the eponymic credit to Parry, whose description should indeed take precedence over that of Graves. In our view, the condition *should* be termed Parry's disease. However, it is probably too late to stem the tide of history, and we will thus continue with common usage. Graves', it is!

THE NATURE OF THE TOXIC GOITER

The idea that hypersecretion of a ductless gland , such as the thyroid, might cause disease in the form of Graves' disease was first put forward by Paul Julius Moebius (24) (1853-1907) in 1886, and supported by William Smith Greenfield (25) (1846-1919) who described histological hyperplasia of the thyroid in 1893. Ludwig Rehn (26) (1847-1930) in 1884 also proposed increased glandular activity as the basis for Graves' disease as a result of the following considerations: the enlargement of the thyroid gland in Graves' disease; the production of symptoms resembling Graves' disease by excessive doses of thyroid gland substance; and the evidence of histological hyperplasia of the thyroid gland. Somewhat later, the recognition that acromegaly represented excess function of the pituitary helped to permit acceptance that excess glandular function did occur.

Other data supported this view. For example, Friedrich von Mueller (27) (1858-1941) in 1893 showed a negative nitrogen balance in Graves' disease, and Adolf Magnus-Levy (28) (1865-1955) in 1895 found that oxygen consumption was increased, but returned to normal after cure.

As to the various theories regarding causation, the reader is referred to the reviews by Sawin (1), Henneman (29), and Solomon (30) who have detailed the evolution of thought regarding etiology of Graves' disease in the nineteenth and early twentieth century. As mentioned above, Parry (9), and separately, Graves' (11,14,15) and Stokes (16), considered the entity to be primarily of cardiac origin. On the other hand, Charcot (20) and Trousseau (21), among others, held to the view that the condition was neural in nature. Indeed , Trousseau thought it to be a neurosis analogous to hysteria. However by the end of the nineteenth century, with the advent of the ideas of Rehn (26), Moebius (24) and Magnus-Levy (28), and the occasional successes of thyroidectomy for Graves' disease, the centrality of the thyroid as the causative factor took hold. The idea that the thyroid made too much thyroid hormone began to prevail, leading to the term 'hyperthyroidism' in the first decade of the twentieth century (31). However, the neural theory died hard, particularly when psychic stress as a precipitating factor was considered (the probable place of stress in the induction of Graves' disease will be mentioned below).

Before the final acceptance of the eponymic designation for Graves' disease, the nineteenth century certainly had been marked by considerable confusion regarding terminology for this entity. Albert H. Iason (32) in 1946 recorded the following collection of terms that had been proposed or utilized for this condition: 1)

Exophthalmus hystericus (Brueck), 1835; 2) Exophthalmos bronchocele (Laycock), 1838; 3) Die Glotzaugen (Basedow), 1848; 4) Glotzaugencachexie (Basedow) 1848; 5) Cachexie exophthalmique (Charcot) 1856; 6) Exophthalmus anemicus (Prael), 1857; 7) Cachexia exophthalmica (Withuisen), 1858; 8) Cardiogmus strumosus s. Morbus Basedowii (Hirsch), 1858; 9) Maladie de Basedow (Charcot), 1859; 10) Goitre exophthalmique (Trousseau), 1860; 11) Morbus Gravesii (Mannheim), 1864; 12) Exophthalmic goitre (Hamill), 1861; 13) Nevrose thyro-exophthalmique (Corlieu), 1863; 14) Struma exophthalmica (Begbie), 1868; 15) Tachycardia strumosa exophthalmica (Lebert), 1872; 16) Morbo del Flajani (Pensutti) 1887; 17) Morbo di Flajani (Bacelli and De Renzi), 1887; 18) Cachexia thyroidienne (Gauthier), 1888; 19) Hystérie thyroidienne (Pader), 1899 and 20) Parry's disease (Osler), 1898. Iason also collected a list of the many theories regarding the etiology of this disease in the nineteenth century, the most important of which have already been discussed.

GRAVES' DISEASE IN THE TWENTIETH CENTURY

In the early twentieth century, while there remained significant morbidity and mortality, thyroidectomy had become a mainstay in the treatment for Graves' disease. Although iodine had been used inconsistently in the treatment of Graves' disease in the nineteenth century, its use did not constitute the consensus of opinion. Indeed Trousseau (33), commenting on this matter, mentioned that he had accidentally prescribed iodine in one case, and it was efficacious; nevertheless he stated that its use was dangerous and could not be recommended. However, by 1924, Plummer and Boothby (34), perhaps acting on prior suggestions by David Marine (see Means' obituary of Marine (35), regularized the use of preoperative iodine before subtotal thyroidectomy for Graves' disease, thus greatly improving the margin of safety.

While, therefore, thyroidectomy remained the focus of treatment for Graves' disease in the early part of this century, new understanding of the role of the pituitary gland was beginning to change the attitude about thyroid gland control. By the mid-1930s, thyrotropin (or thyroid stimulating hormone) was recognized as a separate anterior pituitary hormone,, and it was not long before it was proposed that excess pituitary TSH constitutes the cause of Graves' disease (36). Even so, it did not influence treatment which remained then (and now) thyroid-centered. The idea of a cause external to the thyroid gland persisted, however. Two decades later, in 1956, there was a breakthrough: Adams and Purves (37) were attempting to improve the measurement of TSH, using a bioassay in guinea pigs. They found a stimulator in the serum of patients with Graves' disease, that was initially thought to be an abnormal TSH (38) because it stimulated the thyroid gland for a much longer period than did TSH. This work was confirmed by McKenzie in 1958 (39) using mice as the assay model. The stimulator was initially called Long Acting Thyroid Stimulator (LATS) (40). Kriss et al. in 1964 (41) demonstrated clearly that LATS was an immunoglobulin G, i.e. an antibody. Although LATS could not be demonstrated in all Graves' patients, this proved to be a matter of species specificity and sensitivity, as shown by Onaya et al. (42). These investigations initiated the field of autoimmunity in relation to Graves' disease. For several years, the work was antibody-centered, but in 1972 it was proposed that Graves' disease was a disease of 'delayed hypersensitivity', i.e. a T-lymphocyte disorder in immunoregulation (43). Since that time, studies of Graves' disease have produced a voluminous literature, with innumerable advances in immunology, immunogenetics, experimental models, and immuno-interventions. The role of stress, mentioned earlier in this chapter, may well have its impact on precipitating the disorder by down-regulating the immune system (10,44). The immune nature of Graves' ophthalmopathy is currently under intense investigation.

As for therapeutics in the modern era, the two most important developments took place in the 1940's. In 1938, Hertz and Roberts introduced radioactive iodine (^{131}I) for the diagnosis of Graves' disease (45), and later (1942) for its treatment (46). In 1943, Astwood (47) employed thiourea and thiouracil in the medical treatment of Graves' disease, thus initiating the era of antithyroid drug therapy. Although no new significant therapeutic modalities have been introduced over the last fifty years, we are at least coming to a fuller understanding of the effects, immunological and otherwise, of our current therapy.

While it would appear that the era of Autoimmunity in Graves' disease is now fully ensconced, it is prudent to consider the past, and how we have arrived at this point. Clearly, there has been no straight line progression. The line of the future is unlikely to be any straighter, and, for all we know, new ideas of the cause and cure of Graves' disease may be in the offing.

REFERENCES

1. **Sawin CT.** 1998 Theories of causation of Graves' disease: a historical perspective. Endocr Metab Clin N Amer. 27:63.
2. **Marketos SG, Eftchiadis A, and Koutras DA.** 1983 The first recognition of the association between goiter and exophthalmos. J Endocrinol Invest. 6:401.
3. **de St. Yves C.** 1722 (In English, 1741) Nouveau traité des maladies des yeux, Le mercier, Paris.
4. **Flajani G.** 1802 Sopra un tumor freddo nell'anterior partedell collo detto bronchocele. In: Collezione d'osservazione e riflessioni di chirurgia. Roma 3: 270.
5. **Testa A.** 1800 Collezione d'osservazioni e refflessini di chirurgie, Roma and 1811 Traité des maladies de coeur, Paris.
6. **Rolleston HD.** 1936 The endocrine organs in health and disease, with a historical review. 1936 Oxford University Press, London.
7. **Medvei VC.** 1982 A history of endocrinology. MTP Press, Lancaster, England.
8. **Volpé R.** 1994 The life of Caleb Hillier Parry. Endocrinologist 4:157.
9. **Parry CH.** 1825 Collections from the unpublished medical writings, London, Underwoods 2:110.
10. **Volpé R.** 1999 The immunology of human autoimmune thyroid disease. In: The autoimmune endocrinopathies, Contemporary Endocrinology Series, ed. Volpé R, Humana Press, Totowa, New Jersey, p.218.
11. **Graves RJ.** 1835 Clinical lectures delivered at the Meath Hospital during the session of 1834-5. Lecture XII. London Med Surg J. 7:513.
12. **Taylor S.** 1989 Robert Graves: The golden age of Irish medicine, Roy Soc Med Services Limited, London.
13. **Coakley D.** 1996 Robert Graves: Evangelist of clinical medicine, Irish Endocr Soc, Dublin.
14. **Graves RJ.** 1843 Clinical lectures on the practice of medicine, Dublin, Fannin.

15. **Graves RJ**. 1848 Clinical lectures on the practice of medicine, second edition, ed. Neligan JM, Dublin, Fannin.
16. **Stokes W**. 1854 Diseases of the Heart and Aorta, Dublin, Hodges and Smith.
17. **Pauli FP**. 1837 A case of exophthalmos. Med Ann Heidelberg. 3:218.
18. **Basedow CA**. 1840 Exophthalmos durch Hypertrophie des Zellgewebes in der Augenhohle. Wochenschr Ges Heilk 6:197-204, 220-228.
19. **Legge JW**. 1882 Notes on the history of exophthalmic goitre. St. Bartholomew's Hosp Rep. 18:7.
20. **Charcot JM**. 1857 Memoire sur une affection caracterisé par les palpitation du coeur et les arteres, la tumefaction de la glande thyroide et une double exophthalmie. C R Mem Soc Biol. 3:43.
21. **Trousseau A**. 1862 Discussion sur le goitre exophthalmique, Gazette Hebdomadaire de Medicine et de Chirurgie pp. 472, 492, 554.
22. **Osler W**. 1898 Principles and Practice of Medicine, third edition, D. Appleton and Co., New York. p. 836.
23. **Hoffenberg R**. 1985 The thyroid and Osler. J Roy Coll Phys Lond. 19:80.
24. **Moebius PJ**. 1886 Book Review. Ueber das Wesen der Basedowschen Krankheit. Arch Psychiatrie. 17:301.
25. **Greenfield WS**. 1893 Bradshaw Lecture, Roy Coll Phys. Br Med J. 2:1493 and 1553.
26. **Rehn L**. 1884 Uber die Estirpation des Kropfs bei Morbus basedowii. Berlin Klin Wochenschr. 21:163.
27. **Mueller, F**. 1893 Beitraege zur Kentniss der Basedow'schen Krankheit. Dtsch Arch Klin Med. 51:335.
28. **Magnus-Levy A**. 1895 Ueber den respiratorischen Gaswechsel unter dem Einfluss der Thyroidea sowie unter verschiedenen pathologischen Zustaenden. Berlin Klin Wochenschr. 32:650.
29. **Hennemann G**. 1991 Historical aspects about the development of our knowledge of morbus Basedow. J Endocrinol Invest. 14:617.
30. **Solomon DH, Kleeman KE**. 1976 Concepts of the pathogenesis of Graves' disease. Adv Intern Med. 22:273-299.
31. **Elliott AR**. 1907 Hyperthyroidism. Am J Med Sci. 134:390.
32. **Iason AH**. 1946 The Thyroid Gland in Medical History. Froben Press, New York, p. 85.
33. **Trousseau A**. 1868 Lectures on Clinical Medicine. London, New Sydenham Soc. 2:587.
34. **Plummer HS and Boothby WM**. 1924 The value of iodine in exophthalmic goitre. J Iowa Med Soc. 14:66-73.
35. **Means JH**. 1961 The Association of American Physicians: its first seventy-five years. McGraw-Hill, New York.
36. **Salter WT**. 1940 The Endocrine Function of Iodine, Cambridge, Harvard University Press. p. 86.
37. **Adams DD, Purves HD**. 1956 Abnormal responses to the assay of thyrotrophin. Proc Univ Otago Med Sch. 34:11.
38. **Adams DD**. 1988 Long-acting thyroid stimulator: How receptor autoimmunity was discovered. Autoimmunity. 1:3.
39. **McKenzie JM**. 1958 Delayed thyroid response to serum from thyrotoxic patients. Endocrinology. 62:865.
40. **McKenzie JM**. 1960 Bioassay of thyrotropin in man. Physiol Rev. 40:398.
41. **Kriss JP, Pleshakov V, Chien JR**. 1964 Isolation and identification of the long acting thyroid stimulator and its relation to hyperthyroidism and circumscribed pretibial myxedema. J Clin Endocrinol Metab. 24:1005.
42. **Onaya T, Kotani M, Yamada Y,Ochi Y**. 1973 New in vitro tests to detect the thyroid stimulator in sera from hyperthyroid patients by measuring colloid droplet formation and

cyclic AMP in human thyroid slices. J Clin Endocrinol Metab. 36:859.

43.   **Volpé R, Edmonds MW, Lamki L, Clarke PV, and Row VV.** 1972 The pathogenesis of Graves' disease: A disorder of delayed hypersensitivity? Mayo Clin Proc. 47:824.

44.   **Glaser R and Kiecolt-Glaser JK.** 1994 Handbook of human stress and immunity. Academic Press, London.

45.   **Hertz S, Roberts A, Evans RD.** 1938 Radioactive iodine as an indicator in the study of thyroid physiology. Proc Soc Exp Biol Med. 38:510.

46.   **Hertz S and Roberts A**. 1942 Application of radioactive iodine in therapy of Graves' disease. J Clin Invest. 21:624.

47.   **Astwood EB.** Treatment of hyperthyroidism with thiourea. 1943 J Amer Med Assoc. 122:78.

2

EPIDEMIOLOGY OF GRAVES' DISEASE

David Phillips

INTRODUCTION

It has been estimated that over 3 million Americans currently have Graves' disease of whom over 41,000 are children (1). Graves' disease is associated with considerable morbidity, a decrease in quality of life and sufferers incur considerable health care costs. Yet the disease has been neglected by epidemiologists and as a result relatively little is known about its prevalence in the population and its social or biological antecedents.

EPIDEMIOLOGY

Disease incidence

The incidence of Graves' disease has been estimated by surveys based on the retrospective analysis of medical records or by setting up disease registers in which new cases are detected through endocrine referral services. These studies tend to underestimate the frequency of the disease as patients with mild or subclinical disease who do not get diagnosed will not be included. An additional problem is that surveys based on patients attending endocrine clinics or other referral centers may be misleading as the referral of patients to these services tends to be selective and incomplete. Finally, while there have been a number of studies of the overall incidence of hyperthyroidism, only a few have separated Graves' disease from the other major causes of hyperthyroidism, for example toxic nodular goiter and toxic adenoma. Despite these problems, estimates of the incidence of Graves' disease in a variety of studies in different countries using different methodology are remarkably consistent. They suggest an annual incidence of between 15 and 20 cases of Graves' disease per 100,000 population (Table 1).

In most of the studies, Graves' disease was identified by a case-finding approach. The extensive study from the United States is based on the unified medical care system for Olmsted County, Minnesota which has accumulated comprehensive clinical records for the population of a defined geographical area over many years (2). Several of the other studies used a similar approach, ascertaining new cases by a search of hospital records supplemented by a questionnaire to local medical practitioners. The two United Kingdom studies, however, identified cases through biochemical or nuclear medicine laboratories carrying out thyroid function tests on the basis that the diagnosis of hyperthyroidism would not be reached without measurement of thyroid hormones (3,4). Graves' disease was distinguished from other causes of thyrotoxicosis by the use of thyroid scintiscanning to identify diffuse goiter, the identification of TSH receptor binding antibodies, or a combination of clinical and investigative features suggestive of Graves' disease such as the presence of ophthalmopathy, a diffuse goiter or high titers of antimicrosomal antibody.

Table 1. Estimates of the incidence of Graves' disease

		Annual incidence/100,000			
Country	**Period**	**Total**	**Female**	**Male**	**Reference**
USA	1935-67	19.8	36.8	8.3	Furszfer (2)
Iceland	1938-67	11.4	-	-	Thjodleifsson (5)
Sweden	1970-74	17.7	27.2	7.4	Berglund (6)
Denmark	1980-82	14.8	-	-	Laurberg (7)
Iceland	1980-82	19.3	-	-	Haraldsson (8)
UK	1982	15.4	21.3	7.6	Phillips (4)
New Zealand	1983-85	14.9	23.4	6.2	Brownlie (9)b
UK	1989	15.9	25.8	5.5	Cox (3)

The studies carried out after 1980 are most comparable because of the introduction of specific immunoassay techniques for measuring total and free thyroxine concentrations to establish the diagnosis of hyperthyroidism. A consistent finding of all the studies is the excess disease incidence in women. Incidence rates in women were between 21.3 and 36.8/100,000 compared with 5.5 to 8.3/100,000 in men. Although the disease may occur at any age, Graves' disease presents most commonly between the third and fifth decades of life. The study from Minnesota reported a peak age-specific incidence on the 20-39 year old age group (2). Surveys in the United Kingdom and Europe report somewhat later peaks in the 40-49 and 45-54 year old group respectively (3,4,7).

Seasonality

Several studies have reported a seasonal variation in the presentation of patients with Graves' disease. This was observed in European studies dating back to the 1920's as well as more recent studies from the United States, the United Kingdom, and New Zealand (9-11). These studies suggest that cases tend to present in the spring and early summer months both in the northern and southern hemisphere. The most obvious explanation of this trend is that higher summer temperatures cause the symptoms of hyperthyroidism to be less well tolerated so that patients are more likely to seek medical attention. However, there are other possible explanations. In a study in the United Kingdom it appeared that the onset as well as the presentation of the disease was seasonal with a peak period of onset from January to June (11). It was suggested that a winter increase in the iodine content of the diet could have triggered the disease in some patients. The winter increase in dietary iodine intake is well recognized in northern European countries and is due to the practice of supplementing cattle feed with iodine during the winter months (12).

Time trends

One of the striking features of the earlier literature on thyroid disease are the numerous accounts of epidemics of hyperthyroidism. Although some of these undoubtedly resulted from the introduction of iodine prophylaxis and the precipitation of iodine-induced thyrotoxicosis in people with autonomous thyroid nodules, the phenomenon also affects patients with Graves' disease. The best-described occurred during the Second World War in occupied Denmark. Iversen described a four-fold rise in the incidence of thyrotoxicosis associated with diffuse goiter between 1941-43 (13). There was no apparent cause and, in particular, no evidence of a change in dietary iodine intake before the epidemic. Changes in the incidence of Graves' disease have been observed more recently but again without apparent explanation (3).

Geographical distribution

Very little is known about variations in the incidence of Graves' disease in different countries and in different ethnic groups. It appears to be rare in underdeveloped countries. Trowell encountered only two cases among native Africans during 29 years as a physician in Uganda and Kenya (14). However, there is evidence from a South African study that the incidence of the disease increased markedly in Black Africans during the 1970's (15). The data in **Table 1**, however, suggest that the incidence of this disease is rather similar in Caucasian populations surveyed North and South of the Equator. In a 10 year study of 599 patients with the disease living in Stoke on Trent, United Kingdom, incidence rates tended to be lower in the rural than urban areas but the frequency of the disease was unrelated to social class, population density or overcrowding (3). There was no tendency for cases to cluster geographically or show space-time clustering which would have suggested an infective etiology. Other evidence suggests that differences in dietary iodine intake may be linked with differences in the incidence of Graves' disease. In a comparative study in Iceland and East-Jutland, Denmark, Laurberg and colleagues showed that the incidence of Graves' disease was higher in Iceland (19.7/100,000) than Denmark (14.8/100,000)(7). The difference was particularly marked in the younger age-group among whom the incidence of Graves' disease was two-fold higher in Iceland. As both populations had a similar genetic background and lived in countries with similar medical care provision, the authors suggested that the higher iodine intake of the Icelandic population may have contributed to their higher disease incidence.

Graves' Ophthalmopathy

Until recently very little was known about the epidemiology of Graves' ophthalmopathy. In a recent study based on the case records of residents of Olmsted county, Minnesota, the incidence of this condition was estimated to be 16 cases per 100,000 per year in women and 2.9 per 100,000 in men (16). The age-specific incidence rates were bimodal in both sexes peaking in the 40 to 44 and 60 to 64 year old age groups in women but five years later in men. Hyperthyroidism occurred in over 90 percent of the cases and autoimmune thyroiditis in three percent. Six percent had no evidence of thyroid dysfunction. For reasons which are not clear the severity of the disease increases with the age of presentation. Race also seems to be an important determinant of Graves' ophthalmopathy as Caucasians are six times more likely to develop eye signs in association with Graves' disease compared with Asians (17).

ETIOLOGY

Although much is now understood about the pathogenesis of Graves' disease, the etiology of the disease is still poorly understood. While hereditary factors are important in explaining the susceptibility to Graves' disease there is increasing evidence that environmental factors play an important part in precipitating the disease. There is now evidence for the operation of a number of factors including smoking, stressful life events, infective agents, iodine, and therapeutic radiation of the neck.

Smoking

Hagg and Asplund were the first to describe an association between smoking and Graves' disease (18). They found that 10 out of 12 patients with Graves' ophthalmopathy and 11 out of 24 patients Graves' hyperthyroidism with only minimal or no evidence of ophthalmopathy were smokers compared with 13 out of a group of 42 control subjects. The association between smoking and Graves' disease has now been observed in six studies, the risk of Graves' disease associated with smokers being between 1.5 and 2.4 fold increased (18-23). A metanalysis of the studies (Fig. 1) suggests a combined relative risk of 1.7 (95% CI 1.4 to 2.1). The association is particularly strong in patients with Graves' ophthalmopathy where the relative risk in smokers is estimated at between 2.2 and 10.5 (combined risk 4.2, 95% CI 3.4 to 5.2). Some studies suggest that there is a dose-response relationship with smoking, although this is not a universal finding (21,22). It is striking, however, that autoimmune thyroiditis which shares many common immunological antecedents with Graves' disease is not associated with smoking (19).

The mechanism linking smoking with Graves' disease is not clear. It is possible that smoking merely reflects a behavioral change resulting from the hyperthyroidism in affected subjects. However, where smoking status has been assessed prior to the onset of the disease, the association between smoking and and disease persisted (22). Another possibility is that smoking may mediate it's effects by directly influencing immune function. Evidence from both human studies and animal experiments suggest that smoking is associated with defects in both immune surveillance and cytokine release and activity (19). Finally, it has been suggested that smoking acts to increase the risk of ophthalmopathy in Graves' disease rather than precipitating the disease *per se*. Although a number of studies suggest that the association between smoking and Graves' disease exists in the absence of clinically apparent eye disease, it has been argued that many of these patients have subclinical forms of eye disease. At present this question is not yet resolved.

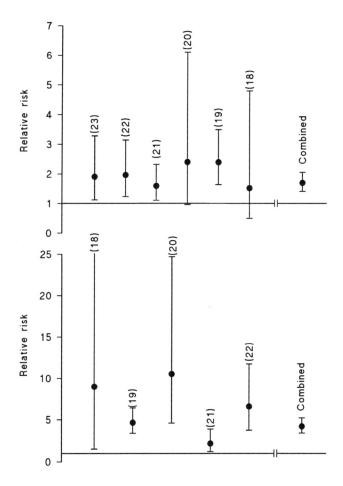

Figure 1. Upper panel – relative risk of Graves' disease in smokers compared with non-smokers in six separate studies. Lower panel - relative risk of Graves' ophthalmopathy in smokers compared with non-smokers in five studies. The combined relative risk is shown in each case.

Stress

Since Caleb Parry's 1825 description of the case of Elizabeth S (24), who two weeks after falling out of a wheel chair went on to develop the classical signs and symptoms of hyperthyroidism, there have been numerous anecdotal reports that stressful events may contribute to the etiology of Graves' disease (25). In practice, however, the role of stress in the etiology of Graves' disease has been difficult to prove and the problem of demonstrating cause and effect remains. Earlier studies failed to show associations between stress and the development of Graves' disease (26). However a recent study from Sweden showed that in 208 newly diagnosed Graves' disease, patients had more negative life events in the year preceding the onset of their hyperthyroidism and significantly higher life event scores than the control group (27). Similar findings were reported in a studies from Italy, the United Kingdom, Hong Kong and Japan, although in the latter study the associations were restricted to women (23,28-30). A major difficulty in these studies is the problem of recall bias. It is well known that patients will tend to assume that negative life events immediately preceding a disease were the cause of that disease. Thus at present no firm conclusions can be drawn although the increasing realization of the existence of neuroendocrine immunological interactions makes the possibility more likely.

Infective agents

A 10-year large-scale study of patients with Graves' disease in the United Kingdom showed that there was no evidence of clustering in space and time, suggesting that infections which occur in an epidemic manner are unlikely to be important precipitators of the disease (3). Nevertheless a body of evidence has suggested that infection could trigger the development of Graves' disease. Some of the strongest evidence relates to an association with *Yersinia enterocolitica* infection. A number of studies have demonstrated the presence of thyroid antibodies in patients with *Y. enterocolitica* infection (31). In addition, significant antibody titres to *Y. enterocolitica* have been reported in patients with Graves' disease (32) although this association is not present in all populations studied (33). The idea is also encouraged by the finding that *Y. enterocolitica* has a hormone-specific binding site for mammalian TSH which resembles the TSH receptor in the human thyroid gland (34). This finding raises the possibility that *Yersinia* infection could precipitate Graves' disease by a process of molecular mimicry. At present, however, the question as to whether infectious agents contribute to the development of Graves' disease remains unanswered.

Iodine

Increasing evidence suggests that the dietary iodine supply plays an important part in determining the incidence and form of hyperthyroidism in the community. It is well established that regions of the world which were formerly iodine deficient but now have an adequate iodine supply have a high incidence of toxic nodular goiter. Thus in regions where the iodine supply has been historically plentiful, Graves' disease accounts for almost all the cases of hyperthyroidism, whereas in areas with a history of iodine deficiency and endemic goiter, toxic nodular goiter may be the most common form of hyperthyroidism (35).   This difference is illustrated by data from the United

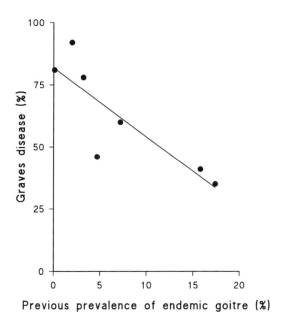

Figure 2. Percentage of cases of thyrotoxicosis due to Graves' disease (as indicated by TSH-receptor antibody positivity) in seven English towns according to the prevalence of endemic goiter 60 years previously. In towns which were historically iodine sufficient nearly 100% of cases of hyperthyroidism were due to Graves' disease, whereas in towns with a history of endemic goiter Graves' disease accounted for less than half of the cases (39).

Kingdom (Fig. 2) showing how the current proportion of cases of hyperthyroidism due to Graves' disease is dependent on the previous pattern of iodine deficiency. It is less certain, however, whether the current dietary iodine intake influences the prevalence of Graves' disease.

There is substantial evidence that the change from iodine deficiency to iodine sufficiency is associated with an increase in lymphocytic infiltration of the thyroid gland and an increase in the prevalence of circulating thyroid autoantibodies.   In addition iodine supplementation increases the prevalence of thyroiditis in strains of animals and birds susceptible to spontaneous autoimmune thyroiditis (36). Long term studies of countries with iodine deficiency which have iodized salt have produced conflicting data as to whether iodization alters the prevalence of Graves' disease. In the United States, Furzyfer et al. (2) reported no increase in the prevalence of Graves' disease despite the increasing use of iodized salt. In contrast, a more recent study from Austria reported a twofold increase following salt iodization in 1990 (37). The idea is also supported by a comparison of hyperthyroidism in Iceland and Denmark which suggested that historically iodine–replete Iceland has a higher incidence of Graves' disease than Denmark which has lower iodine intakes (7). There is, however, much more evidence that iodine may affect the rate of recurrence of Graves' disease. Patients with Graves' disease given iodine supplementation after discontinuation of treatment with antithyroid drugs are more likely to have relapses than patients not given iodine (36). This phenomenon may explain the gradual decrease in the remission rate for Graves' disease in the United States where iodine intakes are now high.

Neck irradiation

In a study of 1787 patients treated for Hodgkin's disease and followed for up to 25 years after diagnosis, 30 patients developed Graves' hyperthyroidism of which 17 had ophthalmopathy (38). This corresponds to an increased risk of Graves' disease of 7.2 (95% CI 4.8 to 9.6) based on the normal population incidence data in Olmsted County, Minnesota, and 20.4 (13.5 to 27.3) on the more recent data from Malmo. Most of the patients had received radiation therapy suggesting a link between neck irradiation and Graves' disease.

Concluding remarks

There is a clear need for more information about the epidemiology of Graves' disease. The studies carried out so far have generated some important clues, especially the link between smoking and ophthalmopathy and the possible role of stress. Future etiological studies need to be take account of the role of immunogenetic susceptibility and the interaction between this and environmental determinants. Graves' disease is not only a significant health problem in its own right but is also a fascinating paradigm for the study of other autoimmune disorders.

REFERENCES

1. **Jacobson DL, Gange SJ, Rose NR, Graham NMH**. 1997 Epidemiology and estimated population burden of selected autoimmune diseases in the United States. Clin Immunol Immunopathol. 84:223-243.
2. **Furszyfer J, Kurland LT, McConahey WM, Elveback LR**. 1970 Graves' disease in Olmsted county, Minnesota. 1935 through 1967. Mayo Clin Proc. 45:636-644.
3. **Cox SP, Phillips DIW, Osmond C**. 1989 Does infection initiate Graves disease?: a population based 10 year study. Autoimmunity. 4:43-49.
4. **Phillips DIW, Barker DJP, Rees Smith B, Didcote S, Morgan D**. 1985 The geographical distribution of thyrotoxicosis in England according to the presence or absence of TSH-receptor antibodies. Clin Endocrinol. 23:283-287.

5. **Thjodleifsson B**. 1975 A study of Graves' disease in Iceland. Acta Med Scand. 198:309-314.
6. **Berglund J, Christensen SB, Hallengren B**. 1990 Total and age-specific incidence of Graves' thyrotoxicosis, toxic nodular goitre and solitary toxic adenoma in Malmö 1970-74. J Int Med. 227:137-141.
7. **Laurberg P, Pedersen KM, Vestergaard H, Sigurdsson G**. 1991 High incidence of multinodular toxic goitre in the elderly population in a low iodine intake area vs. high incidence of Graves' disease in the young in a high iodine intake area: comparative surveys of thyrotoxicosis epidemiology in East-Jutland Denmark and Iceland. J Lab Clin Med. 229: 415-420.
8. **Haraldsson A, Gudmundsson ST, Larusson G, Sigurdsson G**. 1985 Thyrotoxicosis in Iceland 1980 - 1982. Acta Med Scand. 217:253-258.
9. **Brownlie BEW, Wells JE**. 1990 The epidemiology of thyrotoxicosis in New Zealand: incidence and geographical distribution in North Canterbury. Clin Endocrinol. 33:249-259.
10. **Westphal SA**. 1994 Seasonal variation in the diagnosis of Graves' disease. Clin Endocrinol. 41:27-30.
11. **Phillips DIW, Barker DJP, Morris JA**. 1985 Seasonality of thyrotoxicosis. J Epidem Commun Health. 39:72-74.
12. **Phillips DIW**. 1997 Iodine, milk and the elimination of endemic goitre:the story of an accidental public health triumph. J Epidem Commun Health. 51:391-393.
13. **Iversen K**. 1948 Temporary rise in the frequency of thyrotoxicosis in Denmark. Copenhagen: Rosenkilde & Bagger.
14. **Trowell HC**. Non-infective disease in Africa. 1960 London: Edward Arnold, p286
15. **Kalk WJ**. 1981 Thyrotoxicosis in urban black Africans: a rising incidence. S Afr J Med. 52:109-116.
16. **Bartley GB, Fatourechi V, Kadrmas EF, et al**. 1995 The incidence of Graves' ophthalmopathy in Olmsted County, Minnesota. Amer J Ophthal. 120:511-517.
17. **Tellez M, Cooper J, Edmonds C**. 1992 Graves' Ophthalmopathy in relation to cigarette smoking and ethnic origin. Clin Endocrinol. 36:291-294.
18. **Hagg E, Asplund K**. 1987 Is endocrine ophthalmopathy related to smoking? Brit Med J. 295:634-635.
19. **Bartalena L, Bogazzi F, Tanda ML, Manetti L, Dell'Unto E, Martino E**. 1995 Cigarette smoking and the thyroid. Eur J Endocrinol. 133:507-512.
20. **Shine B, Fells P, Edwards OM, Weetman AP**. 1990 Association between Graves' ophthalmopathy and smoking. Lancet. 335:1261-1263.
21. **Winsa B, Mandahl A, Karlsson FA**. 1993 Graves' disease, endocrine ophthalmopathy and smoking. Acta Endocrinol (Copenh). 128:156-160.
22. **Prummel MF, Wiersinga WM**. 1993 Smoking and risk of Graves' disease. JAMA. 269:479-482.
23. **Yoshiuchi K, Kumano H, Nomura S, et al**. 1998 Stressful life events and smoking were associated with Graves' disease in women, but not in men. Psychosom Med. 60:182-185.
24. **Caleb Hillier Parry**. 1932 Hyperthyroidism. In: Major RH, ed. Classic descriptions of disease. Oxford: Blackwell, pp 275-279.
25. **Hobbs JR**. 1992 Stress and Graves' disease. Lancet. 339:427-428.
26. **Gray J, Hoffenberg R**. 1985 Thyrotoxicosis and stress. Q J Med. 54:153-160.
27. **Winsa B, Adami HO, Bergstrom R, et al**. 1991 Stressful life events and Graves' disease. Lancet. 338:1475-1479.
28. **Sonino N, Girelli ME, Boscaro M, Fallo F, Busnardo B, Fava GA**. 1993 Life events in the pathogenesis of Graves' disease. A controlled study. Acta Endocrinol (Copenh).

128:293-296.

29. **Kung.A.W.** 1995 Life events, daily stresses and coping in patients with Graves' disease. Clin Endocrinol. 42:303-308.

30. **Harris T, Creed F, Brugha TS**. 1992 Stressful life events and Graves' disease. Br J Psychiatry. 161:535-541.

31. **Gripenberg M, Miettinen A, Kurki P, Linder E**. 1978 Indirect immunofluorescence and anti-epithelial antibodies in Yersinial infections. Arthritis Rheum. 21:904-908.

32. **Shenkman L, Bottone EJ**. 1976 Antibodies to Yersinia enterocolitica in thyroid disease. Ann Int Med. 85:735-739.

33. **Keddie N, Metcalfe-Gibson C, Tooth JA**. 1977 Yersinia and thyroid disease. Lancet. (ii):1368

34. **Weetman AP, McGregor AM**. 1994 Autoimmune thyroid disease: further developments in our understanding. Endocr Rev. 15:788-830.

35. **Barker DJP, Phillips DIW**. 1984 Current incidence of hyperthyroidism and past prevalence of endemic goitre in 12 British towns. Lancet. (ii):567-570.

36. **Safran M, Paul TL, Roti E, Braverman LE**. 1987 Environmental factors affecting autoimmune thyroid disease. Endocrinol Metab Clin N Amer. 16:327-342.

37. **Mostbeck A, Galvan G, Bauer P, et al**. 1998 The incidence of hyperthyroidism in Austria from 1987 to 1995 before and after an increase in salt iodization in 1990. Eur J Nucl Med. 25:367-374.

38. **Hancock SL, Cox RS, McDougall IR**. 1991 Thyroid diseases after treatment of Hodgkin's disease. N Engl J Med. 325:599-605.

39. **Phillips DIW**. 1985 The Epidemiology of hyperthyroidism in England and Wales. PhD Thesis, University of Southampton pp 51-52.

3

THE GENETICS OF FAMILIAL AND NON-FAMILIAL HYPERTHYROID GRAVES' DISEASE

Yaron Tomer and Terry F. Davies

INTRODUCTION

Graves' disease (GD) is a multifactorial disease that develops as a result of a complex interaction between genetic susceptibility genes and environmental factors (1). Pathologically, the thyroid gland is infiltrated by T cells and B cells reactive with thyroid antigens, including the thyrotropin receptor (TSHR). This infiltration is associated with the production of antibodies which stimulate the thyroid via the TSHR causing hyperthyroidism and diffuse goiter as well as evidence of an ongoing thyroiditis associated with antibodies to thyroglobulin (Tg) and thyroid peroxidase (TPO)(1). Hence, the characterization of GD as autoimmune thyroiditis Type 3 (2). However, the cause of the immune response to thyroid antigens in GD remains unknown. Research into the pathogenesis of GD has focused on the possible precipitating environmental insults (such as infection)(3) and on under-standing the genetic predisposition to the disease. The recent advances in our under-standing of the genetic susceptibility to GD is the focus of this chapter.

A genetic predisposition to the development of GD was first suggested by observations of multiple occurrences of the disease within the same family. These early observations were later confirmed by population studies, family studies and twin studies. However, identifying the susceptibility genes for GD has been extremely difficult. GD, like other autoimmune diseases, is a polygenic disease lacking an overall easily discernable Mendelian pattern of inheritance. It is most likely caused by many genes of variable penetrance. However, recent advances in gene mapping techniques have allowed us to further our understanding of the genetics of GD and it is hoped that these will ultimately lead to the identification of the GD susceptibility genes.

THE ETIOLOGY OF GRAVES' DISEASE AS A COMPLEX DISEASE

Even though the exact etiologic factors causing Grave's disease are still unknown the sequence of events leading to the development of the disease is believed to involve several steps which are probably common to many autoimmune diseases (Figure 1).

The first step is the inborn genetic susceptibility. A genetic susceptibility is required for an individual to develop familial GD. However, there may also be a sporadic form of GD which is less influenced by genetic factors, and low penetrance

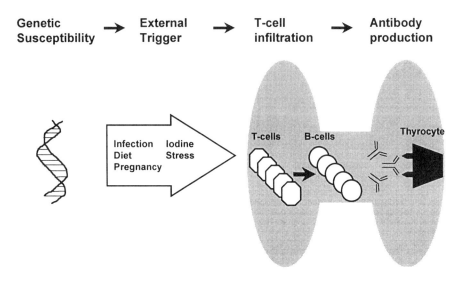

| Genetic Susceptibility | → | External Trigger | → | T-cell infiltration | → | Antibody production |

Figure 1. Four steps involved in the development Graves' disease.

may hide the familial nature of every case. Therefore, studies on the genetic susceptibility to GD should differentiate familial GD from sporadic GD. This is not an easy task since the disease is quite common, with up to 0.5% of the general population having GD (4). Thus, two sporadic cases could occur by chance in the same family and be mistaken for the familial form of the disease.

The second step is an encounter with an environmental triggering factor. Possible triggering factors include infection (3) exposure to high doses of iodine (5), pregnancy (6,7) and stressful life events (8,9). The third step is infiltration of the thyroid gland by thyroid specific T-lymphocytes (10). The normal control mechanisms which prevent such cells from causing disease must be inhibited by the precipitating events. The infiltrating T-cells activate B cells with the help of co-stimulatory molecules (e.g. CD40) expressed on antigen presenting cells and thyroid epithelial cells. The last step is the generation of TSHR antibodies by activated B cells; these antibodies stimulate thyroid growth and production of thyroid hormones which leads to thyrotoxicosis. While the last two steps have been well studied, the genetic susceptibility to GD and the mechanisms by which the environmental factors trigger the disease are only now beginning to be understood.

A brief note on the evidence for environmental triggers of Graves' disease

Cox et al. (11) found seasonality in the diagnosis of GD, and Phillips et al. (12) found that the incidence of thyrotoxic patients who had TSHR and anti-microsomal antibodies varied markedly between towns in England. These observations suggested an infectious etiology in the development of GD but they remain to be confirmed. In another study Valtonen and co-workers found serological evidence for a recent bacterial or viral infection in 36% of newly diagnosed Graves' patients and in only 10% of controls (13). However, to date, only one report of "clustering" of GD patients exists (14). The possibility of Yersinia as the infectious agent triggering GD has received much attention. Studies on patients with Yersinia enterocolitica infections have demonstrated that the sera of these patients contained autoantibodies to thyroid epithelium (15,16) and many different Yersinia antigens cross-react with thyroid antigens although with uncertain affinity (17). In addition, Weiss et al. demonstrated a saturable binding site for TSH on Yersinia enterocolitica (18), and the binding of radiolabeled TSH to Yersinia has been shown to be inhibited by Graves' immunoglobulins (19). One study has shown that lymphocytic thyroiditis can be induced in experimental animals by immunization with the Yersinia enterocolitica purified outer membrane protein (20), but these results were not confirmed by other studies. The possibility of Yersinia-specific immune responses being merely reflective of the "natural" immune response deserves serious consideration in view of the low affinity interactions and lack of predictability in the published studies. Moreover, most patients with Yersinia infection (including those who produce anti-TSHR antibodies) do not develop GD. Other infectious agents implicated in the pathogenesis of GD include retroviruses (21), but data supporting this view remain unsubstantiated. Therefore, even though an infection is a likely environmental trigger of GD (3), the responsible infectious agent has not yet been identified. Other possible environmental triggers of GD include exposure to iodine (5), pregnancy (7), and stressful life events (8).

Evidence for genetic susceptibility to Graves' disease

Abundant epidemiological data point to a strong genetic contribution to the development of GD. These epidemiologic data are derived from studies of unrelated individuals, family studies and twin studies.

Secular trends in the incidence of Graves' disease
Studies from different geographic regions have shown a relatively similar incidence and prevalence of GD in different populations (4,22-24). This similarity suggested a significant genetic effect on the development of the disease because these populations were exposed to different environmental factors. Moreover, the incidence has not changed in the past several decades (25), again pointing to a strong genetic influence on disease development. The incidence rates of diseases with strong environmental influences are expected to change over time while the incidence rates of diseases with strong genetic influences should not change as much.

Variations in the incidence of GD with age
The changes in the incidence of a disease with age can point to the relative influence of genetics and the environment on the pathogenesis of the disease. The incidence of GD was shown to peak in the fifth decade of life in both males and females with subsequent declines to a zero incidence in the eighth decade (26). These data suggested that, in genetically predisposed individuals, the probability of developing the disease increased with age until 80 years when all susceptible people have developed the disease (i.e. the lifetime penetrance of the disease approached 100%). In view of these data, it has been suggested that GD and Hashimoto's thyroiditis develop

at random in a genetically predisposed population (26). However, other interpretations of the data are possible (e.g. an environmental effect peaking at the fifth decade of life).

Familial clustering of GD

The familial occurrence of GD has been recognized for many years. More than 50 years ago it was recognized that a familial predisposition occurred in approximately 60% of cases with GD (27). Martin (28) found that 20 of 90 (22%) of patients with GD had relatives with GD. Moreover, several thyroid abnormalities have been reported in relatives of patients with GD (29-31); most commonly thyroid autoantibodies which were reported in up to 50% of the siblings of patients with GD (26,30,32). Hall and Stanbury (33) found clinical thyroid disease in 33% of siblings of patients with GD or Hashimoto's disease. Additionally, they found 56% of siblings to be thyroid antibody positive and in almost all cases the parents of an affected individual were also positive (33). While the sibling risk of developing autoimmune thyroid disease (λ_s) has not been calculated directly, it can be estimated for GD from published data. For that calculation we can assume (based on several studies) that 10%-15% of siblings of GD patients have GD (33,34) and that the population prevalence of GD is about 0.3%-0.5% (22,35,24). Thus, the sibling risk ratio for GD (i.e. the ratio of the risk for developing GD in a GD sibling over the general population risk for GD - λ_s) can be estimated to be at least 15. Even though only a rough estimate, this relatively high value suggests a strong genetic contribution to the development of GD.

Twins studies

Twin studies can provide information concerning the inheritance of a disease and may yield certain quantitative evaluations on the role of heredity in relation to exogenous factors. The twin method is based upon comparison of the concordance (simultaneous occurrence) of a given disease among monozygotic (MZ) twins and among dizygotic (DZ) twins. MZ twins have similar genetic makeup, whereas DZ twins share an average of ½ of the genes (like siblings). Therefore, a concordance higher in MZ twins than in DZ twins suggests that the disease has an inherited component. Any discordance among the MZ twin pairs is usually interpreted to mean that the gene(s) concerned has reduced penetrance. One cause of reduced penetrance is environmental factors present before the disease becomes manifest. The concordance rate in MZ twins may, therefore, be used as an estimate of the penetrance of the disease up to the ages examined in that particular twin set. For example, a 50% concordance rate among MZ twins can be interpreted to mean that penetrance of the disease genes is approximately 50%. It must be emphasized that MZ twins are not identical in their immune repertoires due to somatic recombinations which T and B cells undergo throughout life as well as individual immune experiences which influence the immune repertoire. Therefore, part of the observed discordance between MZ twins may also be due to the discordance in their immune repertoires. In the largest twin study of GD, performed in Denmark, the concordance rate for MZ twins was 36%, and for DZ twins the concordance rate was 0 (36). In other studies similar results were obtained, with the concordance rate of GD in dizygotic twins reported to be about 3% to 9%, while in monozygotic twins the concordance rate was 30-60% (37). Thus, the twin data have indicated that despite differences in their immune repertoire, there remains a substantial inherited susceptibility to GD, presumably related to both immune and non-immune genes.

Thyroid autoantibodies

Autoantibodies to thyroglobulin (Tg) and thyroid peroxidase (TPO, the microsomal antigen) have been widely used to detect the population at most risk for the development of autoimmune thyroid disease (AITD). Anti-Tg and anti-TPO autoantibodies have been found in up to 50% of the siblings of patients with AITD (26,30,38,39), in contrast to a prevalence of 7-20% in the general population (22). These findings have also been found in different populations such as Japanese (40) and British (33). In one study, it was found that thyroid autoantibodies were almost always present in one parent of an affected individual with AITD (33). Indeed, segregation analysis of families with thyroid antibodies suggested a Mendelian dominant pattern of inheritance for the tendency to develop anti-thyroid antibodies (41). Moreover, complex segregation analysis of TPO autoantibody epitopic 'fingerprints' in multiplex families indicated a major inherited locus on a polygenic background (42).

Graves' ophthalmopathy

The milder form of Graves' ophthalmopathy (GO), better referred to as an orbitopathy, affects about 80% of patients with GD. However, the severe form of ophthalmopathy occurs in less than 10% of GD patients (43). GO is considered pathognomonic of GD even when the individual is not hyperthyroid. It has been suggested that the genetic influence on the development of GO may be more pronounced because GO represents the most severe form of the disease. We, therefore recently performed a segregation analysis in patients selected for severe GO. A segregation analysis is a method for examining if a disease has a genetic component, and for identifying the mode of inheritance (as explained above). This analysis showed that GO was not hereditary even in families where there was definite evidence for a genetic influence on the development of GD. In other words, while GD develops as a result of genetic susceptibility, the ophthalmopathy associated with GD more likely results from an environmental insult occurring in individuals predisposed to develop GD.

Susceptibility genes for Graves' disease

While the susceptibility genes for GD are unknown, the epidemiological data point to the involvement of several genes with varying penetrance in the pathogenesis of the disease. Based on current knowledge of genetic influences in simple and complex diseases, it can be speculated that several classes of genes can operate to induce susceptibility to GD:

Class I genes

These are genes making the individual more susceptible to certain infections. This influence could contribute to the development of autoimmunity by increasing the chance of triggering autoimmune responses. For example, individuals with IgA deficiency are more susceptible to certain type of infections (mostly Gram positive bacteria) (44) and they also have a greater incidence of autoimmunity (45). Moreover, there are reports of associations between IgA deficiency and autoimmune thyroid disease (46). Some genetic variations can alter the susceptibility to specific infectious agents. For example a 32 base deletion in the CCR5 gene significantly decreased susceptibility to HIV infection (47). It is possible that the genetic susceptibility to GD may reflect genetic polymorphic variations that increase susceptibility to infectious organisms that are capable of inducing autoimmune responses.

Class II genes

These are the immune response genes whose polymorphic variations may contribute to the development of autoimmunity. Such variations could augment immune responses to self antigens thus preventing immune tolerance and resulting in auto-immunity. For example, there is now ample evidence that certain HLA polymorphisms (DR4-DQA1*0301-DQB1*0302 and DR3-DQA1*0501-DQB1*0201) are strongly associated with type I diabetes mellitus (IDDM) (48). It is thought that these HLA alleles cause susceptibility to IDDM by allowing lower affinity binding of autoantigens to the HLA molecules. This, in turn, permits autoreactive T cells to survive the apoptosis normally induced by self-antigens which bind with high affinity (see below).

Class III genes

Genes that increase immune responsiveness cannot explain the tissue specificity of certain autoimmune diseases such as GD. For an autoimmune reaction to be directed towards a certain tissue (e.g. thyroid) there may be modifying factors in the target tissue. Class III genes are genes that modify the expression of autoantigens which make them more immunogenic to T cells. An example for such a gene is the insulin VNTR in IDDM. The insulin VNTR has been shown unequivocally to be a susceptibility gene in IDDM (49). The insulin VNTR controls the expression of the insulin gene in different tissues (50). Recently two groups have reported that the VNTR alleles which protected from the development of IDDM (class III alleles) were associated with significantly higher insulin mRNA levels in human fetal thymus (51,52). It was postulated that higher levels of thymic insulin expression in individuals with class III alleles promoted the negative selection of insulin-specific T lymphocytes thus facilitating immune tolerance induction and protection from IDDM (51).

Methods for identifying the Graves' disease genes

Several approaches are being taken to identify the susceptibility genes for GD. The two popular approaches are candidate gene analysis and whole genome screening.

Analysis of candidate genes

Candidate genes are genes of known sequence and location which could, theoretically be involved in disease pathogenesis. If a candidate gene is the cause of the disease, then markers close to that gene should segregate with the disease within a family. The candidate gene approach has already been used successfully; most notable was maturity onset diabetes of the young (MODY)(53). Because the basic abnormality in GD is an immune response against thyroid cells, candidate genes for GD include genes that control antibody responses (e.g. the immunoglobulin gene complexes and genes responsible for B cell growth factors), genes that control T cell responses (e.g. the HLA region, the T-cell receptor genes and genes responsible for T cell growth factors), and genes encoding the target autoantigens (Tg, TPO and the TSHR). All of these genes have now been studied for their possible role in the genetic susceptibility to GD (see below).

Candidate genes can be analyzed by association studies and/or linkage studies. Association studies are based on comparisons of the frequencies of specific alleles of a marker near the candidate gene in patients and controls in an ethnically similar population. If the frequency of a certain allele is significantly increased in patients compared to controls this points to possible involvement of the gene in the disease. In linkage studies a marker inside or near a candidate gene is tested for co-segregation with the disease in families. If a tested marker is close to a disease susceptibility gene, it will co-segregate with the disease in families. The LOD score is the measure of the likelihood of linkage between a disease and a genetic marker (54). A LOD score of >3 is considered strong evidence for linkage and a LOD score of > 2.0 is suggestive of linkage (55). A LOD score of < -2.0 may help to exclude linkage.

Whole genome screens

Linkage studies can also be used for genome-wide genetic screening. The technique of whole genome screening involves typing of individuals in large families with GD for polymorphic markers. These markers are then analyzed for linkage with GD in the tested families. If linkage to one or more markers is established it can be concluded that a susceptibility gene for the disease is located near that marker. The markers chosen may span the whole human genome at distances that will enable detection of linkage to susceptibility genes located between any two of them. The polymorphic markers most often used in genome-wide scans are the microsatellites, which are regions in the genome composed of short repetitive units (e.g. CA-repeats). Microsatellites are abundant and uniformly distributed throughout the genome at distances of less than 1 million base pairs (56). A set of 400 microsatellite markers is now commercially available and they span the whole human genome at distances short enough (< 10 centimorgan) to detect linkage between any two of them. Once a suspected gene region is located, it can be further narrowed using markers that are more closely spaced, and the gene region identified. It is difficult to perform whole genome screening in complex diseases, such as GD, because the gene penetrance may be relatively low and may not manifest until later in life. It would, therefore, be unclear who in the family was yet to develop the disease. Another difficulty is the likelihood that the gene being studied may be present in healthy persons since it may not be an "obligatory" gene. Further difficulties in complex diseases include the definitions of such disease. The phenotype definitions can be complicated, and there is a possibility of genetic heterogeneity, i.e. different genotypes causing a similar phenotype. Therefore, in order to identify complex disease genes it has been necessary to use large numbers of families and to use strict conservative phenotype definitions. A linkage to a gene can be considered confirmed only if two independent groups have identified significant linkage at the same locus.

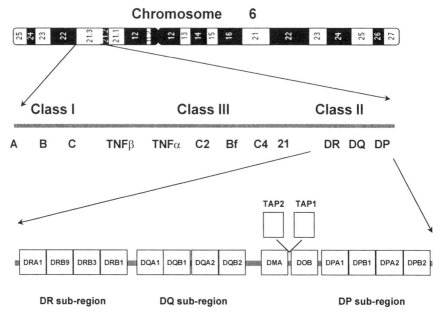

Figure 2. The HLA region is located on chromosome 6p21. It is a complex genetic region which consists of several loci, all of which code for proteins which influence the different arms of the immune system. Depicted are the major loci.

IMMUNE RESPONSE GENES AND GRAVES' DISEASE

The HLA genes

Population and family studies in Graves' disease
    The major histocompatibility complex (MHC) region encoding the HLA glyco-proteins consists of a complex of genes located on chromosome 6p21 (Figure 2). The MHC region also encodes additional proteins associated with immune responsiveness. The genes in the MHC region are grouped into 3 classes: (1) Class I genes include the HLA antigens A, B, and C, (2) Class II genes include the HLA-DR, DP, and DQ genes, and (3) Class 3 genes include several complement components (e.g. C4), tumor necrosis factor α, heat shock protein 70, and several others (57,58). Because the HLA region is highly polymorphic, and contains many immune response genes, it was the first candidate genetic region to be studied in GD, as well as in many other autoimmune diseases. Indeed, associations to the HLA regions have been found in almost all autoimmune diseases, and in some diseases (e.g. type I diabetes) the HLA genes are believed to be of utmost importance (59). This general association of HLA with various autoimmune diseases points to a generalized mechanism by which certain HLA molecules help generate autoimmunity. Evidently, the HLA genes could not explain the tissue specificity of different autoimmune disease such as GD. GD was initially found to be associated with HLA-B8 in Caucasians (60). This finding was then confirmed in a wide number of studies, mostly examining Caucasian populations (Table 1).

Table 1. Some of the important HLA association studies in Graves' disease performed in Caucasians.

Country	Ethnic group	Patient number	HLA allele	Relative risk	Reference
Canada	Caucasians	175	B8	3.1	(74)
			DR3	5.7	
England	Caucasians	127	B8	2.77	(78)
			DR3	2.13	
France	Caucasians	94	B8	3.4	(77)
			DR3	4.21	
Hungary	Caucasians	256	B8	3.48	(72)
			DR3	4.80	
Ireland	Caucasians	86	B8	2.5	(134)
			DR3	2.6	
Newfound-land	Caucasians	133	DR3	4.57	(71)
Sweden	Caucasians	78	B8	4.4	(135)
			DR3	3.9	
USA	Caucasians	65	DR3	3.38	(62)
England	Caucasians	120	DQA1 *0501	3.8	(65)
USA	Caucasians	94	DQA1 *0501	3.71	(66)

In these early studies HLA-B8 was associated with relative risks for GD ranging from 1.5 to 3. Subsequently, GD was found to be more strongly associated with HLA-DR3, which is now known to be in linkage disequilibrium with HLA-B8 (61,62). On the average the frequency of DR3 in GD patients was 40-55% and in the general population 20-30% giving a relative risk for people with HLA-DR3 of 2.1-3.7 (37,62). Even though the frequency of HLA-DR3 was increased in Caucasians with GD, there were also HLA-DR3 negative associations with GD, and the HLA associations were found to be different in other ethnic groups. For example, in the Japanese population GD was associated with HLA-B35 (63), and in the Chinese population an increased frequency of HLA-Bw46 has been reported (64). In addition, HLA-DQA1*0501 has also been found to be associated with GD in Caucasians (relative risk 3.8)(Table 1) (65,66).

There have been several HLA linkage studies in GD, most showing no linkage. In a study of 10 GD families from Hong-Kong, no linkage was demonstrated between

HLA alleles and GD (67). Our laboratory also performed linkage studies between the HLA region and GD using different techniques. In all of these studied we were able to reject linkage between GD and HLA genes. We tested for linkage using both traditional HLA serotyping (68) and DNA restriction fragment polymorphisms (69). The results showed negative LOD scores for both recessive and dominant modes of inheritance at various penetrances (68,69). More recently, we have performed another HLA linkage study using the microsatellite TNFα, which is located inside the HLA region (70). Our study, again failed to demonstrate linkage between GD and TNFα. Only one study has reported evidence for linkage between GD and HLA using classical analyses (71), but there was a strong possibility of selection bias in that particular study. In addition, the risk of developing GD in HLA-identical siblings has been shown to be only 7% (72), which was not significantly different from the general risk in siblings, and was much lower than the 30% concordance for MZ twins described earlier. Therefore, we concluded that the HLA genes were not the primary GD genes, and conferred only a small increase in the risk for the development of GD. Consequently, other genes outside the HLA region are more likely to confer most of the genetic susceptibility to GD.

HLA and Graves' ophthalmopathy (GO)

The more severe form of GO occurs in less than 10% of GD patients (43). GO has been studied for HLA associations in order to determine if the genetic predisposition to eye disease is distinct from that of Graves' thyroid disease. However, to date, studies of HLA associations in GO have produced conflicting results. Schleusener et al. (73) reported a significantly higher prevalence of HLA-B8 and DR3 in patients with GO and/or TSHR antibodies compared to GD patients who had neither ophthalmopathy nor TSHR antibodies. In the same study the patients without TSHR antibodies and without clinical eye signs who relapsed, had a significantly higher prevalence of HLA-DR5 than the control group. Similarly, Farid et al. (74) reported a higher incidence of HLA-DR3 in GD patients with ophthalmopathy. In two studies performed in Hungary and Newfoundland, Canada, Frecker et al. (75,76) reported that HLA-DR7 enhanced the risk for ophthalmopathy in the presence of B8 but had a protective influence in its absence. In contrast, others have found no difference in the distribution of HLA-DR alleles between GD patients with and without ophthalmopathy (74,66,77-80). These conflicting results are not surprising in view of our segregation analysis, described above, which showed no genetic influence on the development of GO. In our own studies we found an association between GO and HLA-DR3 giving a relative risk similar to that of GD in general (74). In summary, although certain HLA alleles have been consistently shown to be elevated in GD patients compared to control populations (mainly HLA-DR3 and DQA1*0501 in Caucasians), there is no specific association between certain HLA polymorphisms and severe GO itself.

Mechanisms of HLA influences

The mechanisms by which HLA associations confer disease susceptibility in GD are now beginning to be understood. In order for T cells to recognize and respond to an antigen there has to be recognition of a complex between the antigenic peptide and an HLA class II molecule (81). It is thought that different HLA alleles have different affinities to autoantigens (e.g. thyroid antigens) which are recognized by T cell receptors (82). Thus, certain alleles may permit the autoantigen to fit in the antigen binding groove inside the HLA molecule and to be recognized by the T-cell receptor while others may not (83). Furthermore, such fits may be of variable ease. It has been postulated that if a certain HLA allele allowed only weak (low affinity) binding of an autoantigen to the HLA molecule then the autoantigen would not be presented to T cells in the thymus during embryonic life. The result would be that the T cell clone recognizing this autoantigen would not be deleted and would survive able to induce an autoimmune condition later in life. Conversely, HLA alleles that confer strong binding to a specific autoantigen will allow its presentation to T cells in the thymus and these autoreactive T cells would be deleted by apoptosis and would not be able to induce an autoimmune condition.

Even if an autoreactive T-cell clone was not deleted it cannot react with thyroid antigens unless these antigens are presented to it in sufficient concentration. Thus, some mechanism of autoantigen presentation must exist within the thyroid gland of Graves' patients or the draining lymph nodes of the gland. One potential intrathyroidal mechanism not utilizing professional antigen presenting cells (APC's) may be through aberrant expression of HLA class II molecules on thyrocytes (84-86). Unlike normals, thyroid epithelial cells from patients with GD have been shown to express HLA class II antigen molecules which are normally expressed only on APC's such as macrophages and dendritic cells (84,85). This aberrant expression of HLA molecules on thyroid cells, could initiate thyroid autoimmunity via direct thyroid autoantigen presentation (85,87). Consistent with this observation was the fact that thyroid cell MHC class II antigen expression has also been shown in response to certain viral infections in vitro (88,89). Indeed, co-culture of PBMC from GD patients with homologous thyrocytes induced T cell activation (90) as well as interferon-γ production and thyroid cell HLA class II antigen expression (91).

Other possible explanations for HLA involvement in GD exist. The HLA region harbors several other important immune regulatory genes (Figure 2). It is possible that the HLA susceptibility to GD is mediated by non-HLA immune regulatory genes in this complex genetic region. For example, two important immune regulatory genes in the HLA gene complex are the TAP1 and TAP2 genes located near the HLA DQB region. These genes encode molecules which transport peptides across membranes and are intimately involved in antigen processing prior to their association with HLA molecules (92). Much has been written about the potential role of these molecules in susceptibility to IDDM (83).

The CTLA-4 gene region

Population and family studies

CTLA-4 is an important co-stimulatory molecule that is necessary for T cell stimulation. Recently, several reports have demonstrated an association between the CTLA-4 gene and the AITDs (Table 2). Earlier studies found an association between a microsatellite marker located near the CTLA-4 gene and GD, giving a relative risk of 2.1 to 2.8 (93,95). With the identification of an alanine/threonine (G/A) polymorphism inside the CTLA-4 leader peptide, this polymorphism was tested for association with the AITDs. The ala (G) polymorphism was found to be associated with GD with

Table 2. Some of the important CTLA-4 association studies in Graves' disease.

Polymorphism/ Marker	Country	Ethnic Group	Dis.	No.	RR[*] / P value	Reference
CTLA-4(AT)	USA	Caucasians	GD	133	2.82	(93)
CTLA-4 (AT)	Hong-Kong	Chinese	GD	94	p = 0.037	(94)
CTLA-4(AT)	UK	Caucasians	GD	112	2.1	(95)
CTLA-4(AT)	Japan	Japanese	GD	62	NS[*]	(96)
Thr/Ala $(A/G)_{49}$	Germany	Caucasians	GD	305	2.0	(97)
Thr/Ala $(A/G)_{49}$	Japan	Japanese	GD	153	2.64	(98)
Thr/Ala $(A/G)_{49}$	UK	Caucasians	GD	94	p=0.003	(99)
C-T (-318)	UK	Caucasians	GD	188	NS	(100)
	Hong-Kong	Chinese	GD	98	NS	

[*]RR-relative risk, NS-not significant

a relative risk of 2.0 (97). These reports have been consistent in several (93,95), although not all (100), populations. Recently, Pearce et al.(101) reported linkage to the CTLA-4 gene region in families with GD. The linkage became stronger when families with AITD, rather than just GD, were included in the study suggesting a more general role for CTLA-4 in thyroid autoimmunity and not a specific predisposition to GD. However, it is unclear if the susceptibility gene in this region is CTLA-4 itself or another gene. Indeed, this region is replete with candidate genes for thyroid autoimmunity (e.g. CD28, STAT1, and 4, and Caspase 8 and 10). In keeping with the possibility that the CTLA-4 region harbors a gene associated with thyroid autoimmunity rather than one specific disease we have recently found evidence that the CTLA-4 gene region is linked with the production of autoantibodies rather than Graves' or Hashimoto's diseases. These observations may suggest that a gene in the CTLA-4 region confers susceptibility to thyroid autoimmunity and that clinical disease (Graves' or Hashimoto's diseases) requires the participation of other disease-specific genes (see below) and triggering environmental factors.

Mechanisms

APC's activate T cells by presenting to the T cell receptor an antigenic peptide bound to an HLA class II protein on the cell surface. However, a second signal is also required for T cell activation and these co-stimulatory signals may be provided by the APC's themselves or by other local cells (102). Co-stimulatory signals are provided by a variety of proteins (e.g. B7-1, B7-2, CD-40) expressed on APC's which interact with receptors (CD28, CTLA-4, and CD-40L) on the surface of CD4+ T-lymphocytes during antigen presentation (102). Whereas, the binding of B7 to CD28 on T cells co-stimulates T cell activation, the binding of B7 to CTLA-4 is thought to down regulate T-cell activation and induce tolerance. The suppressive effects of CTLA-4 on T cell activation have raised the possibility that mutations altering CTLA-4 function could lead to the development of autoimmunity. Indeed, treatment of female NOD (autoimmune diabetes prone) mice with a soluble CD28 antagonist suppressed the development of diabetes (103). Co-stimulator molecules may also influence the resulting Th1 or Th2 T cell phenotype helping to direct the pattern of the autoimmune reaction (104,105). B7-1 has been reported on thyroid cells in Hashimoto's thyroiditis and not in normal thyroid, but CD-40, another co-stimulatory molecule, has been shown to be expressed on all thyroid epithelial cells (106-108).

T cell receptor genes

The initiation of GD involves infiltration of the thyroid by T-cells reactive with thyroid antigens. These T-cells are oligoclonal and are restricted by their T-cell receptor V gene use (10). Thus, the T-cell receptor seemed a likely candidate gene for thyroid autoimmunity and has, therefore, been studied extensively. Earlier studies reported an association between a restriction fragment length polymorphism (RFLP) of the T cell receptor β chain and GD (109). However, these results were not confirmed by other groups (110,62). We have also studied the T-cell receptor α genes (on chromosome 14) and β genes (on chromosome 7) by linkage studies. We were able to conclusively exclude linkage of GD to both of these genes, thus ruling them out as susceptibility genes for GD (111). Therefore, it can be concluded that the T-cell receptor genes are not involved in the specific genetic predisposition to GD.

Other immune related genes

Several other immune related genes have been studied for possible roles in GD. One of the first studied genes was the IgG heavy chain gene (IgH). Early studies found associations between IgG heavy chain Gm allotypes and GD in the Japanese population (112). However, we were unable to confirm linkage between the IgH gene and GD in a primarily Caucasian population (70). Others have examined the interleukin-1 (IL-1) receptor antagonist gene for associations with GD. These studies produced conflicting results (113,114), and at present there is no data to support the IL1 receptor antagonist as a susceptibility gene in GD.

THYROID ANTIGEN GENES AND GRAVES' DISEASE

The hallmark of autoimmune thyroid diseases is the production of antibodies and T-cell responses to thyroid specific antigens (115,116). There are four major proteins which are characteristic of thyroid tissue: the TSHR, TPO, Tg and the sodium-iodide symporter (NIS). Antibodies to all four thyroid antigens have been demonstrated in autoimmune thyroid disease (117,118). Therefore, the genes controlling the expression of the thyroid antigens in the thyroid were likely candidates for inducing susceptibility to GD, just as the insulin gene was a likely target in IDDM.

The thyrotropin receptor

The TSHR gene was a candidate gene for GD susceptibility gene because the most distinctive feature of the disease is the production of TSHR antibodies. A single nucleotide polymorphism in the ectodomain of the TSHR in codon 52 (coding for either threonine of proline) has been described (119). However, early reports of an association between this polymorphism and GO (120) have not been confirmed (121,122). Recent reports on Japanese populations, however, have found a weak association between the TSHR and GD (96). The identification of polymorphic microsatellites inside the TSHR gene (123) enabled two linkage studies in Caucasians: De Roux et al (124) and our own laboratory (125). Both studies failed to show linkage between the TSHR gene and GD. The LOD scores obtained in both studies were extremely negative (< -2) and therefore linkage of GD to the TSHR gene can be ruled out in Caucasian patients.

The TPO and Tg genes

Only one group has tested the TPO gene for an association with GD and Hashimoto's thyroiditis. They found no association between a microsatellite marker inside the TPO gene and these two diseases (126). Similarly, we found no evidence for linkage between the TPO gene and Graves' and Hashimoto's diseases (70). We studied 19 families (107 individuals, 32 with Hashimoto's disease and 14 with GD) using the same marker inside the TPO gene. We were able to exclude linkage between either GD or Hashimoto's disease and the Tg gene (70). These results suggested that thyroid antigen polymorphisms did not contribute significantly to the genetic susceptibility to GD or Hashimoto's disease. This conclusion contrasts with type I diabetes in which the insulin VNTR gene is a major susceptibility gene for the disease (49).

THE X CHROMOSOME AND GRAVES' DISEASE

Autoimmune thyroid diseases are 5-10 times more common in females than in males (22). The increased female preponderance of AITD may be secondary to sex steroid effects or X chromosome effects. Some data support the notion that estrogens promote induction of autoimmunity. Autoimmunity is most common in fertile women (22) and there are animal studies showing induction of autoimmunity in males by estrogens (127-129). Another possibility is that the increased female susceptibility to AITD is related to the X chromosome. There are a number of possible mechanisms whereby the X chromosome could influence the development of AITD. One mechanism is probabilistic. Females have two X chromosomes (one paternal and one maternal) while males have only one X chromosome (maternal). Therefore, females are twice as likely to inherit an X chromosome AITD susceptibility gene as males. Another mechanism relates to the phenomenon of X chromosome inactivation. Even though females have two X chromosomes, only one X chromosome gene is expressed in female somatic cells. This is due to suppression of one of the X chromosomes by a process called X-chromosome inactivation. X-chromosome inactivation occurs early in embryonic life and, thereafter, in each cell either the maternal or paternal chromosome is inactivated. This results in a tissue mosaic of paternally and maternally expressed X-chromosomal alleles, with an average distribution of 1:1. Therefore, a female heterozygous for an X-linked gene encoding for a self antigen will have two classes of cells that differ in the transcription of this X-chromosome encoded gene. If these two cell classes extend to the thymic cells responsible for tolerizing T-cells in embryonic life, some lymphocytes may not be tolerized to one of the two self antigens encoded by the X-chromosome. Such lymphocytes would be autoreactive to that antigen and could induce an autoimmune response. While this attractive theory could help explain the female preponderance of autoimmune conditions (since this escape mechanism from tolerance can occur only in females), there are no data to support it (130).

We have studied the X chromosome for possible linkage with GD. We identified a locus (GD-3. see Table 3) on Xq22 that was linked with GD giving a LOD score of 2.5 (131). The Bruton's tyrosine kinase (BTK) gene is located in this region. The BTK controls B cell ontogeny and, therefore, could theoretically be involved in thyroid autoimmunity. However, we have recently tested the BTK gene directly by SSCP and found no evidence that it is the GD susceptibility gene on the X chromosome (132).

Table 3. Two point and multipoint LOD scores at 4 loci found to be linked with GD.

Locus	Marker Name	Chromo-some	2-Point LOD	θ*	Multi-point LOD	Pene-trance/Inheri-tance	NPL
AITD-1	D6S257	6p21	2.2	0.01	2.9	0.3/Rec	2.3
GD-1	D14S81	14q31	2.1	0.01	2.5	0.3/Rec	1.9
GD-2	D20S195	20q11.2	3.2	0.01	3.5	0.3/Rec	2.4
GD-3	DXS8020	Xq21	1.9	0.01	2.5	0.4/Rec	1.8

* θ denotes the recombination fraction between the marker and the disease gene.

WHOLE GENOME SCREENING IN GRAVES' DISEASE

We have recently completed the first whole genome screening in GD in a dataset of 56 multiplex families (354 individuals)(133). The whole genome screening revealed three new loci which were linked to GD (Table 3): GD-1 on chromosome 14 gave a maximum LOD score (MLS) of 2.5; GD-2 on chromosome 20 (MLS of 3.5); and GD-3 on chromosome X (MLS of 2.5). These loci were not linked with Hashimoto's thyroiditis or to AITD (GD together with Hashimoto's disease). Another locus (AITD-1) was linked with both Graves' and Hashimoto's diseases (MLS of 2.9)(134). Thus, we concluded that the genetic contribution to the development of GD involves several genes with varying effects. The three newly identified loci are unique to GD and unlike previously identified loci (HLA and CTLA-4) confer susceptibility only to GD and not to autoimmunity in general. GD-1 is the site of MNG-1 which has been linked to familial multinodular goiter (135). GD-2 has recently been confirmed in another data set by Pearce et al. (Pearce, personal communication). The genes responsible for these linkages remain to be identified.

CONCLUSIONS AND FUTURE PROSPECTS

GD is a multifactorial disease caused by genetic susceptibility and environmental triggers. Various epidemiological and genetic techniques can be employed to study the genetic contribution to disease development. Most epidemiologic data support an important genetic contribution to the development of GD, and the twin data suggest that penetrance of GD susceptibility genes is greater than 30%. The genetic susceptibility to GD involves several genes with varying effects. Some GD susceptibility genes are most likely immune modifying genes which increase the susceptibility to autoimmunity in general (e.g. HLA, CTLA-4) while others are specific to GD (e.g. GD-1,2,3). These genes probably act in concert to increase the autoimmune responses in susceptible individuals and direct these responses towards the thyroid. There is also evidence to support a GD susceptibility gene on the X chromosome which may partly explain the increased female preponderance of the disease. It is hoped that in the future all the susceptibility genes for GD will be identified and the mechanisms by which they operate deciphered.

REFERENCES

1.   **Davies TF.** The pathogenesis of Graves' disease. 1996 In: Braverman LE, Utiger RD, ed. Werner and Ingbar's The Thyroid: a fundamental and clinical text. Philadelphia: Lippincott-Raven, pp525-536.
2.   **Davies TF, Amino N.** 1993 A new classification for human autoimmune thyroid disease. Thyroid 3:331-333.
3.   **Tomer Y, Davies TF.** 1993 Infection, thyroid disease and autoimmunity. Endocr Rev. 14:107-120.
4.   **Vanderpump MPJ, Tunbridge WMG, French JM, Appleton D, Bates D, Clark F, Grimley Evans J, Hasan DM, Rodgers H, Tunbridge F, Young ET.** 1995 The incidence of thyroid disorders in the community: a twenty-year follow-up of the Whickham survey. Clin Endocrinol. 43:55-68.
5.   **Jansson R, Safwenberg J, Dahlberg PA.** 1985 Influence of HLA DR4 antigen and iodine status on the development of autoimmune thyroiditis. J Clin Endocrinol Metab. 60:168-174.
6.   **Jansson R, Dahlberg PA, Winsa B, Meirik O, Safwenberg J, Karlsson A.** 1987 The postpartum period constitutes an important risk for the development of clinical Graves' disease in young women. Acta Endocrinol. 116:321-325.
7.   **Tada H, Hidaka Y, Tsuruta E, Kashiwai T, Tamaki H, Iwatani Y, Amino N.** 1994 Prevalence of postpartum onset of disease within patients with Graves' disease of child-bearing age. Endocr J. 41:325-327.
8.   **Sonino N, Girelli M, Boscaro M, Fallo F, Busnardo B, Fava GA.** 1993 Life events in the pathogenesis of Graves' disease. A controlled study. Acta Endocrinol. 128:293-296.

9. Winsa B, Adami H-O, Bergstrom R, Gamstedt A, Dahlberg PA, Adamson U, Jansson R, Karlsson A. 1991 Stressful life events and Graves' disease. Lancet 338:1475-1479.

10. Davies TF, Martin A, Concepcion ES, Graves P, Cohen L, Ben-Nun A. 1991 Evidence of limited variability of antigen receptors on intrathyoidal T cells in autoimmune thyroid disease. N Engl J Med. 325:238-244.

11. Cox SP, Phillips DI, Osmond C. 1989 Does infection initiate Graves disease? A population based 10 year study. Autoimmunity 4:43-49.

12. Phillips DI, Barker DJ, Rees Smith B, Didcote S, Morgan D. 1985 The geographical distribution of thyrotoxicosis in England according to the presence or absence of TSH-receptor antibodies. Clin Endocrinol. 23:283-287.

13. Valtonen VV, Ruutu P, Varis K, Ranki M, Malkamaki M, Makela PH.. 1986 Serological evidence for the role of bacterial infections in the patho-genesis of thyroid diseases. Acta Med Scand. 219:105-111.

14. Segal RL, Fiedler R, Jacobs DR, Antrobus J. 1976 Mini-epidemic of thyrotoxicosis occurring in physicians. Am J Med Sci. 271:55-57.

15. Lidman K, Eriksson U, Norberg R, Fagraeus A. 1976 Indirect immunofluorescence staining of human thyroid by antibodies occurring in Yersinia enterocolitica infections. Clin Exp Immunol. 23:429-435.

16. Shenkman L, Bottone EJ. 1976 Antibodies to Yersinia enterocolitica in thyroid disease. Ann Int Med. 85:735-739.

17. Wenzel BE, Heesemann J, Wenzel KW, Scriba PC. 1988 Antibodies to plasmid-encoded proteins of enteropathogenic Yersinia in patients with autoimmune thyroid disease (letter). Lancet 1:56

18. Weiss M, Ingbar SH, Winblad S, Kasper DL. 1983 Demonstration of a saturable binding site for thyrotropin in Yersinia enterocolitica. Science 219:1331-1333.

19. Heyma P, Harrison LC, Robins-Browne R. 1986 Thyrotropin (TSH) binding sites on Yersinia enterocolitica recognized by immunoglobulins from humans with Grave's disease. Clin Exp Immunol. 64:249-254.

20. Ebner S, Alex S, Klugnam T, Appel M, Heesemann J, Wenzel B. 1991 Immunization with Yersinia enterocolitica purified outer membrane protein induces lymphocytic thyroiditis in the BB/WOR rat (abstract). Thyroid 1 (Suppl):S28.

21. Ciampolillo A, Mirakian R, Schulz T, Vittoria M, Buscema M, Pujol Borrell R, Bottazzo GF. 1989 Retrovirus-like sequences in Graves' disease: implications for human autoimmunity. Lancet 1:1096-1099.

22. Tunbridge WMG, Evered DC, Hall R, Appleton D, Brewis M, Clark F, Evans JG, Young E, Bird T, Smith PA. 1977 The spectrum of thyroid disease in a community: the Whickham survey. Clin Endocrinol. 7:481-493.

23. Furszyfer J, Kurland LT, McConahey WM, Elveback LR. 1970 Graves' disease in Olmsted County, Minnesota, 1935 through 1967. Mayo Clin Proc. 45:636-644.

24. Mogensen EF, Green A. 1980 The epidemiology of thyrotoxicosis in Denmark. Incidence and geographical variation in the Funen region 1972-1974. Acta Med Scand. 208:183-186.

25. Furszyfer J, Kurland LT, McConahey WM, Woolner LB, Elveback LR. 1972 Epidemiologic aspects of Hashimoto's thyroiditis and Graves' disease in Rochester, Minnesota (1935-1967), with special reference to temporal trends. Metabolism 21:197-204.

26. Volpe R. 1985 Autoimmune thyroid disease. In: Volpe R, ed. Autoimmunity and endocrine disease. New York: Marcel Dekker, pp109-285.

27. Bartels ED. 1941 Twin Examinations: Heredity in Graves' disease. Copenhagen: Munksgaad 32-36.

28. Martin L. 1945 The heredity and familial aspects of exophathalmic goitre and nodular goitre. Q J Med. 14:207-219.

29.   **Tamai H, Ohsako N, Takeno K, Fukino O, Takahashi H, Kuma K, Kumagai LF, Nagataki S.** 1980 Changes in thyroid function in euthyroid subjects with family history of Graves' disease; a followup study of 69 patients. J Clin Endocrinol Metab. 51:1123-1128.

30.   **Chopra IJ, Solomon DH, Chopra U, Yodhihara E, Tersaki PL, Smith F.** 1977 Abnormalities in thyroid function in relatives of patients with Graves' disease and Hashimoto's thyroiditis: lack of correlation with inheritance of HLA-B8. J Clin Endocrinol Metab. 45:45-54.

31.   **Tamai H, Kumagai LF, Nagataki S.** 1986 Immunogenetics of Graves' disease. In: McGregor AM, editor. Immunology of endocrine diseases. Lancaster, U.K.: MTP Press pp123-141.

32.   **Burek CL, Hoffman WH, Rose NR.** 1982 The presence of thyroid autoanti-bodies in children and adolescents with AITD and in their siblings and parents. Clin Immunol Immunopathol. 25:395-404.

33.   **Hall R, Stanbury JB.** 1967 Familial studies of autoimmune thyroiditis. Clin Exp Immunol. 2:719-725.

34.   **Vyse TJ, Todd JA.** 1996 Genetic analysis of autoimmune disease. Cell 85:311-318.

35.   **Haraldsson A, Gudmundsson ST, Larusson G, Sigurdsson G.** 1985 Thyrotoxicosis in Iceland 1980-1982. An epidemiological survey. Acta Med Scand. 217:253-258.

36.   **Brix TH, Christensen K, Holm NV, Harvald B, Hegedus L.** 1998 A population-based study of Graves' diseases in Danish twins. Clin Endocrinol. 48:397-400.

37.   **Volpe R.** 1990 Immunology of human thyroid disease. In: Volpe R, editor. Autoimmunity in endocrine disease. Boca Raton: CRC Press p73.

38.   **Hall R, Dingle PR, Roberts DF.** 1972 Thyroid antibodies: a study of first degree relatives. Clin Genet. 3:319-324.

39.   **Burek CL, Hoffman WH, Rose NR.** 1982 The presence of thyroid autoantibodies in children and adolescents with AITD and in their siblings and parents. Clin Immunol Immunopathol. 25:395-404.

40.   **Aho K, Gordin A, Sievers K, Takala J.** 1983 Thyroid autoimmunity in siblings: a population study. Acta Endocrinol; Suppl. 251:11-15.

41.   **Phillips DIW, Prentice L, McLachlan SM, Upadhyaya M, Lunt PW, Rees Smith B.** 1991 Autosomal dominant inheritance of the tendency to develop thyroid autoantibodies. Exp Clin Endocrinol. 97:170-172.

42.   **Jaume JC, Guo J, Pauls DL, Zakarija M, McKenzie JM, Egeland JA, Burek CL, Rose NR, Hoffman WH, Rapoport B, McLachlan SM.** 1999 Evidence for genetic transmission of thyroid peroxidase autoantibody epitopic "fingerprints". J Clin Endocrinol Metab. 84:1424-1431.

43.   **Weetman AP.** Thyroid-associated ophthalmopathy. 1992 Autoimmunity 12:215-222.

44.   **Koskinen S.** Long-term follow-up of health in blood donors with primary selective IgA deficiency. J Clin Immunol. 16:165-170.

45.   **Liblau RS, Bach JF.** 1992 Selective IgA deficiency and autoimmunity. Int Arch Allergy Immunol. 99:16-27.

46.   **Mano T, Kawakubo A, Yamamoto M.** 1992 Isolated IgA deficiency accompanied by autoimmune thyroid disease. Int Med. 31:1201-1203.

47.   **Michael NL, Chang G, Louie LG, Mascola JR, Dondero D, Birx DL, Sheppard HW.** 1997 The role of viral phenotype and CCR-5 gene defects in HIV-1 transmission and disease progression. Nat Med. 3:338-340.

48.   **Kockum I, Wassmuth R, Holmberg E, et al.** 1993 HLA-DQ protection and HLA-DR susceptibility in Type 1 (insulin-dependent) diabetes studied in population-based affected families and controls. Am J Hum Genet. 42:150-167.

49.   **Lucassen AM, Julier C, Beressi JP, Boitard C, Froguel P, Lathrop M, Bell JI.** 1993

Susceptibility to insulin-dependent diabetes mellitus maps to a 4.1 kb segment of DNA spanning the insulin gene and associated VNTR. Nat Genet . 4:305-310.

50. **Kennedy GC, German MS, Rutter WJ.** 1995 The minisatellite in the diabetes susceptibility locus IDDM2 regulates insulin transcription. Nat Genet. 9:293-298.

51. **Puglise A, Zeller M, Fernandez Jr. A, Zalcberg LJ, Bartlett RJ, Ricordi C, Pietropaolo M, Eisenbarth GS, Bennett ST, Patel DD.** 1997 The insulin gene is transcribed in the human thymus and transcription levels correlate with allelic variation at the INS VNTR-IDDM2 susceptibility locus for type 1 diabetes. Nat Genet. 15:293-297.

52. **Vafiadis P, Bennett ST, Todd JA, Nadeau J, Grabs R, Goodyer CG, Wickramasinghe S, Colle E, Polychronakos C.** 1997 Insulin expression in human thymus is modulated by INS VNTR alleles at the IDDM2 locus. Nat Genet.15:289-292.

53. **Permutt MA, Chiu KC, Tanizawa Y.** Glucokinase and NIDDM. 1992 A candidate gene that paid off. Diabetes 41:1367-1372.

54. **Ott J.** 1996 Analysis of human genetic linkage. Baltimore: Johns Hopkins University Press..

55. **Lander E, Kruglyak L.** 1995 Genetic dissection of complex traits: guidelines for interpreting and reporting linkage results. Nature Genet. 11:241-247.

56. **Weber JL.** 1990 Human DNA polymorphisms based on length variations in simple-sequence tandem repeats. Genome Anal 1:159-181.

57. **Nelson JL, Hansen JA.** 1990 Autoimmune disease and HLA. CRC Crit Rev Immunol. 10:307-328.

58. **Campbell RD, Trowsdale J.** 1993 Map of the human MHC. Immunol Today 14:349-352.

59. **Todd JA.** 1995 Genetic analysis of type 1 diabetes using whole genome approaches. Proc Natl Acad Sci USA 92:8560-8565.

60. **Bech K, Lumholtz B, Nerup J, Thomsen M, Platz P, Ryder LP, Svejgaard A, Siersbaek-Nielsen K, Hansen JM, Larse JH.** 1977 HLA antigens in Graves' disease. Acta Endocrinol. 86:510-516.

61. **Farid NR, Sampson L, Noel EP, Barnard JM, Mandeville R, Larsen B, Marshall WH, Carter ND.** 1979 A study of human D locus related antigens in Graves' disease. J Clin Invest. 63:108-113.

62. **Mangklabruks A, Cox N, DeGroot LJ.** 1991 Genetic factors in autoimmune thyroid disease analyzed by restriction fragment length polymorphisms of candidate genes. J Clin Endocrinol Metab. 73:236-244.

63. **Kawa A, Nakamura S, Nakazawa M, Sakaguch S, Kawabata T, Maeda Y, Kanehisa T.** 1977 HLA-BW35 and B5 in Japanese patients with Graves' disease. Acta Endocrinol. 86:754-757.

64. **Chan SH, Yeo PP, Lui KF, Wee GB, Woo KT, Lim P, Cheah JS.** 1978 HLA and thyrotoxicosis (Graves' disease) in Chinese. Tissue Antigens 12:109-114.

65. **Barlow ABT, Wheatcroft N, Watson P, Weetman AP.** 1996 Association of HLA-DQA1*0501 with Graves' disease in English caucasian men and women. Clin Endocrinol. 44:73-77.

66. **Yanagawa T, Mangklabruks A, Chang YB, Okamoto Y, Fisfalen M-E, Curran PG, DeGroot LJ.** 1993 Human histocompatibility leukocyte antigen-DQA1*0501 allele associated with genetic susceptibility to Graves' disease in a caucasian population. J Clin Endocrinol Metab. 76:1569-1574.

67. **Hawkins BR, Ma JT, Lam KS, Wang CC, Yeung RT.** 1985 Analysis of linkage between HLA haplotype and susceptibility to Graves' disease in multiple-case Chinese families in Hong Kong. Acta Endocrinol. 1985; 110:66-69.

68. **Roman SH, Greenberg DA, Rubinstein P, Wallenstein S, Davies TF.** 1992 Genetics of autoimmune thyroid disease: lack of evidence for linkage to HLA within families. J Clin Endocrinol Metab.74:496-503.

69. **O'Connor G, Neufeld DS, Greenberg DA, Concepcion L, Roman SH, Davies TF.** 1993 Lack of disease associated HLA-DQ restriction fragment length polymorphisms in families with autoimmune thyroid disease. Autoimmunity 14:237-241.

70. **Tomer Y, Barbesino G, Keddache M, Greenberg DA, Davies TF.** 1997 Mapping of a major susceptibility locus for Graves' disease (GD-1) to chromosome 14q31. J Clin Endocrinol Metab. 82:1645-1648.

71. **Payami H, Joe S, Thomson G.** 1989 Autoimmune thyroid disease in Type 1 diabetes. Genet Epidem. 6:137-141.

72. **Stenszky V, Kozma L, Balazs C, Rochlitz S, Bear JC, Farid NR.** 1985 The genetics of Graves' disease: HLA and disease susceptibility. J Clin Endocrinol Metab. 61:735-740.

73. **Schleusener H, Schernthaner G, Mayr WR, Kotulla P, Bogner U, Finke R, Meinhold H, Koppenhagen K, Wenzel KW.** 1983 HLA-DR3 and HLA-DR5 associated thyrotoxicosis--two different types of toxic diffuse goiter. J Clin Endocrinol Metab. 56:781-785.

74. **Farid NR, Stone E, Johnson G.** 1980 Graves' disease and HLA: clinical and epidemiologic associations. Clin Endocrinol. 13:535-544.

75. **Frecker M, Stenszky V, Balazs C, Kozma L, Kraszits E, Farid NR.** 1986 Genetic factors in Graves' ophthalmopathy. Clin Endocrinol. 25:479-485.

76. **Frecker M, Mercer G, Skanes VM, Farid NR.** 1988 Major histocompatibility complex (MHC) factors predisposing to and protecting against Graves' eye disease. Autoimmunity 1:307-315.

77. **Allannic H, Fauchet R, Lorcy Y, Gueguen M, Le Guerrier AM, Genetet B.** 1983 A prospective study of the relationship between relapse of hyperthyroid Graves' disease after antithyroid drugs and HLA haplotype. J Clin Endocrinol Metab. 57:719-722.

78. **Kendall-Taylor P, Stephenson A, Stratton A, Papiha SS, Perros P, Roberts DF.** 1988 Differentiation of autoimmune ophthalmopathy from Graves' hyperthyroidism by analysis of genetic markers. Clin Endocrinol 28:601-610.

79. **Weetman AP, So AK, Warner CA, Foroni L, Fells P, Shine B.** 1988 Immunogenetics of Graves' ophthalmopathy. Clin Endocrinol 28:619-628.

80. **Weetman AP, Ratanachaiyavong S, Middleton GW, Love W, John R, Owen GM, Darke C, Lazarus JH, Hall R, McGregor AM.** 1986 Prediction of outcome in Graves' disease after carbimazole treatment. Q J Med. 59:409-419.

81. **Buus S, Sette A, Grey HM.** 1987 The interaction between protein-derived immunogenic peptides and Ia. Immunol Rev. 98:115-141.

82. **Nelson JL, Hansen JA.** 1990 Autoimmune disease and HLA. CRC Crit Rev Immunol. 10:307-328.

83. **Faas S, Trucco M.** 1994 The genes influencing the susceptibility to IDDM in humans. J Endocrinol Invest. 17:477-495.

84. **Londei M, Lamb JR, Bottazzo GF, Feldmann M.** 1984 Epithelial cells expressing aberrant MHC class II determinants can present antigen to cloned human T cells. Nature 312:639-641.

85. **Hanafusa T, Pujol Borrell R, Chiovato L, Russell RC, Doniach D, Bottazzo GF.** 1983 Aberrant expression of HLA-DR antigen on thyrocytes in Graves' disease: relevance for autoimmunity. Lancet 2:1111-1115.

86. **Davies TF.** 1985 Co-culture of human thyroid monolayer cells and autologous T cells: impact of HLA class II antigen expression. J Clin Endocrinol Metab. 61:418-422.

87. **Davies TF, Piccinini LA.** 1987 Intrathyroidal MHC class II antigen expression and thyroid autoimmunity. Endocrinol Metab Clin North Am. 16:247-268.

88. **Neufeld DS, Platzer M, Davies TF.** 1989 Reovirus induction of MHC class II antigen in rat thyroid cells. Endocrinology 124:543-545.

89. **Belfiore A, Mauerhoff T, Pujol Borrell R, Badenhoop K, Buscema M, Mirakian R,**

Bottazzo GF. 1991 De novo HLA class II and enhanced HLA class I molecule expression in SV40 transfected human thyroid epithelial cells. J Autoimmunity. 4:397-414.

90. **Davies TF, Bermas B, Platzer M, Roman SH.** 1985 T-cell sensitization to autologous thyroid cells and normal non- specific suppressor T-cell function in Graves' disease. Clin Endocrinol. 22:155-167.

91. **Eguchi K, Otsubo T, Kawabe K, Ueki Y, Fukuda T, Mayumi M, Shimomura C, Ishikawa N, Nakao H, Ito K, Morimoto C, Nagataki S.** 1987 The remarkable proliferation of helper T cell subset in response to autologous thyrocytes and intrathyroidal T cells from patients with Graves' disease. Isr J Med Sci 70:403-410.

92. **Jackson DG, Capra JD.** 1993 TAP1 alleles in insulin-dependent diabetes mellitus: a newly defined centromeric boundary of disease susceptibility. Proc Natl Acad Sci USA 90:11079-11083.

93. **Yanagawa T, Hidaka Y, Guimaraes V, Soliman M, DeGroot LJ.** 1995 CTLA-4 gene polymorphism associated with Graves' disease in a caucasian population. J Clin Endocrinol Metab. 80:41-45.

94. **Nistico L, Buzzetti R, Pritchard LE, et al.** 1996 The CTLA-4 gene region of chromosome 2q33 is linked to, and associated with, type 1 diabetes. Belgian Diabetes Registry. Hum Mol Genet. 5:1075-1080.

95. **Kotsa K, Watson PF, Weetman AP.** 1997 A CTLA-4 gene polymorphism is associated with both Graves' disease and autoimmune hypothyroidism. Clin Endocrinol. 46:551-554.

96. **Sale MM, Akamizu T, Howard TD, Yokota T, Nakao K, Mori T, Iwasaki H, Rich SS, Jennings-Gee JE, Yamada M, Bowden DW.** 1997 Association of autoimmune thyroid disease with a microsatellite marker for the thyrotropin receptor gene and CTLA-4 in a Japanese population. Proc Assoc Am Phys. 109:453-461.

97. **Donner H, Rau H, Walfish PG, Braun J, Siegmund T, Finke R, Herwig J, Usadel KH, Badenhoop K.** 1997 CTLA4 alanine-17 confers genetic susceptibility to Graves' disease and to type 1 diabetes mellitus. J Clin Endocrinol Metab. 82:143-146.

98. **Yanagawa T, Taniyama M, Enomoto S, Gomi K, Maruyama H, Ban Y, Saruta T.** 1997 CTLA4 gene polymorphism confers susceptibility to Graves' disease in Japanese. Thyroid 7:843-846.

99. **Vaidya B, Imrie H, Perros P, Dickinson J, McCarthy MI, Kendall-Taylor P, Pearce SH.** 1999 Cytotoxic T lymphocyte antigen-4 (CTLA-4) gene polymorphism confers susceptibility to thyroid associated orbitopathy (letter). Lancet 354:743-744.

100. **Heward JM, Allahabadia A, Carr-Smith J, Daykin J, Cockram CS, Gordon CBAH, Franklyn JA, Gough SCL.** 1998 No evidence for allelic association of human CTLA-4 promoter polymorphism with autoimmune thyroid disease in either population-based case-control or family-based studies. Clin Endocrinol. 49:331-334.

101. **Vaidya B, Imrie H, Perros P, Young ET, Kelly WF, Carr D, Large DM, Toft AD, McCarthy MI, Kendall-Taylor P, Pearce SH.** 1999 The cytotoxic T lymphocyte antigen-4 is a major Graves' disease locus. Hum Mol Genet. 8:1195-1199.

102. **Reiser H, Stadecker MJ.** 1996 Costimulatory B7 molecules in the pathogenesis of infectious and autoimmune diseases. N Engl J Med. 335:1369-1377.

103. **Lenschow DJ, Ho SC, Sattar H, Rhee L, Gray G, Nabavi N, Herold KC, Bluestone JA.** 1995 Differential effects of anti-B7-1 and anti-B7-2 monoclonal antibody treatment on the development of diabetes in the nonobese diabetic mouse. J Exp Med. 181:1145-1155.

104. **Lenschow DJ, Herold KC, Rhee L, Patel B, Koons A, Qin HY, Fuchs E, Singh B, Thompson CB, Bluestone JA.** 1996 CD28/B7 regulation of Th1 and Th2 subsets in the development of autoimmune diabetes. Immunity 5:285-293.

105. **Abbas AK, Murphy KM, Sher A.** 1996 Functional diversity of helper T lymphocytes. Nature 383:787-793.

106. **Smith TJ, Sciaky D, Phipps RP, Jennings TA.** 1999 CD40 expression in human thyroid

tissue: evidence for involvement of multiple cell types in autoimmune and neoplastic diseases. Thyroid 9:749-755.

107. **Metcalfe RA, McIntosh RS, Marelli-Berg F, Lombardi G, Lechler R, Weetman AP.** 1998 Detection of CD40 on human thyroid follicular cells: analysis of expression and function. J Clin Endocrinol Metab. 83:1268-1274.

108. **Faure GC, Bensoussan-Lejzerowicz D, Bene MC, Aubert V, Leclere J.** 1997 Coexpression of CD40 and class II antigen HLA-DR in Graves' disease thyroid epithelial cells. Clin Immunol Immunopathol. 84:212-215.

109. **Demaine A, Welsh KI, Hawe BS, Farid NR.** 1987 Polymorphism of the T cell receptor beta-chain in Graves' disease. J Clin Endocrinol Metab. 65:643-646.

110. **Weetman AP, So AK, Roe C, Walport MJ, Foroni L.** 1987 T-cell receptor alpha chain V region polymorphism linked to primary autoimmune hypothyroidism but not Graves' disease. Human Immunol. 20:167-173.

111. **Barbesino G, Tomer Y, Concepcion ES, Davies TF, Greenberg DA.** 1998 Linkage analysis of candidate genes in autoimmune thyroid disease: I. Selected immunoregulatory genes. J Clin Endocrinol Metab. 83:1580-1584.

112. **Nakao Y, Matsumoto H, Miyazaki T, Nishitani H, Takatsuki K, Kasukawa R, Nakayama S, Izumi S, Fujita T, Tsuji K.** 1980 IgG heavy chain allotypes (Gm) in atrophic and goitrous thyroiditis. Clin Exp Immunol. 42:20-26.

113. **Blakemore AIF, Watson PF, Weetman AP, Duff GW.** 1995 Association of Graves' disease with an allele of the interleukin-1 receptor antagonist gene. J Clin Endocrinol Metab. 80:111-115.

114. **Cuddihy RM, Bahn RS.** 1996 Lack of an association between alleles of interleukin-1 alpha and interleukin-1 receptor antagonsit genes and Graves' disease in a north American Caucasian population. J Clin Endocrinol Metab. 81:4476-4478.

115. **Weetman AP, Gunn C, Hall R, McGregor AM.** 1985 Thyroid autoantigen-induced lymphocyte proliferation in Graves' disease and Hashimoto's thyroiditis. J Clin Lab Immunol. 17:1-6.

116. **Weetman AP.** 1992 Autoimmune thyroiditis: predisposition and pathogenesis. Clin Endocrinol. 36:307-323.

117. **Rosenbaum D, Davies TF.** 1992 The clinical use of thyroid autoantibodies. The Endocrinologist 2:55-62.

118. **Raspe E, Costagliola S, Ruf J, Mariotti S, Dumont JE, Ludgate M.** 1995 Identification of the thyroid Na+/I- cotransporter as a potential autoantigen in thyroid autoimmune disease (see comments). Eur J Endocrinol. 132:399-405.

119. **Bohr URM.** 1993 A heritable point mutation in an extracellular domain of the TSHR involved in the interaction with Graves' disease. Biochem Biophys Acta 1216:504-508.

120. **Bahn RS, Dutton CM, Heufelder AE, Sarkar G.** 1994 A genomic point mutation in the extracellular domain of the TSHR in patients with Graves' ophthalmopathy. J Clin Endocrinol Metab. 78:256-260.

121. **Ahmad MF, Stenszky V, Juhazs F, Balzs G, Farid NR.** 1994 No mutations in the translated region of exon 1 in the TSHR in Graves' thyroid glands. Thyroid 4:151-153.

122. **Watson PF, French A, Pickerill AP, McIntosh RS, Weetman AP.** 1995 Lack of association between a polymorphism in the coding region of the thyrotropin receptor gene and Graves' disease. J Clin Endocrinol Metab. 80:1032-1035.

123. **De Roux N, Misrahi M, Chatelain N, Gross B, Milgrom E.** 1996 Microsatellites and PCR primers for genetic studies and genomic sequencing of the human TSHR gene. Mol Cell Endocrinol. 117:253-256.

124. **De Roux N, Shields DC, Misrahi M, Ratanachaiyavong S, McGregor AM, Milgrom E.** 1996 Analysis of the thyrotropin receptor as a candidate gene in familial Graves' disease. J Clin Endocrinol Metab. 81:3483-3486.

125. **Tomer Y, Barbesino G, Greenberg DA, Concepcion ES, Davies TF.** 1998 Linkage analysis of candidate genes in autoimmune thyroid disease: 3. Detailed analysis of chromosome 14 localizes GD-1 close to MNG-1. J Clin Endocrinol Metab. 83:4321-4327.

126. **Pirro MT, De Filippis V, Di Cerbo A, Scillitani A, Liuzzi A, Tassi V.** 1995 Thyroperoxidase microsatellite polymorphism in thyroid disease. Thyroid 5:461-464.

127. **Paavonen T.** Hormonal regulation of immune responses. Ann Med 1994; 26:255-258.

128. **Van Griensven M, Bergijk EC, Baelde JJ, De Heer E, Bruijn JA.** 1997 Differential effects of sex hormones on autoantibody production and proteinuria in chronic graft-versus-host disease-induced experimental lupus nephritis. Clin Exp Immunol. 107:254-260.

129. **Grossman CJ, Roselle GA, Mendenhall CL.** 1991 Sex steroid regulation of autoimmunity. J Steroid Biochem Mol Biol. 40:649-659.

130. **Stewart JJ.** 1998 The female X-inactivation mosaic in systemic lupus erythematosus. Immunol Today 19:352-357.

131. **Barbesino G, Tomer Y, Concepcion ES, Davies TF, Greenberg D.** 1998 Linkage analysis of candidate genes in autoimmune thyroid disease: 2. Selected gender-related genes and the X-chromosome. J Clin Endocrinol Metab. 83:3290-3295.

132. **Villanueva RB, Tomer Y, Tucci S, Greenberg DA, Concepcion ES, Davies TF.** 1999 Analysis of the BTK gene on chromosome X as a candidate gene in Graves' disease. Endocrine Society 81st Annual Meeting; San Diego, CA.

133. **Tomer Y, Barbesino G, Greenberg DA, Concepcion ES, Davies TF.** 1998 A new Graves disease-susceptibility locus maps to chromosome 20q11.2. Am J Hum Genet. 63:1749-1756.

134. **Tomer Y, Barbesino G, Greenberg DA, Concepcion ES, Davies TF.** 1999 Mapping the major susceptibility loci for familial Graves' and Hashimoto's diseases: Evidence for genetic heterogeneity and gene interactions. J Clin Endocrinol Metab. In press.

135. **Bignell GR, Canzian F, Shayeghi M, et al.** 1997 A familial non-toxic multinodular thyroid goiter locus maps to chromosome 14q but does not account for familial non-medullary thyroid cancer. Am J Hum Genet. 61:1123-1130.

136. **McKenna R, Kearns M, Sugrue D, Drury MI, McCarthy CF.** 1982 HLA and hyperthyroidism in Ireland. Tissue Antigens 19:97-99.

137. **Dahlberg PA, Holmlund G, Karlsson FA, Safwenberg J.** 1981 HLA-A, -B, -C and -DR antigens in patients with Graves' disease and their correlation with signs and clinical course. Acta Endocrinol. 97:42-47.

4

THYROID AUTOANTIBODIES IN GRAVES' DISEASE

Basil Rapoport and Sandra M. McLachlan

INTRODUCTION

Graves' hyperthyroidism is caused by autoantibodies to the TSH receptor (TSHR) that mimic the stimulatory effects of TSH (reviewed in 1). At the other extreme is Hashimoto's thyroiditis, in which autoantibodies to thyroid peroxidase (TPO) and sometimes to thyroglobulin (Tg), are associated with (but do not necessarily cause) destruction of thyroid follicular cells and hypothyroidism. Less commonly, atrophic thyroiditis can be caused by TSH receptor antibodies that block TSH action (reviewed in 1). Occasionally, in the same patient, the balance may shift from hyperthyroidism to hypothyroidism, and vice versa.

Although phenotypically quite different, Graves' and Hashimoto's diseases have overlapping immunological characteristics. In particular, lymphocytic infiltrates are present in Graves' thyroid glands, albeit to a lesser extent than in Hashimoto's thyroiditis. Moreover, besides TSHR autoantibodies, TPO autoantibodies are present in ~75 % of Graves' patients (2,3). Tg autoantibodies occur in a smaller proportion of Graves' patients (~25%)(2,3). Although there is some evidence for the presence in autoimmune thyroid disease of autoantibodies to the sodium/iodide symporter, the major autoimmune response in Graves' disease is directed towards the TSHR and TPO. Consequently, the focus of this chapter is the structure of these two fascinating, complex glycoproteins and the interaction with their respective autoantibodies.

TSHR STRUCTURE

Relationship to other G protein coupled receptors

The TSHR is a member of the G-protein coupled receptor family with seven transmembrane regions. Like the related LH/CG and FSH receptors, but unlike most other members of this superfamily, the N-terminal ectodomain represents nearly half of the TSHR mass (397 of 764 amino acid residues)(Fig. 1). The glycoprotein hormone receptors have different ligands yet similar signaling pathways and their transmembrane and cytoplasmic regions are more homologous than their ectodomains. Within the ectodomains, homology is greatest in the mid-regions which contain leucine rich repeats. The TSHR contains 9 such repeats between TSHR amino acid residues 54-254. The less conserved N-terminal and C-terminal regions of the TSHR contain two

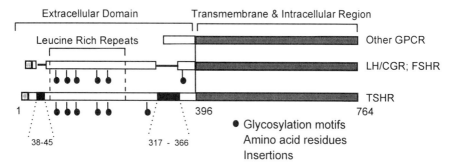

Figure 1. Schematic comparison of TSHR with LH/CGR and other G-protein coupled receptors (GPCR) with 7 transmembrane regions which have small ectodomains.

clusters of additional residues compared to the gonadotropin receptors, giving the appearance of two "insertions"; one of 8 amino acids at approximately residues 38-45 and the other of 50 amino acids at approximately residues 317-366. The relatively low homology between receptors in these regions make the exact localization of these insertions imprecise.

Cleavage of the TSHR

In 1982, covalent crosslinking of radiolabeled TSH to thyroid cell membranes indicated that the TSHR is a 80 kDa heterodimer with a 50 kDa hormone-binding A subunit linked by disulfide bonds to a membrane-spanning 30 kDa B subunit (4). The molecular cloning of the TSHR in 1989 confirmed the existence of A and B subunits (5,6). Moreover, the presence of a single mRNA encoding both subunits indicated that these subunits must be formed by intramolecular cleavage. In addition to a two subunit form, uncleaved, single chain TSHR with high affinity for TSH were also observed on the surface of intact transfected non-thyroidal cells (5). Whether or not single chain TSHR exist on thyrocytes in vivo is an unknown issue.

Surprisingly, intramolecular cleavage of the TSHR does not occur at a single site but involves the removal of a "C peptide region" which corresponds, approximately, to the 50 amino acid 'insertion' (7,8)(Fig. 2). Cleavage probably occurs first at upstream Site 1, which is between TSHR residues 303 and 317 (8,9). The C peptide region is then excised either by cleavage at a downstream Site 2 or by progressive N-terminal degradation of the B subunit downstream to the Site 2 region (at approximately residue 370)(8,10). Intact C peptide cannot be recovered from the medium of cultured cells, suggesting that this region is degraded (8,11). A factor contributing to the difficulty in precisely localizing the TSHR cleavage site(s) is that all amino acid residues with the cleavage regions can be substituted without reducing cleavage (9,10). Such 'relaxed' specificity is consistent with cleavage being produced by a matrix metalloprotease (MMP), although evidence for the involvement of such an enzyme is conflicting (8,12).

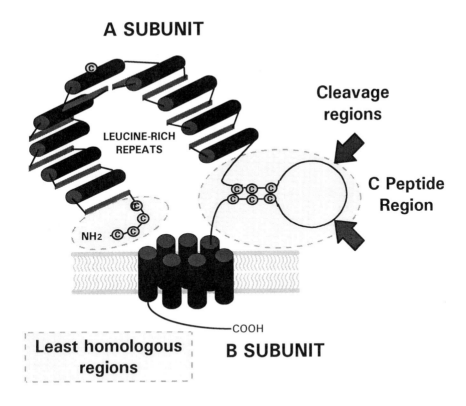

A SUBUNIT

Cleavage regions

LEUCINE-RICH REPEATS

C Peptide Region

NH2

Least homologous regions

B SUBUNIT

COOH

Figure 2. Present concept of the three dimensional structure of the TSHR.

Disulfide bonds

As for any large protein, disulfide bonding is essential for the correct folding and conformation of the TSHR (reviewed in 1). Of the 13 cysteine (Cys) residues in the TSHR, two Cys in the first and second *extracellular loops* are conserved in the G-protein coupled receptor family and are likely to be paired with each other. The 11 Cys in the TSHR *ectodomain* could form 5 pairs with one residue remaining as the orphan. Although there are no direct data to indicate which of the other Cys are paired, indirect evidence (reviewed in 1) provides the basis for the model shown in Fig.2). Of the cluster of four cysteines at the N-terminus of the A subunit, Cys41 is particularly important, either through its influence on the autoantibody binding site or on protein expression and folding.

Carbohydrate moieties on the TSHR

The human TSHR ectodomain contains 6 potential N-linked glycosylation sites, all on the A subunit. The presence of ~25 kDa of glycan on the TSHR ectodomain suggests that most, if not all, of these potential sites contain glycan. However, only

Asn302 of the TSHR has been determined directly to contain glycan (9). The mature TSHR on the cell surface (both single chain and cleaved) contains complex carbohydrate (reviewed in 1). The potential role of glycan in autoantibody binding to the TSHR is discussed below.

RECOMBINANT TSHR EXPRESSION

The small number of TSHR in thyroid tissue, perhaps only 5,000 receptors per thyrocyte (13), and protein instability has made purification of receptor from this source difficult. Consequently, a large effort has been made to generate recombinant TSHR. Two major questions need to be addressed:- which expression system to use and whether to express the TSH holoreceptor (743 amino acids without the 21 residue signal peptide), the more hydrophilic ectodomain (397 amino acids) or smaller ectodomain fragments. Expression systems used include (i) prokaryotic bacteria; (ii) cell-free translation; (iii) eukaryotic insect cells and (iv) stably transfected eukaryotic mammalian cells. As described below, the generation of effective TSHR antigen has been extraordinarily difficult (Table 1).

Prokaryotic TSHR expression

Because it is technically more easy and because high levels of expression may be attained, numerous groups have expressed the TSHR ectodomain in bacteria (reviewed in1). In some systems, the TSHR ectodomain has been generated, at least in part, in soluble form, rather than as insoluble inclusion bodies that require dissolving in chaotropic agents. However, it is controversial as to whether the non-glycosylated TSHR ectodomain of bacterial origin specifically binds TSH and/or TSHR autoantibodies is (reviewed in 1).

Cell-free translation of TSHR or synthetic TSHR peptides

Cell-free translation of TSHR mRNA using microsomal preparations is straightforward and generates products lacking glycan. The system can be modified to generate glycosylated material, but not with the quantity and quality of glycoproteins expressed by mammalian cells. Both the TSHR holoreceptor and the TSHR ectodomain have been expressed in cell-free translation systems. Results obtained with this approach have been controversial (reviewed in 1).

Synthetic TSHR polypeptide synthesis is a technically demanding but routine procedure performed by commercial or specialized laboratories. The practical advantages of generating peptides is counterbalanced by their limited ability to reconstitute the binding sites on a native, conformational and glycosylated protein (reviewed in 1).

Eukaryotic insect cell expression

High levels of glycosylated proteins can be expressed in insect cells. The TSHR ectodomain, but not the holoreceptor, has been expressed using this approach (reviewed

Table 1. Expression of recombinant TSHR and properties of proteins generated.

System	Soluble/ Secreted	Glycan	TSH/ Antibody binding
Bacteria			
Ectodomain	Insoluble	None	Controversial
In vitro transcription/translation			
Holoreceptor	Soluble?	None	TSH
Ectodomain	Soluble	None/some	Controversial
Synthetic TSHR peptides			
Various	Variable	None	TSH; antibody (low affinity)
Insect cell (TSHR ectodomain)			
With signal peptide	Insoluble	None	Controversial
Without signal peptide	Intracellular	High mannose	Antibody (ELISA)
Ectodomain; earlier promoter	Intracellular (trace, soluble)	High mannose	Antibody only (neutralization)
Denaturation & refolding	Insoluble	Present	Antibody (western)
Baculovirus signal peptide	Insoluble (most)	Present	Antibody (neutralization)
Mammalian Cells			
Holoreceptor (overexpression)	Soluble	Complex	TSH; Autoantibodies (FACS)
Ectodomain	Intracellular, soluble	High mannose	Autoantibodies
Ectodomain	Secreted (low levels)	Complex	Autoantibodies (neutralization)
TSHR-261, -289, -301 (overexpression)	Secreted	Complex	Autoantibodies (neutralization)
GPI-anchored ectodomain	Cell surface	Complex	Autoantibodies (FACS)

in 1). Initial reports that the TSHR ectodomain expressed without its signal peptide is glycosylated and is recognized by TSH and autoantibodies have now been refuted. However, when generated *with* a signal peptide and shown to contain 14 kDa of glycan, TSHR autoantibody (but not TSH) binding to the ectodomain is observed.

A number of technical modifications have been used to improve the quality of the TSHR ectodomain produced in insect cells, including the use of promoters that are active at an earlier stage after baculovirus infection, refolding of insoluble material and replacement of the mammalian TSHR signal peptide with an insect cell signal peptide. Several provocative conclusions have been made from some studies using this material (14,15) including that TSHR conformation and glycosylation are not major factors in autoantibody recognition and that linear epitopes are clearly recognized by many TSHR autoantibodies. We suggest caution in drawing these conclusions because of the very high concentration at which sera were studied. In addition, *qualitative* recognition by a serum of a particular form of antigen does not indicate what proportion of the antibodies in the serum interact with this antigenic form. Quantitative adsorption studies are required to address this issue.

TSHR expression in mammalian cells

Gradually, it is now being appreciated that TSHR expression in mammalian cells provides the optimal antigen for studying autoantibodies in Graves' disease.

Holoreceptor
Stable expression of the human TSH holoreceptor has been reported in numerous non-thyroidal cell lines, including Chinese hamster ovary (CHO) and SP2/0 mammalian cells. Unlike with other expression systems, there is no question that the TSHR expressed in mammalian cells is completely functional. Mammalian cells expressing the TSHR transduce a signal following stimulation by TSH and by TSHR autoantibodies (reviewed in 1). TSHR expression in such cells is typically ~90,000 receptors per cell, as in the commonly used JPO9 line (16). Even at this level of expression, purification of significant amounts of TSHR would be a formidable task. Recently, overexpression of greater numbers (~ 2 million TSHR per cell) has been attained using a dihydrofolate reductase minigene system (17).

Ectodomain
Lacking the hydrophobic transmembane regions of the holoreceptor, the more hydrophilic ectodomain (much of it the ligand binding A subunit) has become the focus of attempts to generate TSHR antigen. Unfortunately, even when expressed in mammalian cells, the TSHR ectodomain is retained within the cell in a form containing immature, high mannose carbohydrate (18). However, unlike in insect cells, the retained ectodomain in mammalian cells is largely soluble, even when overexpressed by transgenome amplification (18). Glycoproteins contain immature, high mannose carbohydrate when they leave the endoplasmic reticulum. Transfer to the Golgi complex, where the glycan matures to complex form, occurs only after folding is satisfactorily completed. Therefore, it is likely that the immature glycan on the TSHR ectodomain within the endoplasmic reticulum is the consequence, rather than the cause,

of abnormal folding and trafficking. Indeed, recent expression of TSHR in mutant CHO cell lines deficient in different stages of glycan maturation indicates that autoantibody and TSH binding to cell surface receptors is not dependent on the presence of complex carbohydrate (19).

The TSHR ectodomain has been converted into a secreted antigen by progressive C-terminal truncations at amino acid residues 309, 289 and 261 (20). The secreted TSHR ectodomain variants contain complex carbohydrate, like the mature holoreceptor (21) and, although they do not bind TSH, they are extremely potent in neutralizing functional autoantibodies in Graves' sera (20). Another successful maneuver has been the production of a bioactive TSHR ectodomain inserted into the plasma membrane by a glycosylphosphatidylinositol anchor (22,23).

TSHR AUTOANTIBODY ASSAYS

In 1956, Graves' disease was found to be caused by a serum stimulator with a duration of action longer than that of TSH, the "long acting thyroid stimulator" (LATS) (24). LATS was determined to be an IgG (25,26) and was renamed thyroid *stimulatory* antibodies or immunoglobulins (TSAb or TSI). Sera from some hypothyroid patients contained IgG that inhibited TSH activation of thyroid adenylate cyclase (27), now referred to as TSH *blocking* autoantibodies (TBAb). In our opinion, this nomenclature is preferable to TSH stimulating blocking antibodies (TSBAb), a confusing term in common use. Autoantibodies that stimulate thyroid growth independent of the adenylate cyclase pathway have been reported (28,29). However, available evidence indicates that "growth" antibodies are not a separate species from conventional TSAb/TSI (which also induce thyroid growth)(30,31).

TSHR autoantibody assays are of three types; bioassays, indirect binding assays and direct binding assays. The principles of these assays, as well as future potential developments, are summarized in Table 2 and are outlined below.

Bioassays for thyroid stimulating antibodies (TSAb)

LATS was detected by injecting patients' immunoglobulins into laboratory animals (first guinea pigs and later mice) and measuring radioiodine released *in vivo* (24,32,33). The relatively low sensitivity of the "McKenzie bioassay"in mice was improved by an ingenious modification based on the observation that LATS activity was adsorbed by human thyroid tissue extracts (26). This "LATS protector" assay (34) compensated for the use of human IgG in the mouse bioassay. Subsequently, *in vitro* bioassays for TSAb were established, involving quantification of secretory 'colloid' droplet formation; cAMP production in thyroid tissue slices (35), or adenylate cyclase activation in thyroid plasma membranes (27).

Based on the precision and sensitivity of the cAMP response to TSH in thyroid cell monolayers, a bioassay for TSAb was developed using culture human thyroid cells (36,37). The TSAb assay sensitivity was further improved by incubation of cells in sodium chloride-free medium (38). Although nearly 50% of Graves' sera fail to stimulate the mouse thyroid in the McKenzie bioassay (39), the FRTL5 rat thyroid cell line has proved to be valuable and practical in a bioassay for TSI (40). Establishment of CHO cell lines expressing the human TSHR has been a further advance in the bioassay of TSAb (41,42).

Bioassays for TSH blocking antibodies (TBAb)

TBAb can only be detected by bioassay using monolayers of FRTL5 cells (43) or CHO cells stably transfected with the human TSHR (reviewed in 1). This assay quantitates the ability of autoantibodies to inhibit the increase in cAMP production (44) or iodide transport (45) in response to a standard concentration of TSH.

Indirect, TSH binding inhibition (TBI) assays

The observation that TSHR autoantibodies can compete for radiolabeled TSH binding to the TSHR (46) is the basis for the TBI assay. The ability to use a detergent extract of *porcine* thyroid membranes in solution and the development of highly potent, affinity-purified TSH (47) led to the present popularity of the TBI assay. Soluble, recombinant *human* TSHR (hTSHR) extracted from non-thyroidal mammalian cells has recently become available and is replacing the use of porcine TSHR (48,49). Recent data suggest improved sensitivity with TBI assays utilizing human, rather than porcine, TSHR (50).

Future TBI assays are likely to involve use of both human (h) TSHR and human TSH rather than bovine TSH. However, hTSH is a less effective ligand than bTSH, even with the human TSHR. 'Superanalogs' of human TSH may provide the ligand needed for an homologous, totally human TBI assay (51). However, even when hTSHR and hTSH are used, the limitations of the TBI assay will still include a relatively poor correlation with the TSAb assay (reviewed in 1) and lack of discrimination between TSAb and TBAb autoantibodies.

Direct assays for TSHR autoantibodies (DTAb)

Two major factors contributed to the difficulty in directly detecting autoantibody binding to the TSHR. Technical advances in generating recombinant mammalian TSHR have largely overcome the first difficulty (see above). The second, remaining problem concerns the very low concentration of TSHR autoantibodies in patients' sera (52). Thus, unlike TPO autoantibody levels that can reach 1 mg/ml (53), only rare, highly potent Graves' sera contain TSHR autoantibody levels as high as 1-5 µg/ml (20,54). Despite these problems, five different DTAb assays have been described recently for Graves' sera: (i) immunoprecipitation of ^{35}S-TSHR cell free translates (55); (ii) immunoprecipitation of ^{125}I-labeled, recombinant mammalian TSHR (56); (iii) detection by ELISA of recombinant, mammalian cell TSHR ectodomain (57); (iv) protein A capture of patients' serum IgG and detection of ectodomain variant TSHR-289 using a biotinylated murine monoclonal antibody to the poly-histidine tail engineered into the antigen and (v) protein A precipitation of TSHR-radiolabeled using the Fab fragment of murine monoclonal antibody to the TSHR C-terminus (58). Significant problems are associated with some of these assays. As yet, no DTAb assay has been introduced into clinical use.

Table 2. Principles of assays for detecting TSHR autoantibodies in Graves' disease and atrophic thyroiditis.

Assay & Antibody	Source of TSHR	Detection system(s)
Bioassays		
LATS; LATS-P	In vivo mouse assay	Release of ^{131}I from thyroid gland
TSAb (TSI)	Human thyroid cells Rat FRTL5 cells CHO cells (human TSHR)	cAMP generation Iodide transport Chemiluminescence
TBAb (TSBAb)	Human thyroid cells Rat FRTL5 cells CHO cells (human TSHR)	Inhibition of cAMP release (or iodide uptake) by standard TSH concentration
Indirect, TSH inhibition assays		
TBI	Thyroid membranes CHO cells (human TSHR) Soluble TSHR (porcine; human)	Inhibition of ^{125}I-bovine TSH binding
Direct binding assays		
DTAb	^{35}S-TSHR cell free translates	Immunoprecipitation
	^{125}I-labeled hTSHR	Immunoprecipitation
	TSHR-ectodomain-His tail	ELISA
	TSHR-289-6 His tail	Protein A capture of antibodies; detection by anti-His antibody
	TSHR labeled with Fab to C-terminus	Protein A precipitation of antibodies

As with the TBI assay, TSHR autoantibody *function* cannot be determined with present DTAb. Available data (methods ii, iv and v, above) indicate that DTAb assays correlate better with the TBI than with the TSAb assay. One conclusion from this correlation is that most autoantibodies that bind to the TSHR also inhibit TSH binding. Discrimination between TSAb and TBAb will require the expression of a variety of TSHR variants. Selected chimeric TSH-LH/CG receptors (59-61) are ideal candidates for this purpose. Recent reports on the use of chimeric receptors to determine the clinical outcome of therapy in Graves' patients are provocative and potentially important (62,63) and await confirmation.

BINDING OF TSHR AUTOANTIBODIES TO THE TSHR

General principles of antibody binding

Two principles regarding antibodies in general are helpful in understanding TSHR autoantibody binding. *First*, the majority of antibodies to large polypeptide molecules recognize conformational epitopes. *Second*, recognition of linear and conformational epitopes is not mutually exclusive. Thus, if three discontinuous segments contribute to an epitope, binding to one segment may be sufficient for ELISA detection. However, the affinity of this interaction is likely to be lower than with the entire antigen.

Binding to the holoreceptor or ectodomain?

Detection of TSHR autoantibodies using the TSHR ectodomain (rather than the more difficult to generate holoreceptor) has been criticized on the basis that autoantibodies to other regions of the receptor may be overlooked.   While this possibility cannot be entirely excluded, the ability of truncated forms of the TSHR ectodomain to neutralize essentially all TSHR autoantibodies in individual Graves' sera indicates that the TSHR ectodomain is a satisfactory antigen (20,64).

TSH and TSHR autoantibodies primarily recognize conformational epitopes

Strong evidence for the conformational nature of the *TSH* binding site is that when the TSHR ectodomain is divided into five arbitrary segments, every segment can be replaced with the corresponding segment of the LH/CGR without compromising high affinity TSH binding (65,66). Similarly, studies with chimeric TSH-LH/CG receptors indicate that *TSHR autoantibodies* interact with multiple regions of the TSHR ectodomain (59,60). The epitopes of both TSH and TSHR autoantibodies are, therefore, discontinuous and conformational. The inability of autoantibodies to recognize TSHR fragments expressed in a TSHR cDNA fragment library (67) is consistent with, but does not prove, the conformational nature of TSHR autoantibodies. This is because Graves' sera do not recognize the *entire* TSHR expressed in the same system.

In our view, the use of synthetic linear peptides to define TSHR autoantibody epitopes is problematic (reviewed in 1).   Thus, although some linear epitopic determinants are detected, these small segments are likely to be components of larger, conformational epitopes (see above). The affinity of TSHR autoantibody binding to synthetic peptides is orders of magnitude lower than to the holoreceptor. At such low levels of affinity, it is difficult to discriminate between specific and non-specific signals. Finally, if all published studies utilizing synthetic peptides are taken at face value, TSHR epitopes would comprise a large portion of the ~ 400 amino acid TSHR ectodomain, not a reasonable conclusion.

The role of carbohydrate in binding by TSHR autoantibodies

The role of glycan moieties in autoantibody binding is a subject of present interest. Two points should be emphasized. First, regarding the debate on linear TSHR epitopes, synthetic peptides and polypeptides generated in bacteria are not glycosylated. Many previous peptide studies are now considered "non-definitive" (68). Second, observations of a relationship between TSHR glycan and autoantibody binding do *not* establish whether the glycan moieties comprise part of the epitope or whether glycosylation is a determinant of TSHR autoantigenicity (69). As mentioned above, incomplete glycosylation is likely to be *secondary* to abnormal TSHR folding (18). Complex glycan is not essential for TSHR autoantibody recognition (19).

TSHR amino acid residues in the binding site TSHR autoantibodies

Two main approaches have been used to define the binding site(s) for TSHR autoantibodies; synthetic peptides and TSHR mutagenesis.

Synthetic peptides
TSHR peptides have been used in four ways (reviewed in 1):- Direct binding of patients' IgG to TSHR peptides; peptide inhibition ("neutralization") of TSHR autoantibody binding or activity; affinity enrichment of TSHR autoantibodies using immobilized peptides and study of the consequences of immunizing animals with TSHR peptides. In our opinion, confidence in interpreting these data is reduced for the following reasons:- (i) TSHR autoantibodies in serum comprise a very small proportion of the total IgG. Use of patients' sera at high concentrations in binding or enrichment studies can contribute to high background binding values; (ii) Exceptionally high peptide concentrations are required for autoantibody neutralization (typically 10^{-5} to 10^{-4} M); (iii) As mentioned above, although an epitope typically involves only ~ 20 amino acids, studies using peptides have implicated more than 180 and 330 amino acids for stimulating and blocking autoantibodies, respectively (reviewed in 1).

One peptide that has generated great interest is the "immunogenic peptide" (TSHR residues 352-366/367)(reviewed in 1). This peptide is highly immunogenic when injected into rabbits and is reportedly recognized by the majority of TSHR autoantibodies. However, the immunogenic peptide lies within the C peptide region which is excised following intramolecular cleavage (see above). Peptide 352-366 has not been used to absorb out TSHR autoantibody activity in Graves' sera, a critical experiment.

Mutagenesis of the TSHR
The principle of these studies is that alteration of the amino acid residues in the TSHR autoantibody binding site should reduce autoantibody binding. Three approaches have been used; deletion of TSHR residues, replacement of TSHR residues with irrelevant (non-homologous) substitutions, and replacement of TSHR residues with the corresponding residues from the LH/CGR (homologous substitutions) to

generate "chimeric" receptors. Based on mutagenesis studies, a number of major conclusions can be made (reviewed in 1)(Fig. 3). Thus, the epitopes for *TSAb*:- (i) overlap with, but are not precisely the same as, the TSH binding site (59,60); (ii) the N-terminal third of the TSHR ectodomain is necessary for TSHR autoantibody stimulation (59,60); (iii) stimulatory autoantibodies bind to discontinuous segments in both the N-terminal *and* the C-terminus (59); (iv) several N-terminal amino acid residues are involved in the activity of (at least some) stimulatory autoantibodies; namely, Ser 25-Glu 30 (70) and Thr 40 (71).

The epitopes for *TBAb*:- (i) overlap with, but are not precisely the same as, the TSH binding site and the TSAb epitope (59,60). Overlap between the TBAb, TSAb and TSH binding sites is greatest in the *C-terminal region* of the TSHR ectodomain (59); (ii) residues in the TSHR C-terminus that appear to be involved in TSH binding (in particular residues 295-302, 385 and 387-395)(72) are also important in TBAb activity (71); (iii) the emphasis on blocking autoantibody binding to the C-terminus of the TSHR ectodomain (reviewed in 73) should not obscure the finding that these autoantibodies also bind to the *N-terminus* or *mid-region* of the TSHR ectodomain (residues 1-261)(59).

- Highly conformational

- Multiple, discontinuous contact points throughout the ectodomain

- TSH binding site - Important elements identified in mid-region (domain C) and in C-terminal region (domains D and E)

- TSAb epitope - biased more towards the N terminus than TSH, but also contains elements in C-terminal regions

- TBAb epitope - overlaps with, but not identical to, the TSH binding site

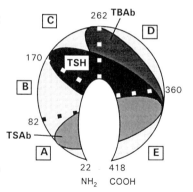

Figure 3. Summary of major concepts regarding TSH and TSHR autoantibody binding sites, as determined from chimeric TSH-LH/CGR data. The ectodomain of the TSHR, subdivided into 5 arbitrary units, A through E, is depicted in semicircular form, with the – and C-termini close to one another (see Fig. 2). TSAb, Thyroid stimulating autoantibodies; TBAb, TSH blocking autoantibodies. Reproduced with permission from Rapoport et al. (1).

MOLECULAR MIMICRY

An unresolved issue is whether autoantibodies to the TSHR arise in response to a foreign protein that "mimics" an epitope on the human TSHR (reviewed in 74). Although antigenic cross-reactivity between the TSHR and a variety of infectious agents has been reported, the most intriguing observations involve the gram negative bacterium *Yersinia enterocolitica.* Thus there are reports of:- (i) an association between *Y. enterocolitica* antibodies and thyroid disease in countries with a low incidence of infections to this bacterium (75,76); (ii) an interaction between Yersinia antibody-positive sera and thyroid epithelium (77); (iii) a saturable TSH binding site on Yersinia organisms (78) that could be competed for by sera with TSHR autoantibodies (79) and (iv) an interaction between antibodies in mice immunized with *Y. enterocolitica* and the TSHR (80). The nature of the *Y. enterocolitica* protein(s) cross-reacting with TSHR autoantibodies is controversial (81-83).

Several difficulties exist regarding the relationship between the TSHR and *Yersinia enterocolitica,* including:- (i) the " TSH binding site" on Yersinia (and other organisms) is of low affinity, comparable to plastic; (ii) antibodies induced by immunization with Yersinia were tested with non-glycosylated TSHR (80) shown subsequently not to interact with TSHR autoantibodies (69); (iii) cross-reactivity between purified Yersinia lipoprotein and the TSHR has not been studied with autoantibodies in Graves' sera and there is no amino acid homology between this lipoprotein and the TSHR; (iv) other studies have found no unique pattern of serological reactivity against Yersinia membrane proteins in patients with autoimmune thyroid disease, raising the possibility that cross-reactivity with Yersinia in Graves' disease may occur at the T cell epitope level rather than via autoantibodies (84); (v) molecular mimicry between *Y. enterocolitica* and the TSHR does not explain the frequent detection of autoantibodies to TPO and, to a lesser extent, Tg in Graves' disease.

HUMAN MONOCLONAL AUTOANTIBODIES TO THE TSHR

A variety of approaches have been used since the early 1980s to obtain murine and human monoclonal antibodies (mAb) to the TSHR. *Murine* mAb are invaluable reagents for identifying and characterizing the receptor. Prior to the molecular cloning of the TSHR it is unclear whether effective or specific murine mAb were obtained. In contrast, immunization with recombinant TSHR preparations has generated unequivocally effective mAb (reviewed in 1).

Human mAb are representative of the repertoire of TSHR autoantibodies in the sera of patients with autoimmune thyroid disease (primarily Graves' disease) and are, therefore essential for:- (i) mapping the TSHR epitopes recognized by functionally different populations of serum autoantibodies (the epitopes of mouse mAb may not be the same as those of naturally occurring autoantibodies); (ii) determining the three-dimensional structure of TSHR autoantibodies and, if feasible, crystallization of autoantibody-TSHR complexes to provide the structure of the epitopes recognized by TSHR autoantibodies; (iii) identifying and characterizing the heavy (H) and light (L) chain genes coding for TSHR autoantibodies. Besides permitting investigation of a possible association between immunoglobulin germline gene usage and TSHR epitope specificity (particularly relevant for stimulatory and blocking antibodies), this information may also contribute to understanding the genetic basis for Graves' disease.

Approaches for isolating human mAb

It is considerably more difficult to isolate human mAb of IgG class than mouse mAb and the following approaches have been used to obtain human TSR monoclonal antibodies representative of those in Graves' disease:-

Fusion of human B cells with a myeloma cell partner

Early reports on the generation of B cells clones secreting TSHR-specific mAb involved fusing peripheral blood mononuclear cells (PBMC) from Graves' patients with either mouse or human myeloma cell lines (reviewed in 1). Human-human fusions are frequently unstable and there have been no further reports on the clones with weak or ambiguous specificity that were obtained. In 1982, fusion of human B cells with a mouse myeloma partner was reported to be successful in obtaining clones representative of TSAb and TBAb (85), a feat recently repeated by the same laboratory (86). Independent confirmation is awaited.

Epstein Barr virus (EBV) infection to immortalize human B cells

In the mid-1980s, numerous laboratories attempted to obtain human TSHR mAb from patients' PBMC using EBV immortalization. A handicap with EBV-transformed B cells is the predominant secretion of IgM, a large, sticky molecule that provide false positives. Although many IgM mAb were produced, some were IgG and successful production of TSHR mAb with TSAb, TBAb or mixed activities was reported (reviewed in 1). Removal of IgM secreting B cells, has greatly facilitated the cloning of EBV-immortalized B cells of IgG class (87,88).

Source of B cells used to obtain human TSHR monoclonal autoantibodies

The exceptionally low concentration of TSHR autoantibodies in patients' sera indicates that the B cells responsible for producing these autoantibodies are likely to be very rare. All published attempts to generate human mAb to the TSHR have used peripheral blood lymphocytes (PBMC) from patients with autoimmune thyroid disease. PBMC contain naive and memory B cells, which are appropriate for EBV transformation. However, in autoimmune thyroid disease it is the thyroid gland that is enriched with thyroid autoantibody secreting B lymphocytes (reviewed in 13). Moreover, thyroidal B cells (unlike PBMC) are activated, spontaneously secrete TSHR autoantibodies (89), and are likely to be most appropriate for cell fusion. Incidentally, the debate as to whether or not TSHR autoantibodies are secreted by the Graves' thyroid revolves around the detection of an autoantibody arterio-venous (A-V) gradient across the thyroid bed. It should be appreciated that detection of an A-V gradient for IgG, a molecule with a very long half-life (up to three weeks) and a very large pool size, is a near impossibility (reviewed in 1).

Information from studies on the cloning of putative human TSHR autoantibodies

A number of important observations or conclusions have been made from the above studies:-(i) human mAb obtained can have TSAb activity, TBAb activity, or both activities; (b) TSAb can be obtained that do not inhibit TSH binding (86,90).

Conversely, some TBAb do not compete well for TSH binding (87); © TSAb secreting B cells can be isolated from patients with myxedema and TBAb secreting B cells from hyperthyroid patients (88); (d) the H and L chain genes for a number of mAb have been sequenced, characterized and expressed (91,92). However, these data have not yet fulfilled the following criteria (93) that, in our view, are necessary to confirm the specificity of the TSHR autoantibodies.

Thus, monoclonal human TSHR autoantibodies should be (i) of IgG class; (ii) functional at nanogram per ml concentrations (the concentration of human TSHR autoantibodies in serum (20); (iii) activity should be adsorbed with specific, but not control, antigen; (iv) active after IgG purification (cAMP stimulation assays are influenced by non-immunoglobulin factors in serum and high concentrations of normal IgG can inhibit TSH binding); (v) the H and L chain genes of the TSHR autoantibody should be expressed and the purified, recombinant proteins should be functional at nanogram/ml concentrations.

For these reasons, uncertainty remains about the specificity of the *human* TSHR mAb generated, none of which presently meet all of the suggested criteria (reviewed in 1). For example:- (i) the specificity of some human TSHR autoantibodies secreted in culture may now be doubted because the TSHR antigen used for screening was shown later not to be recognized by TSHR autoantibodies in patients' sera; (ii) the reported very high frequency of TSHR autoantibody B cells in peripheral blood should be viewed with caution because of the subsequent determination of the very low concentration of TSHR autoantibodies in patients' sera (20); and (iii) the specificity of some human mAb tested by immunoblotting is less certain in the light of new information on TSHR structure.

TPO AUTOANTIBODIES IN GRAVES' DISEASE

As mentioned above, TPO autoantibodies also occur in the great majority of Graves' patients. The goal of this section is to highlight the similarities and differences between TPO and TSHR autoantigens and their respective autoantibodies.

TPO structure and expression of recombinant protein

TPO, like the TSHR, is a membrane bound glycoprotein. Located primarily at the *apical* surface of the thyrocyte, TPO consists of two identical ~100 kDa subunits with a heme prosthetic group. Although TPO is more abundant than the TSHR in the thyroid, limited amounts can be purified from this source. Recombinant TPO expressed in eukaryotic cells (not in bacteria) is recognized by human TPO autoantibodies to the same extent as thyroid-derived TPO (reviewed in94). Unlike the TSHR, the full extracellular region of TPO is readily secreted and is suitable for studies of human TPO autoantibodies (95).

Immunological characteristics of TPO autoantibodies

Unlike TSHR autoantibodies that are *oligoclonal,* TPO autoantibodies are *polyclonal* as reflected in the presence in the same serum of kappa and lambda L chains and multiple IgG subclasses (96,97). Moreover, as mentioned above, TPO autoantibody levels are much higher than those for TSHR autoantibodies. Unlike the difficulties experienced with human TSHR mAbs, TPO autoantibody abundance, together with the relative ease of obtaining effective TPO autoantigen, has facilitated the generation of panels of human monoclonal TPO autoantibodies. Most of these human mAb were isolated from patients' thyroid tissue using the immunoglobulin gene combinatorial library approach (reviewed in 98). These recombinant human monoclonal TPO autoantibodies, expressed as Fab, closely resemble serum TPO autoantibodies in terms of the predominance of kappa over lambda L chains and the presence of subclasses IgG1 and IgG4. Importantly, the affinities for TPO of serum autoantibodies and most Fab are high (Kd $\sim 10^{-10}$ M)(reviewed in 98).

The relative ease of isolating human TPO-specific Fab permits comprehensive analysis of the variable region (V) genes encoding these autoantibodies. There are no unusual features of the H or L chain V genes encoding TPO Fab. Some L chain V regions are in germline conformation, whereas somatic mutation is apparent in most VH genes (reviewed in 98). Such mutations are anticipated for antigen-driven, high affinity antibodies.

Preferential recognition of conformational epitopes in an immunodominant region

As for TSHR autoantibodies, TPO autoantibodies and TPO-specific Fab preferentially bind to *conformational* epitopes (reviewed in 98). Moreover, unlike a panel of mouse monoclonals which recognize *diverse* epitopes, serum TPO autoantibodies interact with a *restricted* region on TPO (99,100).

The human TPO-specific Fab bind to overlapping epitopes in two domains (A and B) in an "immunodominant region" that is recognized by sera from all individuals and comprises >80% of TPO autoantibodies in the sera of each individual patient. Competition studies with individual Fab have been used to produce quantititative autoantibody epitopic "fingerprints" for TPO autoantibodies in patients' sera (101). Although unrelated to thyroid status (102), these fingerprints are conserved, regardless of fluctuations in autoantibody levels as in the postpartum period (103). Such conservation even up to 13 years (104) suggested that TPO autoantibody epitopic fingerprints may be inherited and segregation analysis of fingerprints has confirmed genetic transmission of the TPO B domain (105).

The conformational epitopes within the immunodominant region cannot be analyzed using peptides or polypeptide fragments. As for the TSHR, one approach used to circumvent this problem is the construction of *chimeric molecules* between TPO and an homologous protein, in this case myeloperoxidase (MPO). From these studies, as well from analysis of antibody binding to monomeric and dimeric TPO, several areas on the molecule have been excluded from containing the immunodominant region (106), including the mAb47/C21 linear epitope (amino acid residues 713-721) recognized by some patients' autoantibodies, the contact region between the homodimers and the N-terminal 121 amino acids. The C-terminus of the TPO extracellular region is a strong candidate region (107,108). Localization of the TPO immunodominant region will be difficult and may require crystallization of a TPO-Fab complex. One TPO-specific human Fab has been crystallized and its three-dimensional structure determined (109).

POTENTIAL ROLE OF B CELLS AND AUTOANTIBODIES IN ANTIGEN PRESENTATION TO T CELLS

Production of IgG class thyroid autoantibodies, like antibodies to other proteins, requires "help" from thyroid -specific T cells. Unlike antibodies that interact with primarily conformational epitopes, T cells recognize linear peptides (~ 20 amino acids in length) "processed" from large protein antigens and subsequently bound to major histocompatibility complex (MHC) class II molecules on antigen presenting cells (APC). Professional APC include macrophages and dendritic cells that play an important role in *initiating* T cell responses. In this connection, it should be appreciated that thyrocytes "aberrantly" express MHC class II molecules (110) and have been shown to function as antigen-presenting cells (111,112).

In *secondary* T cell responses, antibodies may play a critical role in antigen presentation to T cells. Thus, macrophages internalize and process antigen/antibody complexes by phagocytosis and/or binding to Fc receptors. Alternatively, and potentially more important, membrane-bound antibodies on B lymphocytes provide a powerful system for specific antigen capture (reviewed in 113). Antibodies may also modulate antigen processing and thereby enhance or suppress presentation of different T cell determinants (114).

Evidence is gradually accumulating for the role of B cells/antibodies in thyroid autoimmunity. Thus, a recombinant TPO-specific autoantibody has been shown to capture and present TPO *in vitro* (115). Moreover, in a mouse model for the induction of TPO antibodies resembling those arising spontaneously in human thyroid autoimmunity, evidence was obtained for TPO-specific B cells in antigen presentation to autologous T cells (116). The potentially important role of TSHR autoantibodies in antigen presentation to T cells has yet to be explored.

REFERENCES

1. **Rapoport B, Chazenbalk GD, Jaume JC, McLachlan SM.** 1998 The thyrotropin receptor: Interaction with thyrotropin and autoantibodies. Endocr Rev. 19:673-716.
2. **Karlsson FA, Dahlberg PA, Jansson R, Westermark K, Enoksson P.** 1989 Importance of TSH receptor activation in the development of severe endocrine ophthalmopathy. Acta Endocrinol. (Copenh) 121(Suppl.2):132-141.
3. **McLachlan SM, Bahn R, Rapoport B**. 1992 Endocrine ophthalmopathy: A re-evaluation of the association with thyroid autoantibodies. Autoimmunity 14:143-148.
4. **Buckland PR, Rickards CR, Howells RD, Jones ED, Rees Smith B.** 1982 Photo-affinity labelling of the thyrotropin receptor. FEBS Letters 145:245-249.
5. **Russo D, Chazenbalk GD, Nagayama Y, Wadsworth HL, Seto P, Rapoport B.** 1991 A new structural model for the thyrotropin (TSH) receptor as determined by covalent crosslinking of TSH to the recombinant receptor in intact cells: Evidence for a single polypeptide chain. Mol Endocrinol. 5:1607-1612.
6. **Loosfelt H, Pichon C, Jolivet A et al.** 1992 Two-subunit structure of the human thyrotropin receptor. Proc Natl Acad Sci USA 89:3765-3769.
7. **Chazenbalk GD, Tanaka K, Nagayama Y et al.** 1997 Evidence that the thyrotropin receptor ectodomain contains not one, but two, cleavage sites. Endocrinology 138:2893-2899.
8. de **Bernard S, Misrahi M, Huet J-C et al.** 1999 Sequential cleavage and excision of a

segment of the thyrotropin receptor ectodomain. J Biol Chem. 274:101-107.

9.   **Tanaka K, Chazenbalk GD, McLachlan SM, Rapoport B.** 1998 Thyrotropin receptor cleavage at site 1 does not involve a specific amino acid motif but instead depends on the presence of the unique, 50 amino acid insertion. J Biol Chem. 273:1959-1963.

10.   **Kakinuma A, Chazenbalk GD, Tanaka K, Nagayama Y, McLachlan SM, Rapoport B.** 1997 An N-linked glycosylation motif from the non-cleaving luteinizing hormone receptor substituted for the homologous region (Gly-367 to Glu-369) of the thyrotropin receptor prevents cleavage at its second, downstream site. J Biol Chem. 272:28296-28300.

11.   **Tanaka K, Chazenbalk GD, McLachlan SM, Rapoport B.** 1999 Subunit structure of thyrotropin receptors expressed on the cell surface. J Biol Chem. In press.

12.   **Couet J, Sokhavut S, Jolivet A, Vu Hai M-T, Milgrom E, Misrahi M.** 1996 Shedding of human thyrotropin receptor ectodomain: Involvement of a matrix metalloprotease. J Biol Chem. 271:4545-4552.

13.   **Rees Smith B, McLachlan SM, Furmaniak J.** 1988 Autoantibodies to the thyrotropin receptor. Endocr Rev. 9:106-121.

14.   **Graves PN, Vlase H, Davies TF.** 1995 Folding of the recombinant human thyrotropin (TSH) receptor extracellular domain: identification of folded monomeric and tetrameric complexes that bind TSH receptor autoantibodies. Endocrinology 136:521-527.

15.   **Vlase H, Graves PN, Magnusson RP, Davies TF.** 1995 Human autoantibodies to the thyrotropin receptor: recognition of linear, folded, and glycosylated recombinant extracellular domain. J Clin Endocrinol Metab. 80:46-53.

16.   **Costagliola S, Swillens S, Niccoli P, Dumont JE, Vassart G, Ludgate M.** 1992 Binding assay for thyrotropin receptor autoantibodies using the recombinant receptor protein. J Clin Endocrinol Metab. 75:1540-1544.

17.   **Chazenbalk GD, Kakinuma A, Jaume JC, McLachlan SM, Rapoport B.** 1996 Evidence for negative cooperativity among human thyrotropin receptors overexpressed in mammalian cells. Endocrinology 137:4586-4591.

18.   **Rapoport B, McLachlan SM, Kakinuma A, Chazenbalk GD.** 1996 Critical relationship between autoantibody recognition and TSH receptor maturation as reflected in the acquisition of mature carbohydrate. J Clin Endocrinol Metab. 81:2525-2533.

19.   **Nagayama Y, Namba H, Yokoyama N, Yamashita S, Niwa M.** 1998 Role of asparagine-linked oligosaccharides in protein folding, membrane targetting, and thyrotropin and autoantibody binding of the human thyrotropin receptor. J Biol Chem. 273:33423-33428.

20.   **Chazenbalk GD, Jaume JC, McLachlan SM, Rapoport B.** 1997 Engineering the human thyrotropin receptor ectodomain from a non-secreted form to a secreted, highly immunoreactive glycoprotein that neutralizes autoantibodies in Graves' patients' sera. J Biol Chem. 272:18959-18965.

21.   **Misrahi M, Ghinea N, Sar S et al.** 1994 Processing of the precursors of the human thyroid-stimulating hormone receptor in various eukaryotic cells (human thyrocytes, transfected L cells and baculovirus-infected insect cells). Eur J Biochem. 222:711-719.

22.   **Da Costa CR, Johnstone AP.** 1998 Production of the thyrotropin receptor extracellular domain as a glycosylphosphatidylinositol-anchored membrane protein and its interaction with thyrotropin and autoantibodies. J Biol Chem. 273:11874-11880.

23.   **Costagliola S, Khoo D, Vassart G.** 1998 Production of bioactive amino-terminal domain of the thyrotropin receptor via insertion in the plasma membrane by a glycosylphosphatidylinositol anchor. FEBS Lett. 436:427-433.

24.   **Adams DD, Purves HD.** Abnormal responses in the assay of thyrotropins. Proc Univ Otago Sch Med. 1956; 34:11-12.

25.   **Meek JC, Jones AE, Lewis UJ, Vanderlaan WP.** 1964 Characterization of the long-

acting thyroid stimulator of Graves' disease. Proc Natl Acad Sci USA 52:342-349.

26. **Kriss JP, Pleshakov V, Chien JR.** 1964 Isolation and identification of the long-acting thyroid stimulator and its relation to hyperthyroidism and circumscribed pretibial myxedema. J Clin Endocrinol Metab. 24:1005-1028.

27. **Orgiazzi J, Williams DE, Chopra IJ, Solomon DH.** 1976 Human thyroid adenyl cyclase-stimulating activity in immunoglobulin G of patients with Graves' disease. J Clin Endocrinol Metab. 42:341-354.

28. **Drexhage HA, Bottazzo GF, Doniach D, Bitensky L, Chayen J.** 1980 Evidence for thyroid-growth-stimulating immunoglobulins in some goitrous thyroid diseases. Lancet ii:287-292.

29. **Yavin E, Yavin Z, Schneider MD, Kohn LD.** 1981 Monoclonal antibodies to the thyrotropin receptor: Implications for receptor structure and the action of autoantibodies in Graves disease. Proc Natl Acad Sci USA 78:3180-3184.

30. **Dumont JE, Roger PP, Ludgate M.** 1987 Assays for thyroid growth immunoglobulins and their clinical implications: methods, concepts and misconceptions. Endocr Rev. 8:448-452.

31. **Zakarija M, Jin S, McKenzie JM.** 1988 Evidence supporting the identity in Graves' disease of thyroid-stimulating antibody and thyroid growth-promoting immunoglobulin G as assayed in FRTL5 cells. J Clin Invest. 81:879-884.

32. **Adams DD.** 1958 The presence of an abnormal thyroid stimulator in the serum of some thyrotoxic patients. J Clin Endocrinol. 18:699-712.

33. **McKenzie JM.** 1958 Delayed thyroid response to serum from thyrotoxic patients. Endocrinology 62:865-868.

34. **Adams DD, Kennedy TH.** 1967 Occurrence in thyrotoxicosis of a gamma globulin which protects LATS from neutralization by an extract of thyroid gland. J Clin Endocrinol Metab. 27:173-177.

35. **Onaya T, Kotani K, Yamada T, Ochi Y.** 1973 New in vitro tests to detect the thyroid stimulator in sera from hyperthyroid patients by measuring colloid droplet formation and cyclic AMP in human thyroid slices. J Clin Endocrinol Metab. 36:859-866.

36. **Toccafondi R, Aterini S, Medici MA, Rotella CM, Tanini A, Zonefrati R.** 1980 Thyroid-stimulating antibody (TSAb) detected in sera of Graves' patients using human thyroid cell cultures. Clin Exp Immunol. 40:532-539.

37. **Hinds WE, Takai N, Rapoport B, Filetti S, Clark OH.** 1981 Thyroid-stimulating immunoglobulin bioassay using cultured human thyroid cells. J Clin Endocrinol Metab. 52:1204-1210.

38. **Kasagi K, Konishi J, Iida Y et al.** 1982 A new in vitro assay for human thyroid stimulator using cultured thyroid cells: Effect of sodium chloride on adenosine 3',5'-monophosphate increase. J Clin Endocrinol Metab. 54:108-114.

39. **Chopra IJ, Solomon DH, Limberg NP.** 1970 Specific and non-specific responses in the bioassay of long-acting thyroid stimulator (LATS). J Clin Endocrinol Metab. 31:382-390.

40. **Vitti P, Rotella CM, Valente WA et al.** 1983 Characterization of the optimal stimulatory effects of Graves' monoclonal and serum immunoglobulin G on adenosine 3',5'- monophosphate production in FRTL-5 thyroid cells: a potential clinical assay. J Clin Endocrinol Metab. 57:782-791.

41. **Vitti P, Elisei R, Tonacchera M et al.** 1993 Detection of thyroid-stimulating antibody using Chinese hamster ovary cells transfected with cloned human thyrotropin receptor. J Clin Endocrinol Metab. 76:499-503.

42. **Michelangeli VP, Munro DS, Poon CW, Frauman AG, Colman PG.** 1994 Measurement of thyroid stimulating immunoglobulins in a new cell line transfected with a functional human TSH receptor (JP09 cells), compared with an assay using FRTL-5 cells. Clin Endocrinol. 40:645-652.

43. **Chiovato L, Vitti P, Lombardi A et al.** 1987 Detection and characterization of autoantibodies blocking the TSH-dependent cAMP production using FRTL-5 cells. J Endocrinol Inves.t 10:383-388.

44. **Konishi J, Iida Y, Endo K et al.** 1983 Inhibition of thyrotropin-induced adenosine 3'5'-monophosphate increase by immunoglobulins from patients with primary myxedema. J Clin Endocrinol Metab. 57:544-549.

45. **Takasu N, Mori T, Koizumi Y, Takeuchi S, Yamada T.** 1984 Transient neonatal hypothyroidism due to maternal immunoglobulins that inhibit thyrotro-pin-binding and post-receptor processes. J Clin Endocrinol Metab. 59:142-146.

46. **Rees Smith B, Hall R.** Thyroid-stimulating immunoglobulins in Graves' disease. Lancet 1974;427-431.

47. **Shewring GA, Rees Smith B.** 1982 An improved radioreceptor assay for TSH receptor antibodies. Clin Endocrinol. 17:409-417.

48. **Matsuba T, Yamada M, Suzuki H et al.** 1995 Expression of recombinant human thyrotropin receptor in myeloma cells. J Biochem. 118:265-270.

49. **Kakinuma A, Chazenbalk GD, Jaume JC, Rapoport B, McLachlan SM.** 1997 The human thyrotropin (TSH) receptor in a TSH binding inhibition assay for TSH receptor autoantibodies. J Clin Endocrinol Metab. 82:2129-2134.

50. **Costagliola S, Morgenthaler NG, Hoermann R et al.** 1999 Second generation assay for thyrotropin receptor antibodies has superior diagnostic sensitivity for Graves' disease. J Clin Endocrinol Metab. 84:90-97.

51. **Szkudlinski MW, Teh NG, Grossmann M, Tropea JE, Weintraub BD.** 1996 Engineering human glycoprotein hormone superactive analogues. Nature Biotech. 14:1257-1263.

52. **Jaume JC, Kakinuma A, Chazenbalk GD, Rapoport B, McLachlan SM.** 1997 TSH receptor autoantibodies in serum are present at much lower concentrations than thyroid peroxidase autoantibodies: Analysis by flow cytometry. J Clin Endocrinol Metab. 82:500-507.

53. **Beever K, Bradbury J, Phillips D et al.** 1989 Highly sensitive assays of autoantibodies to thyroglobulin and to thyroid peroxidase. Clin Chem. 35:1949-1954.

54. **De Forteza R, Smith CU, Amin J, McKenzie JM, Zakarija M.** 1994 Visualization of the thyrotropin receptor on the cell surface by potent autoantibodies. J Clin Endocrinol Metab. 78:1271-1273.

55. **Morgenthaler NG, Tremble J, Huang G, Scherbaum WA, McGregor AM, Banga JP.** 1996 Binding of antithyrotropin receptor autoantibodies in Graves' disease serum to nascent, in vitro translated thyrotropin receptor: Ability to map epitopes recognized by antibodies. J Clin Endo Metab. 81:700-706.

56. **Minich WB, Loos U.** 1999 Isolation of radiochemically pure 125I-labeled human thyrotropin receptor and its use for the detection of pathological autoantibodies in sera from Graves' patients. J Endocrinol. 160:239-245.

57. **Lee MH, Park JY, Cho BY, Chae C-B.** 1999 Expression of the functional extracellular domain of human thyrotropin receptor using a vaccinia virus system: its purification and analysis of autoantibody binding. J Clin Endocrinol Metab. 84:1391-1397.

58. **Sanders J, Oda Y, Kiddie A.** 1999 The interaction of TSH receptor autoantibodies with 125-I-labelled TSH receptor. J.Endocrinol.Invest. 22 [(Suppl. to No. 6)], 82 (Abstract).

59. **Nagayama Y, Wadsworth HL, Russo D, Chazenbalk GD, Rapoport B.** 1991 Binding domains of stimulatory and inhibitory thyrotropin (TSH) receptor autoantibodies determined with chimeric TSH- lutropin/chorionic gonadotropin receptors. J Clin Invest. 88:336-340.

60. **Tahara K, Ban T, Minegishi T, Kohn LD.** 1991 Immunoglobulins from Graves' disease patients interact with different sites on TSH receptor/LH-CG receptor chimeras

than either TSH or immunoglobulins from idiopathic myxedema patients. Biochem Biophys Res Comm. 179:70-77.

61. **Kosugi S, Ban T, Kohn LD.** 1993 Identification of thyroid-stimulating antibody-specific interaction sites in the N-terminal region of the thyrotropin receptor. Mol Endocrinol. 7:114-130.

62. **Kim WB, Cho BY, Park HY et al.** 1996 Epitopes for thyroid-stimulating antibodies in Graves' sera: a possible link of heterogeneity to differences in response to antithyroid drug treatment. J Clin Endocrinol Metab. 81:1758-1767.

63. **Kim WB, Chung HK, Lee HK, Kohn LD, Tahara K, Cho BY.** 1997 Changes in epitopes for thyroid-stimulating antibodies in Graves' disease sera during treatment of hyperthyroidism: Therapeutic implications. J Clin Endocrinol Metab. 82:1953-1959.

64. **Chazenbalk GD, Wang Y, Guo J et al.** 1999 A mouse monoclonal antibody to a thyrotropin receptor ectodomain variant provides insight into the exquisite antigenic conformational requirement, epitopes and in vivo concentration of human autoantibodies. J Clin Endocrinol Metab. 84:702-710.

65. **Nagayama Y, Russo D, Chazenbalk GD, Wadsworth HL, Rapoport B.** 1990 Extracellular domain chimeras of the TSH and LH/CG receptors reveal the mid-region (amino acids 171-260) to play a vital role in high affinity TSH binding. Biochem Biophys Res Comm. 173:1150-1156.

66. **Nagayama Y, Wadsworth HL, Chazenbalk GD, Russo D, Seto P, Rapoport B.** 1991 Thyrotropin-luteinizing hormone/chorionic gonadotropin receptor extracellular domain chimeras as probes for TSH receptor function. Proc Natl Acad Sci USA 88:902-905.

67. **Libert F, Ludgate M, Dinsart C, Vassart G.** 1991 Thyroperoxidase, but not the thyrotropin receptor, contains sequential epitopes recognized by autoantibodies in recombinant peptides expressed in the pUEX vector. J Clin Endocrinol Metab. 73:857-860.

68. **Prabhakar BS, Fan J-L, Seetharamaiah GS.** 1997 Thyrotropin-receptor-mediated diseases: a paradigm for receptor autoimmunity. Immunol Today 18:437-442.

69. **Seetharamaiah GS, Dallas JS, Patibandla SA, Thotakura NR, Prabhakar BS.** 1997 Requirement of glycosylation of the human thyrotropin receptor ectodomain for its reactivity with autoantibodies in patients' sera. J Immunol. 158:2798-2804.

70. **Nagayama Y, Rapoport B.** 1992 Thyroid stimulatory autoantibodies in different patients with autoimmune thyroid disease do not all recognize the same components of the human thyrotropin receptor: selective role of receptor amino acids Ser25-Glu30. J Clin Endocrinol Metab 75:1425-1430.

71. **Kosugi S, Ban T, Akamizu T, Kohn LD.** 1992 Identification of separate determinants on the thyrotropin receptor reactive with Graves' thyroid-stimulating antibodies and with thyroid-stimulating blocking antibodies in idiopathic myxedema: these determinants have no homologous sequence on gonadotropin receptors. Mol Endocrinol. 6:168-180.

72. **Kosugi S, Ban T, Akamizu T, Kohn LD.** 1991 Site-directed mutagenesis of a portion of the extracellular domain of the rat thyrotropin receptor important in autoimmune thyroid disease and nonhomologous with gonadotropin receptors. Relationship of functional and immunogenic domains. J Biol Chem. 266:19413-19418.

73. **Kohn LD, Shimura H, Shimura Y et al.** 1995 The thyrotropin receptor. Vitam Horm. 50:287-384.

74. **Tomer Y, Davies TF.** 1993 Infection, thyroid disease, and autoimmunity. Endocr Rev. 14:107-120.

75. **Shenkman L, Bottone EJ.** 1976 Antibodies to Yersinia enterocolitica in thyroid disease. Ann Int Med. 85:735-739.

76. **Weiss M, Rubinstein E, Bottone EJ, Shenkman L, Bank H.** 1979 Yersinia enterocolitica antibodies in thyroid disorders. Isr J Med Sci. 15:553-555.

77.   **Lidman K, Eriksson U, Norberg R, Fagraeus A.** 1976 Indirect immunofluorescence staining of human thyroid by antibodies occurring in Yersinia enterocolitica infections. Clin Exp Immunol. 23:429-435.

78.   **Weiss M, Ingbar SH, Winblad S, Kasper DL.** 1983 Demonstration of a saturable binding site for thyrotropin in Yersinia enterocolitica. Science 219:1331-1333.

79.   **Byfield PGH, Davies SC, Copping S, Barclay FE, Borriello SP.** 1989 Thyrotropin (TSH)-binding proteins in bacteria and their cross-reaction with autoantibodies against the human TSH receptor. J Endocrinol. 121:571-577.

80.   **Luo G, Fan J-L, Seetharamaiah GS et al.** 1993 Immunization of mice with Yersinia enterocolitica leads to the induction of antithyrotropin receptor antibodies. J Immunol. 151:922-928.

81.   **Wenzel BE, Heesemann J, Wenzel KW, Scriba PC.** 1988 Antibodies to plasmid-encoded proteins of enteropathogenic Yersinia in patients with autoimmune thyroid disease. Lancet i:56.

82.   **Zhang H, Kaur I, Niesel DW et al.** 1997 Lipoprotein from Yersinia enterocolitica contains epitopes that cross-react with the human thyrotropin receptor. J Immunol. 158:1976-1983.

83.   **Luo G, Seetharamaiah GS, Niesel DW et al.** 1994 Purification and character-ization of Yersinia enterocolitica envelope proteins which induce antibodies that react with human thyrotropin receptor. J Immunol. 152:2555-2561.

84.   **Arscott P, Rosen ED, Koenig RJ et al.** 1992 Immunoreactivity to Yersinia enterocolitica antigens in patients with autoimmune thyroid disease. J Clin Endocrinol Metab. 75:295-300.

85.   **Valente WA, Vitti P, Yavin Z et al.** 1982 Monoclonal antibodies to the thyro-tropin receptor: Stimulating and blocking antibodies derived from the lympho-cytes of patients with Graves disease. Proc Natl Acad Sci USA 79:6680-6684.

86.   **Kohn LD, Suzuki K, Hoffman WH et al.** 1997 Characterization of monoclonal thyroid-stimulating and thyrotropin binding-inhibiting autoantibodies from a Hashimoto's patient whose children had intrauterine and neonatal thyroid disease. J Clin Endocrinol Metab. 82:3998-4009.

87.   **Okuda J, Akamizu T, Sugawa H, Matsuda F, Hua L, Mori T.** 1994 Preparation and characterization of monoclonal antithyrotropin receptor antibodies obtained from peripheral lymphocytes of hypothyroid patients with primary myxedema. J Clin Endocrinol Metab. 79:1600-1604.

88.   **Morgenthaler NG, Kim MR, Tremble J et al.** 1996 Human IgG autoantibodies to the thyrotropin receptor from Epstein Barr virus transformed B lymphocytes: characterization by immunoprecipitation with recombinant antigen and biological activity. J Clin Endocrinol Metab. 81:3155-3161.

89.   **McLachlan SM, Pegg CAS, Atherton MC, Middleton SM, Clark F, Rees Smith B.** 1986 TSH receptor antibody synthesis by thyroid lymphocytes. Clin Endocrinology 24:223-230.

90.   **Li H, Akamizu T, Okuda J et al.** 1995 Isolation of Epstein-Barr-virus-transformed lymphocytes producing IgG class monoclonal antibodies using a magnetic cell separator (MACS): Preparation of thyroid-stimulating IgG antibodies from patients with Graves' disease. Biochem Biophys Res Comm. 207:985-993.

91.   **Shin EK, Akamizu T, Matsuda F et al.** 1994 Variable regions of Ig heavy chain genes encoding antithyrotropin receptor antibodies of patients with Graves' disease. J Immunol. 152:1485-1492.

92.   **Akamizu T, Moriyama K, Miura M, Saijo M, Matsuda F, Nakao K.** 1999 Characterization of recombinant monoclonal antithyrotropin receptor antibodies (TSHRAbs) derived from lymphocytes of patients with Graves' disease: epitope and

binding study of two stimulatory TSHRAbs. Endocrinology 140:1594-1601.

93. **McLachlan SM, Rapoport B**. 1996 Editorial: Monoclonal human autoantibodies to the TSH receptor: the holy grail, and why are we looking for it? J Clin Endocrinol Metab. 81:3152-3154.

94. **McLachlan SM, Rapoport B**. 1992 The molecular biology of thyroid peroxidase: cloning, expression and role as autoantigen in autoimmune thyroid disease. Endocr Rev. 13:192-206.

95. **Foti D, Kaufman KD, Chazenbalk GD, Rapoport B**. 1990 Generation of a biologically-active, secreted form of human thyroid peroxidase by site-directed mutagenesis. Mol Endocrinol. 4:786-791.

96. **Parkes AB, McLachlan SM, Bird P, Rees Smith B.** 1984 The distribution of microsomal and thyroglobulin antibody activity among the IgG subclasses. Clin Exp Immunol. 57:239-243.

97. **Weetman AP, Black CM, Cohen SB, Tomlinson R, Banga JP, Reimer CB.** 1989 Affinity purification of IgG subclasses and the distribution of thyroid auto-antibody reactivity in Hashimoto's thyroiditis. Scand J Immunol. 30:73-82.

98. **McLachlan SM, Rapoport B**. 1995 Genetic and epitopic analysis of thyroid peroxidase (TPO) autoantibodies: markers of the human thyroid autoimmune response. Clin Exp Immunol. 101:200-206.

99. **Ruf J, Toubert M, Czarnocka B, Durand-Gorde J, Ferrand M, Carayon P**. 1989 Relationship between immunological structure and biochemical properties of human thyroid peroxidase. Endocrinology 125:1211-1218.

100. **Chazenbalk GD, Portolano S, Russo D, Hutchison JS, Rapoport B, McLachlan SM.** 1993 Human organ-specific autoimmune disease: molecular cloning and expression of an autoantibody gene repertoire for a major autoantigen reveals an antigenic dominant region and restricted immunoglobulin gene usage in the target organ. J Clin Invest. 92:62-74.

101. **Nishikawa T, Costante G, Prummel MF, McLachlan SM, Rapoport B.** 1994 Recombinant thyroid peroxidase autoantibodies can be used for epitopic "fingerprinting" of thyroid peroxidase autoantibodies in the sera of individual patients. J Clin Endocrinol Metab. 78:944-949.

102. **Jaume JC, Costante G, Nishikawa T, Phillips DIW, Rapoport B, McLachlan SM.** 1995 Thyroid peroxidase autoantibody fingerprints in hypothyroid and euthyroid individuals. I. Cross-sectional study in elderly women. J Clin Endocrinol Metab. 80:994-999.

103. **Jaume JC, Parkes AB, Lazarus JH et al.** 1995 Thyroid peroxidase autoantibody fingerprints. II. A longitudinal study in postpartum thyroiditis. J Clin Endocrinol Metab. 80:1000-1005.

104. **Jaume JC, Burek CL, Hoffman WH, Rose N, McLachlan SM, Rapoport B**. 1996 Thyroid peroxidase autoantibody epitopic 'fingerprints'in juvenile Hashimoto's thyroiditis: Evidence for conservation over time and in families. Clin Exp Immunol. 104:115-123.

105. **Jaume JC, Guo J, Pauls DL et al.** 1999 Evidence for genetic transmission of thyroid peroxidase autoantibody epitopic "fingerprints". J Clin Endocrinol Metab. 84:1424-1431.

106. **Nishikawa T, Rapoport B, McLachlan SM.** 1996 The quest for the autoantibody immunodominant region on thyroid peroxidase: Guided mutagenesis based on a hypothetical 3-dimensional model. Endocrinology 137:1000-1006.

107. **Finke R, Foti D, Rapoport B.** 1992 Importance of the carboxyl terminus of human thyroid peroxidase in the efficient expression of the protein in eukaryotic cells. Molec Cell Endocrinol. 84:73-78.

108. **Estienne V, Duthoit C, Vinet L, Durand-Gorde JM, Carayon P, Ruf J.** A 1998

Conformational B-cell epitope on the C-terminal end of the extracellular part of human thyroid peroxidase. J Biol Chem. 273:8056-8062.

109.   **Chacko S, Padlan E, Portolano S, McLachlan SM, Rapoport B**. 1996 Structural studies of human autoantibodies. Crystal structure of a thyroid peroxidase autoantibody Fab. J Biol Chem. 271:12191-12198.

110.   **Bottazzo GF, Pujol-Borrell R, Hanafusa T, Feldmann M**. 1983 Role of aberrant HLA-DR expression and antigen presentation in induction of endocrine autoimmunity. Lancet ii:1115-1118.

111.   **Londei M, Bottazzo GF, Feldmann M**. 1985 Human T cell clones from autoimmune thyroid glands: Specific recognition of autologous thyroid cells. Science 228:85-89.

112.   **Mackenzie WA, Davies TF.** 1987 An intrathyroidal T-cell clone specifically cytotoxic for human thyroid cells. Immunol. 61:101-103.

113.   **Lanzavecchia A.** 1990 Receptor-mediated antigen uptake and its effect on antigen presentation to class II-restricted T lymphocytes. Ann Rev Immunol. 8:773-793.

114.   **Simitsek PD, Campbell DG, Lanzavecchia A, Fairweather N, Watts C.** 1995 Modulation of antigen processing by bound antibodies can boost or suppress class II major histocompatibility complex presentation of different T cell determinants. J Exp Med. 181:1957-1963.

115.   **Guo J, Quaratino S, Jaume JC et al.** 1996 Autoantibody-mediated capture and presentation of autoantigen to T cells via the Fc epsilon receptor by a recombinant human autoantibody Fab converted to IgE. J Immunol Methods 195:81-92.

116.   **Guo J, Rapoport B, McLachlan SM.** 1999 Evidence for antigen presentation to T cells by thyroid peroxidase (TPO)-specific B cells in mice injected with fibroblasts co-expressing TPO and MHC class II. Clin Exp Immunol. 117:19-29.

5

T CELLS AND THE AUTOIMMUNE RESPONSE TO THE TSH RECEPTOR

Sandra M. McLachlan and Basil Rapoport

INTRODUCTION

Production of IgG class TSH receptor (TSHR) autoantibodies, the direct cause of Graves' disease, requires "help" from CD4+ T cells. However, there is a major difference in the way that T and B cells recognize antigen. Thus, TSHR autoantibodies, like antibodies to other protein antigens, interact predominantly with conformational epitopes on intact antigen (Chapter 4). In contrast, T cells only interact with antigen that has been internalized and degraded into peptides. Peptides (~ 20 amino acids) are presented to T cells within a groove in MHC class II molecules on the surface of the antigen-presenting cell (APC)(Fig.1).

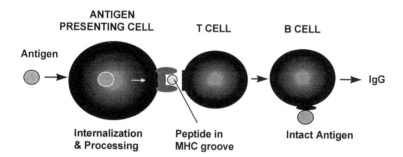

ANTIGEN PRESENTING CELL   **T CELL**   **B CELL**

Antigen

Internalization & Processing   Peptide in MHC groove   Intact Antigen   IgG

Figure 1. Interactions between antigen-presenting cells, T cells and B cells required for the production of antibodies.

The interactions leading to activation of a T cell are extremely complex. Besides the MHC molecule on the APC, a mechanism for uptake and processing of intact protein by the APC and the receptor for the peptide on the T cell ("first signal"), several other interactions are required for co-stimulation via a set of "second signals". For this purpose, the receptor-ligand pairs on the T cell and the APC include the co-stimulatory molecules CD40 and CD40 ligand, CD28 (or CTLA-4) and B7-1 or B7-2 (reviewed in 1). Assuming that the appropriate second signal requirements are fulfill-ed, engagement of an MHC-peptide complex by a specific T cell receptor leads to T cell activation. The activated T cell can then activate a B cell (recognizing the same *intact* antigen by means of its membrane-bound immunoglobulin), causing the B cell to proliferate and its progeny to differentiate into memory cells and/or plasma cells secreting antibody.

APPROACHES TO STUDYING TSHR-SPECIFIC T CELL RESPONSES

T cell responses *in vitro* are typically assessed by their ability to proliferate (measured as ^{3}H thymidine incorporation) or to produce cytokines (such as the autocrine T cell growth factor interleukin, IL-2). Although these techniques are not technically demanding, investigating TSHR specific T cell responses in Graves' patients, as for studies of most other human responses, poses the following problems.

First, only small numbers of TSHR-specific T cells are likely to be present in the peripheral blood, the source of lymphoid tissue most readily available for study. In particular, the very low serum levels of TSHR autoantibodies (2) suggest that the frequency of TSHR-specific T cells is similarly limited. Moreover, T cell studies in rodents, unlike investigations in humans, are performed shortly after immunization using lymphocytes from the draining lymph node or less commonly from the spleen. *Second*, a continuous supply of cells bearing autologous MHC molecules is required to characterize TSHR-specific T cell lines or clones. In man, the most convenient source of autologous antigen-presenting cells is B cells immortalized with Epstein-Barr virus (EBV). Such immortalized B cells can present peptide-MHC complexes but their capacity to internalize intact exogenous antigen for processing is limited.

An advantage in studying human thyroid autoimmunity is the occasional availability of Graves' thyroid tissue, which is enriched (relative to peripheral blood) in thyroid-specific T cells (for example, 3-7). Importantly, thyroid-derived T cells are activated and bear receptors for the growth factor interleukin 2, a characteristic that has been exploited for expansion and cloning of T cells specific for thyroid autoantigens including the TSHR and thyroid peroxidase (TPO)(7,8) as well as for T cells of unknown specificity (5,9,10).

Responses To Synthetic TSHR Peptides

Synthetic, overlapping peptides based on the predicted amino acid sequence of large complex proteins such as the TSHR can bypass the requirement for antigen processing. This approach has been used to investigate T cell responses in lymphocytes from peripheral blood (PBMC)(11-16) as well as to characterize T cell lines and clones generated from PBMC by repeated stimulation with recombinant TSHR-ectodomain (17). In addition to synthetic peptides, some studies have employed larger peptides expressed in bacteria (18,19).

The TSHR peptides recognized by Graves' patients encompass the entire range of the ectodomain including, in some studies, the transmembrane region (Fig. 2). Some of these peptides (12,14,15,20) are located within the "C peptide region" (amino acid residues ~317-366) that is removed from TSHRs on the thyroid cell surface following cleavage and carboxyl terminal degradation (see Chapter 4). It is possible that fragments of the C peptide region are taken up by antigen-presenting cells in the thyroid or in thyroid-draining lymph nodes and presented to T cells. Evidence in favor of this hypothesis comes from studies on insulin dependent diabetes (IDDM). Despite

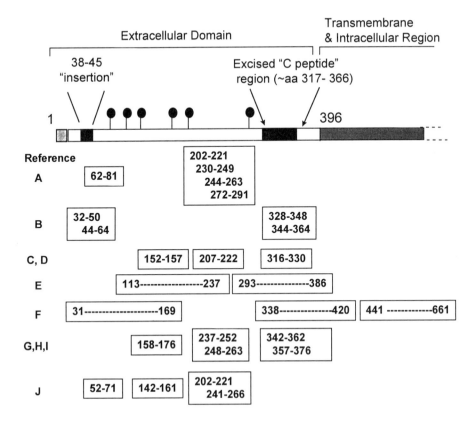

Figure 2. Schematic representation of the location on the TSHR of T cell epitopes identified using synthetic TSHR peptides or bacterial TSHR peptides that stimulate proliferation in Graves' (but not control) peripheral blood mononuclear cells, T cell lines or T cell clones. Included for the TSHR are the position of "insertions" between amino acid residues 38-45 and 317-366 (75) C peptide region" (76) and the 6 potential glycosylation sites. References to the peptides identified are: A (11); B (12); C (14); D (13); E (18); F (19); G (15); H (23); I (22); J (16).

the presence of insulin antibodies in ~50% of patients, it is difficult to demonstrate T cell responses to insulin, possibly because the immunodominant epitope that is present in pre-proinsulin is proteolytically destroyed during maturation of the insulin molecule (21).

In studies from different groups there is some overlap of TSHR peptides recognized by T cells from Graves' patients, but not from control individuals (Fig.2). Particularly striking are responses to peptides covering amino acid residues 202-222 and 244-266 (11,14,16). Also of interest are the observations concerning comparable recognition of TSHR peptide 158-176 in Graves' patients and family members (22), as well as in Graves' patients before and after different types of therapy (23).

As a cautionary note, it should be appreciated noted that many responses to

TSHR synthetic peptides are small and, in some cases, there are no differences between the responses in patients and in controls (24). On the other hand, it is possible that autoimmune responses are unlikely to be of similar magnitude to those observed in animals immunized with antigen and adjuvant. A potentially more disturbing issue arising from the use of synthetic peptides comes from observations for another receptor-antibody mediated disease, myasthenia gravis. Thus, T cell clones generated using synthetic peptides fail to recognize a component of the major autoantigen involved in myasthenia, the acetylcholine receptor α subunit (25). Consequently, it is possible that the most important TSHR-specific T cell epitopes in human autoimmunity have not yet been defined.

Endogenous processing of TSHR by dendritic cells/macrophages versus "non-professional APC"

For the reasons cited above, a more pathophysiological approach is to study T cell epitopes presented by cells that have themselves processed the antigen. The primary cells that ingest and process antigen for presentation to T cells are those that constitutively express class II molecules on their surface. Of these, the best known are dendritic cells and monocytes/macrophages. Dendritic cells may play a role in the initiation of many immune responses (reviewed in 26). Because limited numbers of dendritic cells can be isolated or cultured from peripheral blood (27), investigation of their role in thyroid autoantigen presentation has only been performed for thyroglobulin (28). However, it is possible that dendritic cells may be involved in the responses observed using TSHR-ectodomain (generated in bacteria) to stimulate PBMC and to generate T cell lines and clones (15,23).

"Non-professional" cells may also be involved in antigen presentation. The first recognition of this phenomenon was in autoimmune thyroid disease in which thyrocytes were observed to "aberrantly" express MHC class II molecules (29) and to function as antigen-presenting cells (3,30). These observations provided the impetus for studies using cDNA for TPO and the TSHR to stably transfect immortalized B cells (31-34). TPO-expressing immortalized B cells have been used to derive non-clonal T cell lines (32) and to test previously isolated T cell clones specific for TPO (31). Furthermore, such B cell lines have been used to identify TSHR-specific T cells among a panel of clones isolated from activated intrathyroidal T cells by expansion with IL-2 and anti-CD3 (33).

B cells as antigen-presenting cells

B cells constitutively express MHC class II and also function as professional APC for T cells. There is a major difference between dendritic cells, monocyte/macrophages and B cells in terms of their antigen presenting mechanism. The former cell type is voracious for ingesting cell particles and, via their Fcγ receptors, bind IgG-antigen complexes regardless of the specificity of the antibody involved. On the other hand, B cells express antibodies on their surface that function as an antigen receptor (Fig. 3). Each B cell, by virtue of its unique surface antibody, is antigen specific. Antigen bound to membrane-bound immunoglobulin molecules is internalized, digested

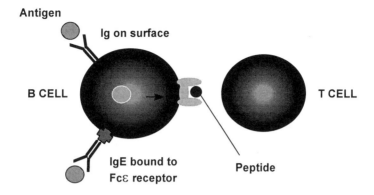

Figure 3. B cells capture, internalize, process and present antigens to T cells via their membrane-bound "immunoglobulin receptors" and also by means of Fc e receptors (CD23).

and presented via MHC molecules to T cells (reviewed in 35,36). In addition, B cells can capture and internalize antigens complexed with IgE (but not with IgG) following binding to the Fcε receptor (also known as CD23)(37)(Fig. 3).

B cells, therefore, compensate for their limited spontaneous phagocytic activity by being able to capture, focus and ingest specific antigen in the surrounding milieu. By this means, they are highly effective APC and function to perpetuate and amplify secondary T cell responses. Moreover, in addition to their ability to capture exceptionally small amounts of antigen, antibodies are able to *modulate* antigen processing and thereby enhance or suppress presentation of different T cell determinants (38-41).

The role of B cells in antigen presentation is increasingly being recognized in a variety of immune responses to infections and parasites, for example hepatitis B (42) and malaria (43) as well as in systemic autoimmunity, namely lupus erythematosus (44). More relevant are findings for an organ-specific autoimmune disease. IDDM type I, long regarded as the archetypal T cell-mediated organ-specific autoimmune disease (45), does not develop in NOD mice in the absence of B cells (46). The reason for this observation is that B cells are required to present islet-cell autoantigens to T cells (47,48).

Turning to thyroid autoimmunity, a recombinant TPO-specific *human* autoantibody converted to an IgE molecule captures and presents TPO to a T cell clone *in vitro* (49). Moreover, the induction in mice of high affinity TPO antibodies resembling patients' autoantibodies by injection of fibroblasts expressing small amounts of TPO, but not using high concentrations of purified protein and adjuvant (50), is consistent with a role for B cells. Similarly, TSHR antibodies induced by DNA vaccination (51) or by injecting TSHR expressing fibroblasts (52-54) may also involve B cells. The reason for this deduction is that when antigen levels are limiting (as is likely to be the case with transfected fibroblasts or following DNA vaccination) only the highest affinity B cells can engage antigen and become activated. More direct evidence for this hypothesis is that in mice that develop TPO antibodies resembling those in patients, TPO specific B cells appear to present antigen to sensitized T cells (55).

Overall, although it is unknown whether TSHR autoantibodies (secreted or as membrane receptors on B cells) are involved as APC in Graves' disease, evidence is accumulating to suggest that B cells play a role in presenting thyroid autoantigens to T cells in humans.

TSHR-SPECIFIC T CELL RECEPTOR GENES

The characteristics of the T cell antigen receptor determine whether the cell can or cannot bind to a peptide presented in the groove of the MHC class II molecule. T-cell antigen receptors are heterodimers and each α-chain and β-chain contains an inner constant region and an outer variable (V) region. (Incidentally, there is no evidence of a role for γδ T cells in autoimmune thyroid disease; 56). Because the thyroid is enriched in thyroid-specific T and B cells (see above), initial studies were directed at comparing the V gene repertoire of T cell receptors in thyroid tissue and peripheral blood from Graves' patients. However, such analyses have yielded controversial results. First, restriction of TCR Vα (but not Vß) has been observed in some (57,58) but not all (59) thyroids from patients with thyroid autoimmunity. Second, this approach cannot establish the antigenic specificity of the T cells because thyroid tissues from different patients contain variable proportions of T cells responding to TPO, Tg, the TSHR, as well as a variety of non-thyroid antigens.

T cell clones are required to characterize the T cell receptor V gene usage for TSHR-specific cells and, to date, only limited information is available. Thus, 5 different T cell receptor Vα genes were expressed by a PBMC-derived line that responded to peptides from the N-terminal and C-terminal portions of the TSHR extracellular domain, as well as to the N-terminal half of the transmembrane region (19). However, based on analysis of TPO-specific T cell clones, it is possible that restricted T cell receptor (TCR) V region usage may not always correspond to identical epitopic recognition. Thus, clones using identical TCR encoded by identical Vß and Vα genes and differing only in their "joining" (Jα) regions recognized different, non-overlapping epitopes of TPO (60).

FUNCTIONAL CHARACTERIZATION OF TSHR-SPECIFIC T CELL LINES AND CLONES

Cytokine Production by TSHR-Specific T Cells

Because the role of cytokines in Graves' disease is addressed in depth in Chapter 6, cytokine production by TSHR-specific T cells will only be briefly outlined. Antibody responses and cell mediated responses are controlled by different subsets of T cells (reviewed in 61). Th1 cells secrete interferon γ (IFN-γ) and little Interleukin 4 (IL-4) and regulate cell-mediated responses. In contrast, Th2 cells secrete IL-4 and little IFN-γ and provide "help" for antibody production.

T cell clones responsive to the TSHR extracellular domain (of bacterial origin) produce IL-4 and IFN-γ and, therefore resemble many other human T cell clones in being " Th0-like" rather than Th1 or Th2 (17). On the other hand, thyroid-derived TSHR-specific T cells, identified using TSHR-expressing autologous B cells, were predominantly of Th2-type (33). Together with observations on the detection of mRNA for IL-4 in numerous Graves' glands (62-64), these findings for TSHR-specific T cells are in accordance with the role of TSHR autoantibodies in causing hyperthyroidism.

Provision of "help" for B cells in antibody synthesis

For Graves' disease, the most meaningful, but the most difficult, "readout" of T cell function is the ability of TSHR-activated T cells to induce specific autoantibody synthesis by autologous B cells. One approach to address this question is the use of SCID mice that accept xenografts of human tissue because they lack mature T and B cells (reviewed in 65). Human IgG class autoantibodies to Tg and TPO develop in SCID mice engrafted with suspensions of Graves' or Hashimoto blood lymphocytes, thyroid lymphocytes, or even intact thyroid tissue (66-70). Moreover, some mice xenografted with Graves' thyroid tissue develop TSHR stimulating activity (TSAb) and transient hyperthyroxinemia (70).

Several problems are associated with SCID mouse models of autoimmunity including the rapid decline in T cell function shortly after lymphocyte transfer (reviewed in 65) and the variability between individual mice (66,71). Even more demanding is the necessity for using MHC class II matched T and B cells in studies designed to analyze the individual components of an immune response. Despite these major hurdles, SCID recipients of TSHR-specific T cell lines (but not control T cell lines) and autologous PBMC developed low but detectable levels of TSAb (72). Moreover, the ability of T cell lines to induce autologous B cells to secrete TSAb in SCID mice was MHC class II restricted and dependent on their cytokine profile (Th0, not Th1) and, most importantly, specificity for the TSHR (73).

CONCLUSIONS

The major goals of studying T cell responses in human thyroid autoimmunity are to characterize the autoantigen specific T cells in terms of the TSHR epitopes recognized, the genes encoding the T cell receptor α and β chains, the MHC molecule(s) and the co-stimulatory molecules involved in antigen presentation and T cell activation, and the effector function of the T cells. Although TSHR-specific T cells are, perhaps, less well characterized than those specific for TPO (reviewed in 74) information is becoming available on proliferation and cytokine production for T cell responses to synthetic peptides as well as to endogenously processed TSHR. Ultimately, this information may provide the basis for the development of an immunospecific form of therapy for Graves' disease and its extrathyroidal manifestations.

REFERENCES

1. **Bluestone JA.** 1995 New perspectives of CD28-B7-mediated T cell costimulation. Immunity 2:555-559.
2. **Jaume JC, Kakinuma A, Chazenbalk GD, Rapoport B, McLachlan SM.** 1997 TSH receptor autoantibodies in serum are present at much lower concentrations than thyroid peroxidase autoantibodies: Analysis by flow cytometry. J Clin Endocrinol Metab. 82:500-507.
3. **Londei M, Bottazzo GF, Feldmann M.** 1985 Human T cell clones from autoimmune thyroid glands: Specific recognition of autologous thyroid cells. Science 228:85-89.
4. **Weetman AP, Volkman DJ, Burman KD et al.** 1986 The production and characterization of thyroid-derived T-cell lines in Graves' disease and Hashimoto's thyroiditis. Clin Immunol Immunopathol. 39:139-150.
5. **Grubeck-Loebenstein B, Londei M, Greenall C et al.** 1988 Pathogenetic relevance of HLA class II expressing thyroid follicular cells in nontoxic goiter and in Graves' disease. J Clin Invest. 81:1608-1614.
6. **Mackenzie WA, Schwartz AE, Friedman EW, Davies TF.** 1987 Intrathyroidal T cell clones from patients with autoimmune thyroid disease. J Clin Endocrinol Metab. 64:818-824.
7. **Dayan CM, Londei M, Corcoran AE et al.** 1991 Autoantigen recognition by thyroid-infiltrating T cells in Graves disease. Proc Natl Acad Sci USA. 88:7415-7419.
8. **Feldmann M, Dayan C, Rapoport B, Londei M.** 1992 T cell activation and antigen presentation in human thyroid autoimmunity. J Autoimmunity 5 (Supplement A):115-121.
9. **Del Prete G, Tiri A, Mariotti S, Pinchera A, Ricci M, Romagnani S.** 1987 Enhanced production of gamma-interferon by thyroid-derived T cell clones from patients with Hashimoto's thyroiditis. Clin Exp Immunol. 69:323-331.
10. **Guo J, Rapoport B, McLachlan SM.** 1997 Cytokine profiles of *in vivo* activated thyroid-infiltrating T cells cloned in the presence or absence of interleukin-4. Autoimmunity 26:103-110.
11. **Tandon N, Freeman MA, Weetman AP.** 1992 T cell responses to synthetic TSH receptor peptides in Graves' disease. Clin Exp Immuno. l 89:468-473.
12. **Sakata S, Tanaka S-I, Okuda K, Miura K, Manshouri T, Atassi MZ.** 1993 Autoimmune T-cell recognition sites of human thyrotropin receptor in Graves' disease. Molec Cell Endocrinol. 92:77-82.
13. **Fan J-L, Desai RK, Dallas JS, Wagle NM, Seetharamaiah GS, Prabhakar BS.** 1994 High frequency of B cells capable of producing anti-thyrotropin receptor antibodies in patients with Graves' disease. Clin Immunol Immunopathol. 71:69-74.
14. **Okamoto Y, Yanagawa T, Fisfalen ME, DeGroot LJ.** 1994 Proliferative responses of peripheral blood mononuclear cells from patients with Graves' disease to synthetic peptides epitopes of human thyrotropin receptor. Thyroid 4:37-42.
15. **Soliman M, Kaplan E, Yanagawa T, Hidaka Y, Fisfalen ME, DeGroot LJ.** 1995 T-cells recognize multiple epitopes in the human thyrotropin receptor extracellular domain. J Clin Endocrinol Metab. 80:905-914.
16. **Martin A, Nakashima M, Zhou A, Aronson D, Werner AJ, Davies TF.** 1997 Detection of major T-cell epitopes on human TSH receptor by overriding immune heterogeneity in patients with Graves' disease. J Clin Endocrinol Metab. 82:3361-3366.
17. **Fisfalen ME, Palmer EM, van Seventer GA et al.** 1997 Thyrotropin-receptor and thyroid peroxidase-specific T cell clones and their cytokine profile in autoimmune thyroid disease. J Clin Endocrinol Metab. 82:3655-3663.
18. **Nagy EV, Morris JC, Burch HB, Bhatia S, Salata K, Burman KD.** 1995 Thyrotropin

receptor T cell epitopes in autoimmune thyroid disease. Clin Immunol Immunopathol. 75:117-124.

19. **Akamizu T, Ueda Y, Okuda J, Mori T.** 1995 Establishment and characterization of an antihuman thyrotropin (TSH) receptor-specific CD4+ T cell line from a patient with Graves' disease: Evidence for multiple T cell epitopes on the TSH receptor including the transmembrane domain. Thyroid 5:259-264.

20. **Fisfalen ME, Soliman M, Okamoto Y, Soltani K, DeGroot LJ.** 1995 Proliferative responses of T-cells to thyroid antigens and synthetic thyroid peroxidase peptides in autoimmune thyroid disease. J Clin Endocrinol Metab. 80:1597-1604.

21. **Congia M, Patel S, Cope AP, De Virgilis S, Sonderstrup G.** 1998 T cell epitopes of insulin defined in HLA-DR4 transgenic mice are derived from preproinsulin and proinsulin. Proc Natl Acad Sci USA. 95:3833-3838.

22. **Soliman M, Kaplan E, Guimaraes V, Yanagawa T, DeGroot LJ.** 1996 T-cell recognition of residue 158-176 in thyrotropin receptor confers risk for development of thyroid autoimmunity in siblings in a family with Graves' disease. Thyroid 6:545-551.

23. **Soliman M, Kaplan E, Abdel-Latif A, Scherberg N, DeGroot LJ.** 1995 Does thyroidectomy, radioactive iodine therapy, or antithyroid drug treatment alter reactivity of patients' T cells to epitopes of thyrotropin receptor in autoimmune thyroid diseases. J Clin Endocrinol Metab. 80:2312-2321.

24. **Kellerman S-A, McCormick DJ, Freeman SL, Morris JC, Conti-Fine BM.** 1995 TSH receptor sequences recognized by CD4+ T cells in Graves' disease patients and healthy controls. J Autoimmunity 8:685-698.

25. **Matsuo H, Batocchi A-P, Hawke S et al.** 1995 Peptide-selected T cell lines from myasthenia gravis patients and controls recognize epitopes that are not processed from whole acetylcholine receptor. J Immunol. 155:3683-3692.

26. **Steinman RM.** 1991 The dendritic cell system and its role in immunogenicity. Annu Rev Immunol. 9:271-296.

27. **Huang YM, Xiao BG, Westerlund I, Link H.** 1999 Phenotypic and functional properties of dendritic cells isolated from human peripheral blood in comparison with mononuclear cells and T cells. Scand J Immunol. 49:177-183.

28. **Farrant J, Bryant AE, Chan J, Himsworth RL.** 1996 Thyroglobulin-treated blood dendritic cells induce IgG anti-thyroglobulin antibody in vitro in Hashimoto's thyroiditis. Clin Immunol Immunopathol. 41:433-442.

29. **Bottazzo GF, Pujol-Borrell R, Hanafusa T, Feldmann M.** 1983 Role of aberrant HLA-DR expression and antigen presentation in induction of endocrine autoimmunity. Lancet ii:1115-1118.

30. **Mackenzie WA, Davies TF.** 1987 An intrathyroidal T-cell clone specifically cytotoxic for human thyroid cells. Immunol. 61:101-103.

31. **Mullins RJ, Chernajovsky Y, Dayan C, Londei M , Feldmann M.** 1994 Transfection of thyroid autoantigens into EBV-transformed B cell lines. J Immunol. 152:5572-5580.

32. **Martin A, Magnusson RP, Kendler DL, Concepcion E, Ben-Nun A, Davies TF.** 1993 Endogenous antigen presentation by autoantigen-transfected Epstein-Barr virus-lymphoblastoid cells. J Clin Invest. 91:1567-1574.

33. **Mullins RJ, Cohen SBA, Webb MC et al.** 1995 Identification of thyroid stimulating hormone receptor-specific T cells in Graves' disease thyroid using autoantigen-transfected Epstein-Barr virus-transformed B cell lines. J Clin Invest. 96:30-37.

34. **McIntosh RS, Mulcahy AF, Hales JM, Diamond AG.** 1993 Use of Epstein-Barr virus-based vectors for expression of thyroid auto-antigens in human B-lymphoblastoid cell lines. J Autoimmunity 6:353-365.

35. **Lanzavecchia A.** 1985 Antigen-specific interaction between T and B cells. Nature 314:537-539.

36.   **Lanzavecchia A**. 1990 Receptor-mediated antigen uptake and its effect on antigen presentation to class II-restricted T lymphocytes. Ann Rev Immunol. 8:773-793.

37.   **Bheeka Escura R, Wasserbauer E, Hammerschmid F, Pearce A, Kidd P**. 1995 Regulation and targeting of T-cell immune responses by IgE and IgG antibodies. Immunol. 86:343-350.

38.   **Manca F, Fenoglio D, Kunkl A, Cambiaggi C, Sasso M, Celada F**. 1988 Differential activation of T cell clones stimulated by macrophages exposed to antigen complexed with monoclonal antibodies. A possible influence of paratope specificity on the mode of antigen processing. J Immunol. 140:2893-2898.

39.   **Davidson HW, Watts C**. 1989 Epitope-directed processing of specific antigen by B lymphocytes. J Cell Biol. 109:85-92.

40.   **Watts C, Lanzavecchia A**. 1993 Suppressive effect of antibody on processing of T cell epitopes. J Exp Med. 178:1459-1463.

41.   **Simitsek PD, Campbell DG, Lanzavecchia A, Fairweather N, Watts C**. 1995 Modulation of antigen processing by bound antibodies can boost or suppress class II major histocompatibility complex presentation of different T cell determinants. J Exp Med. 181:1957-1963.

42.   **Milich DR, Chen M, Schodel F, Peterson DL, Jones JE, Hughes JL.** 1997 Role of B cells in antigen presentation of the hepatitis B core. Proc Natl Acad Sci USA. 94:14648-14653.

43.   **Hirunpetcharat C, Vukovic P, Liu XQ, Kaslow DC, Miller LH, Good MF.** 1999 Absolute requirement for an active immune response involving B cells and Th cells in immunity to Plasmodium yoelii passively acquired with antibodies to the 19-kDa carboxyl-terminal fragment of merozoite surface protein-1. J Immuno.l 162:7309-7314.

44.   **Chan OT, Madaio MP, Shlomchik MJ.** 1999 The central and multiple roles of B cells in lupus pathogenesis. Immunol Rev. 169:107-121.

45.   **Liblau RS, Singer SM, McDevitt HO.** 1995 Th1 and Th2 CD4+ T cells in the pathogenesis of organ-specific autoimmune diseases. Immunol Today 16:34-38.

46.   **Serreze DV, Chapman HD, Varnum DS et al.** 1996 B lymphocytes are essential for the initiation of T cell- mediated autoimmune diabetes: Analysis of a new "speed congenic" stock of NOD.Igm[null] mice. J Exp Med. 184:2049-2053.

47.   **Serreze DV, Fleming SA, Chapman HD, Richard SD, Leiter EH, Tisch RM.** 1998 B lymphocytes are critical antigen-presenting cells for the initiation of T cell-mediated autoimmune diabetes in nonobese diabetic mice. J Immunol. 161:3912-3918.

48.   **Falcone M, Lee J, Patstone G, Yeung B, Sarvetnick N.** 1998 B lymphocytes are crucial antigen-presenting cells in the pathogenic autoimmune response to GAD65 antigen in nonobese diabetic mice. J Immunol. 161:1163-1168.

49.   **Guo J, Quaratino S, Jaume JC et al.** 1996 Autoantibody-mediated capture and presentation of autoantigen to T cells via the Fc epsilon receptor by a recombinant human autoantibody Fab converted to IgE. J Immunol Methods 195:81-92.

50.   **Jaume JC, Guo J, Wang Y, Rapoport B, McLachlan SM.** 1999 Cellular thyroid peroxidase (TPO), unlike purified TPO and adjuvant, induces antibodies in mice that resemble autoantibodies in human autoimmune thyroid disease. J Clin Endocrinol Metab. 84:1651-1657.

51.   **Costagliola S, Rodien P, Many M-C, Ludgate M, Vassart G**. 1998 Genetic immunization against the human thyrotropin receptor causes thyroiditis and allows production of monoclonal antibodies recognizing the native receptor. J Immunol. 160:1458-1465.

52.   **Shimojo N, Kohno Y, Yamaguchi K-I et al.** 1996 Induction of Graves-like disease in mice by immunization with fibroblasts transfected with the thyrotropin repector and a class II molecule. Proc Natl Acad Sci USA. 93:11074-11079.

53. **Kita M, Ahmad L, Marians RC et al.** 1999 Regulation and transfer of a murine model of thyrotropin receptor antibody mediated Graves' disease. Endocrinol. 140:1392-1398.

54. **Jaume JC, Rapoport B, McLachlan SM.** 1999 Lack of female bias in a mouse model of autoimmune hyperthyroidism (Graves' disease). Autoimmunity 29:269-272.

55. **Guo J, Rapoport B, McLachlan SM.** Evidence for antigen presentation to T cells by thyroid peroxidase (TPO)-specific B cells in mice injected with fibroblasts co-expressing TPO and MHC class II. Clin Exp Immunol. In press.

56. **McIntosh RS, Tandon N, Pickerill AP, Davies R, Barnett D, Weetman AP.** 1993 The gamma delta T cell repertoire in Graves' disease and multinodular goitre. Clin Exp Immunol. 94:473-477.

57. **Davies TF, Martin A, Concepcion ES, Graves P, Cohen L, Ben-Nun A.** 1991 Evidence of limited variability of antigen receptors on intrathyroidal T cells in autoimmune thyroid disease. N Engl J Med. 325:238-244.

58. **Davies TF, Martin A, Concepcion ES et al.** 1992 Evidence for selective accumulation of intrathyroidal T lymphocytes in human autoimmune thyroid disease based on T cell receptor V gene usage. J Clin Invest. 89:157-162.

59. **McIntosh RS, Watson PF, Pickerill AP, Davies R, Weetman AP.** 1993 No restriction of intrathyroidal T cell receptor V alpha families in the thyroid of Graves' disease. Clin Exp Immunol. 91 :147-152.

60. **Quaratino S, Feldmann M, Dayan CM, Acuto O, Londei M.** 1996 Human self-reactive T cell clones expressing identical T cell receptor beta chains differ in their ability to recognize a cryptic self-epitope. J Exp Med. 183:349-358.

61. **Mosmann TR, Coffman RL.** 1989 TH1 and TH2 cells: Different patterns of lymphokine secretion lead to different functional properties. Ann Rev Immunol. 7:145-173.

62. **Paschke R, Schuppert F, Taton M, Velu T.** 1994 Intrathyroidal cytokine gene expression profiles in autoimmune thyroiditis. J Endocrinol. 141:309-315.

63. **McLachlan SM, Prummel MF, Rapoport B.** 1994 Cell-mediated or humoral immunity in Graves' ophthalmopathy? Profiles of T-cell cytokines amplified by polymerase chain reaction from orbital tissue. J Clin Endocrinol Metab. 78:1070-1074.

64. **Heuer M, Aust G, Ode-Hakim S, Scherbaum WA.** 1996 Different cytokine mRNA profiles in Graves' disease, Hashimoto's thyroiditis, and nonautoimmune thyroid disorders determined by quantitative reverse transcriptase polymerase chain reaction (RT-PCR). Thyroid 6:97-106.

65. **Vladutiu AO.** 1993 The severe combined immunodeficient (SCID) mouse as a model for the study of autoimmune diseases. Clin Exp Immunol. 93:1-8.

66. **Macht L, Fukuma N, Leader K et al.** 1991 Severe combined immunodeficient (SCID) mice: a model for investigating human thyroid autoantibody synthesis. Clin Exp Immunol. 84:34-42.

67. **Davies TF, Kimura H, Fong P et al.** 1991 The SCID-hu mouse and thyroid autoimmunity: characterization of human thyroid autoantibody secretion. Clin Immunol Immunopathol. 60:319-330.

68. **Martin A, Kimura H, Thung S, Fong P, Shultz LD, Davies TF.** 1992 Characteristics of long-term human thyroid peroxidase autoantibody secretion in scid mice transplanted with lymphocytes from patients with autoimmune thyroiditis. Int Arch Allergy Immunol. 98:317-323.

69. **Akasu F, Morita T, Resetkova E et al.** 1993 Reconstitution of severe combined immunodeficient mice with intrathyroidal lymphocytes of thyroid xenografts from patients with Hashimoto's thyroiditis. J Clin Endocrinol Metab. 76:223-230.

70. **Morita T, Yoshikawa N, Akasu F et al.** 1993 Studies of thyroid xenografts from Graves' disease in severe combined immunodeficient mice. J Clin Endocrinol Metab. 77:255-261.

71. **Saxon A, Macy E, Denis K, Tary-Lehmann M, Witte O, Braun J.** 1991 Limited B cell

repertoire in severe combined immunodeficient mice engrafted with peripheral blood mononuclear cells derived from immunodeficient or normal humans. J Clin Invest. 87:658-665.

72.   **Soliman M, Kaplan E, Straus F et al.** 1995 Graves' disease in severe combined immunodeficient mice. J Clin Endocrinol Metab. 80:2848-2855.

73.   **Fisfalen ME, Soltani K, Kaplan E et al.** 1997 Evaluating the role of Th0 and Th1 clones in autoimmune thyroid disease by use of Hu-SCID chimeras. Clin Immunol Immunopathol. 85:253-264.

74.   **McLachlan SM, Rapoport B.** 1992 The molecular biology of thyroid peroxidase: cloning, expression and role as autoantigen in autoimmune thyroid disease . Endocr Rev. 13:192-206.

75.   **Nagayama Y, Kaufman KD, Seto P, Rapoport B.** 1989 Molecular cloning, sequence and functional expression of the cDNA for the human thyrotropin receptor. Biochem Biophys Res Comm. 165:1184-1190.

76.   **Chazenbalk GD, Tanaka K, Nagayama Y et al.** 1997 Evidence that the thyrotropin receptor ectodomain contains not one, but two, cleavage sites. Endocrinol. 138:2893-2899.

6

CYTOKINES IN GRAVES' DISEASE

R. A. Ajjan, P. F. Watson and A. P. Weetman

INTRODUCTION

Cytokines are a heterogeneous group of water-soluble glycoproteins that play a crucial role in triggering and co-ordinating inflammatory and immune responses. These molecules usually have pleiotropic actions and their effects can be synergistic or antagonistic. Many cytokines are produced by both immune and non-immune cells, often act in an autocrine or paracrine fashion, and thus they infrequently achieve detectable levels in the circulation. In addition to their action on inflammatory cells, cytokines have a wide array of effects on non-immunological cells, thereby potentially modulating organ function.

CYTOKINE PRODUCTION BY INFLAMMATORY CELLS

T cells

T helper cells in mice have been classified according to the pattern of cytokines produced (1). Murine Th1 cells secrete predominantly interferon-γ (IFNγ), tumor necrosis factor-β (TNFβ) and interleukin (IL)-2, whereas Th2 cells predominantly produce IL-4, IL-5, IL-6, IL-10 and IL-13. Some cytokines are produced by both subsets, such as TNFα and IL-3, and some CD4$^+$ clones show combined production of both Th1- and Th2-derived cytokines and these are termed Th0 (2).

In general, cytokines secreted by one class of Th cells exhibit an autocrine positive feedback effect on their own Th class, together with a paracrine negative feedback on the other class. Th1 cells promote inflammation, cytotoxicity and delayed type hypersensitivity, while Th2 cells promote B cell differentiation, antibody formation and IgE-mediated hypersensitivity reactions.

A similar Th1 and Th2 dichotomy has also been identified in human, but it is less well defined. For example, IL-6, IL-10 and IL-13, produced by Th2 cells in mice, are products of both Th1 and Th2 cells in man (3). It should be noted that the separation of cells into Th1 and Th2 subsets is largely an *in vitro* classification and may not reflect the *in vivo* situation. Several studies have indeed failed to show a clear separation into nonoverlapping Th1/Th2 subsets (4,5). Furthermore, some T cell clones produce IL-4 but not IL-5 (and vice versa), and established Th2 clones can transiently express IFNγ, making subset classification misleading if only a single Th1 and a single Th2 cytokine are studied.

Other inflammatory cells

Cytokine production by macrophages, monocytes, B cells and dendritic cells is important for activation of T cells and may play a role in priming towards a Th1 or a Th2 response. For instance, IL-12 (mainly produced by macrophages) is essential for priming towards a Th1 response. On the other hand, IL-4 is important for priming towards a Th2 response, but the source of the initial polarizing IL-4 remains largely unclear and apparently includes naive T cells themselves (6), mast cells and basophils (7). IL-6, probably produced by antigen presenting cells, enhances IL-4 production by naive T cells (6), indicating a key role for this cytokine in Th2 responses. The type of antigen present cell (APC) also seems to be important in committing naive lymphocytes to Th1 or Th2 cells; macrophages and dendritic cells are now regarded as Th1-inducing APC, whereas B cells support the induction of Th2 responses (8). In addition to the role of the primitive immune system and APC, cell-cell interaction, the nature and dose of antigen, the way the antigen is processed and presented are all important determinants of which Th subset is stimulated (9).

CYTOKINE PRODUCTION BY NON-INFLAMMATORY CELLS

Cytokines can be also produced by non-inflammatory cells. For example, endothelial cells can produce IL-1, IL-6 and TNFα, all of which play an important role in the acute phase response. Similarly, IL-1, IL-8, IL-10 and IL-12 are products of keratinocytes, whereas IL-15 is mainly produced by non-inflammatory cells (10). Other sources of cytokines are glandular epithelial cells and fibroblasts, as discussed below.

CYTOKINES AND THE THYROID GLAND

It is now clear that cytokines play a key role in autoimmunity, including Graves' disease (GD). *Ex vivo* studies have examined cytokines in whole thyroid tissue samples and *in vitro* studies have analyzed cytokine production by intrathyroidal lymphocytes (ITL) and thyroid follicular cells (TFC). Studies on cytokine production by ITL and other cells *in vitro* may not reflect the *in vivo* situation, because even short term culture of lymphocytes can radically alter their profile. It is worth bearing in mind that complete separation of ITL and TFC is difficult and contamination with only a few cells highly expressing a particular cytokine can lead to artifacts. There is also a potential for modulation of cytokine profile by antithyroid drugs, steroids and even thyroxine, given to GD patients prior to operation, to further complicate data interpretation.

Cytokine expression in thyroid tissue *ex vivo*

Using immunohistochemistry, IFNγ has been detected in infiltrating lymphocytes in GD tissue (11), and IL-1α, IL-6, TNFα have also been shown to be produced by TFC as well as inflammatory cells (12-14). However, TFC production of TNFα was detected in only a minority of GD tissue (1 of 7 samples) compared with multinodular goiter (MNG) tissue (6 of 7 samples; 14).

IL-1α, IL-1β, IL-6, TNFα and IFNγ mRNA were found in GD tissue by slot-blot analysis (15), and in situ hybridization showed the expression of IL-1, IL-6, TNFα and IFNγ, but not IFNα or IFNβ, in GD tissue sections (12,13,16). Subsequent studies have focused on the reverse transcription-polymerase chain reaction (RT-PCR) as a sensitive and simple method to investigate cytokine gene expression in the thyroid. Indeed, the high sensitivity of this method is a potential drawback, as the signals detected may simply represent illegitimate transcription (17), and quantitation is another problem. Using RT-PCR, variable expression of IL-2, IL-4, IL-10 and IFNγ has been found is GD thyroid tissue (18-20). TNFα has also been analyzed by RT-PCR and has been detected in a minority of GD samples studied (19,21). However, quantitative RT-PCR has shown higher levels of TNFα mRNA in both GD and MNG compared with normal thyroid tissue (22).

High serum thyroid peroxidase (TPO) antibody levels have been associated with a higher tissue mRNA levels of IL-1β, IL-4, IL-8, IL-10 and IFNγ in GD tissue samples (23), suggesting a link between intrathyroidal cytokine and TPO antibody production. As TPO (and other) autoantibody levels fall with antithyroid drug treatment, it is possible that the immunomodulatory effects of these agents are responsible for the differing results between studies. IL-12, IL-13 and IL-15 transcripts have also been detected in GD tissue samples. IL-13 mRNA is more frequently found in GD tissue than Hashimoto's thyroiditis (HT) and MNG (24). All but one of the samples from patients with high TPO antibody titers showed IL-13 expression, suggesting a role for this cytokine in intrathyroidal autoantibody synthesis. In contrast, only a minority of HT patients with high TPO antibody titers showed IL-13 mRNA expression in their thyroid, whereas IL-4 mRNA was expressed in the majority of these samples (24, 25). As IL-4 mRNA has not been consistently detected in GD tissue, it is possible that IL-13, rather than IL-4, mediates antibody production in GD with the situation being reversed in HT. Similarly, others have demonstrated the importance of IL-13, but not IL-4, in mediating a Th2 response that results in gastrointestinal nematode clearance (26).

Cytokine production *in vitro*

Cytokine production by ITL

Although HT-derived T cells have a high potential for TNFα secretion *in vitro* (27), TNFα production by ITL from GD patients does not differ substantially from that seen in MNG-derived ITL, but it is still higher than peripheral blood mononuclear cells (PBMC) from the same patient (22). IFNγ production from GD-derived ITL is similar to that of PBMC (28), in contrast to HT-derived ITL (29). More refined studies on T cell clones (rather than mixed T cell lines) have demonstrated Th1 characteristics in TPO-specific T cell clones, whereas Th2 cells predominated in thyroid stimulating hormone receptor (TSHR)-specific T cell clones (30,31). Others (32) have shown a predominance of the Th1 phenotype in thyroglobulin- (TG) and TPO-specific T cell clones, and Th0 phenotype in TSHR-specific T cell clones. Single cell analysis of ITL has revealed a predominant Th1 and Th2 phenotype in HT and GD respectively, when larger T cells (presumably activated) were analyzed (33).

Moreover, PBMC from GD patients are biased towards Th2 cytokine production (34) and an increase in IL-5 levels has been demonstrated in sera from patients with GD (35), further emphasizing the predominance of a Th2 response in GD. The involvement of a Th2 response in GD is certainly an attractive idea as autoantibody production is paramount in disease pathogenesis. However, thyroid autoantibodies (against TG, TPO and TSHR) are also found in HT, indicating that a Th2 response occurs in autoimmune hypothyroidism. Therefore, the concept of a clear predominance of a Th1 and Th2 response in HT and GD respectively, is almost certainly an over-simplification. This is supported by recent studies demonstrating a mixed Th1/Th2 profile in GD-derived ITL and high serum IL-12 levels in GD patients (36,37), indicating that the predominance of a particular subset is not a feature of the disease.

Cytokine production by TFC

TFC seem to produce more cytokines than any other endocrine cell. IL-1, IL-6 and IL-8 have all been found in TFC culture supernatants, in particular after cytokine treatment (15,38). Low levels of TNFα have been detected in primary TFC cultures but only after IL-1 stimulation (22). TFC also produce transforming growth factor β_1 (TGFβ_1) in culture, which is stimulated by exposure to iodide (39).

Slot blot and RT-PCR analysis have shown IL-1α, IL-6, IL-8, IL-12, IL-13 and IL-15 gene expression in GD-derived TFC cultures, and their expression is modulated by IL-1, IFNγ and TSH (15,24,40). Cytokine production by TFC suggests that these cells probably play an active role in the autoimmune process in GD. It is noteworthy that TNFα protein, but not mRNA, production was enhanced by IL-1 treatment of TFC (22) indicating that mechanisms other than direct gene transcription are involved in the regulation of cytokine production by TFC and emphasizing the importance of complementing mRNA studies with protein production analysis.

Immunological effects of cytokines on TFC

Major histocompatibility complex (MHC) class I expression on TFC is upregulated by IFNγ and TNF treatment *in vitro*, and this upregulation is further enhanced by IL-1 (41), which could augment the inflammatory reaction and tissue destruction via CD8$^+$ T-cell mediated cytotoxicity. The majority of TFC in ATD express MHC class II molecules and hyperinducibility of class II on TFC from GD patients has been demonstrated (42,43). IFNγ, produced by infiltrating lymphocytes in GD, induces class II molecule expression on TFC *in vitro*, which is further enhanced by TNF and TSH (44). Furthermore, the spatial correlation between IFNγ-containing T cells and MHC class II-expressing TFC supports the IFNγ dependence of class II expression *in vivo* (11). MHC class II-expressing TFC has been shown to enhance the activation and proliferation of autologous lymphocytes (45), but recent evidence suggests that class II expression by TFC may, in fact, be protective. This is due to the inability of TFC to express costimulatory signals necessary for naive T cell activation, instead rendering these cells anergic, and thus inducing peripheral tolerance (46). On the other hand, there is still a possible role for TFC as APC in perpetuation of the disease, after autoimmunity is firmly established and B7-dependence is no longer important for continued T cell responses.

IFNγ, TNFα and IL-1 also enhance TFC expression of intercellular adhesion molecule-1 (ICAM-1), Hermes-1, lymphocyte function-associated molecule-3 and neural cell adhesion molecule (10), all of which have a central role in autoimmune disease through leukocyte activation and localization to the inflammatory sites. In addition, cytokines modulate nitric oxide (NO) production by TFC (47), an agent that has pro-inflammatory and destructive potential in experimental autoimmune disease (48).

The involvement of apoptosis in causing tissue destruction in autoimmune thyroid disease has provoked recent interest. A high frequency of apoptotic TFC in thyroid tissue from patients with HT, but not GD, has been demonstrated, which is possibly due to an increased expression of Fas in these cells (49,50). Interaction of Fas with its ligand (FasL), for example on T cells, triggers apoptosis in Fas positive cells. *In vitro* studies have shown that Fas expression in TFC is upregulated by cytokines and inhibited by TSH (49,51). This observation may explain why apoptosis is uncommon in GD as a result of the protective effects of thyroid stimulating antibody (TSAb; mimicking TSH action on Fas expression), which is stronger than any Fas upregulation

Table 1. Potentially pro-inflammatory immunological effects of cytokines on TFC and their role in the pathogenesis of GD.

Cytokine	Effect on TFC	Potential pro-inflammatory role in GD
IFNγ, TNFα	induction of class II expression	proliferation of non B-7 dependent T cells
IL-1, IFNγ, TNFα	increased class I expression	tissue destruction (CD8$^+$ cytotoxicity)
IL-1, IFNγ, TNFα	increased expression of adhesion molecules	leukocyte activation and localization to the inflammatory site
IL-1, IFNγ, TNFα	stimulation of NO production	pro-inflammatory effect
IL-1, IFNγ, TNFα	production of IL-1, IL-6, IL-13, IL-15	perpetuation of the inflammatory reaction
IL-1	production of IL-8, TNFα	perpetuation of the inflammatory reaction
IL-1	increased Fas expression	induction of apoptosis (probably limited or no role in GD; see text)

IFN = interferon; TNF = tumor necrosis factor
TGF = transforming growth factor; NO = nitric oxide

induced by intrathyroidal cytokines. However, a decline in TSAb titers during the course of the disease may result in increased expression of Fas on TFC (loss of protective effect), and could explain the progression of GD to autoimmune hypothyroidism in some patients. The likely proinflammatory effects of cytokines in GD are summarized in Table 1.

Cytokines can also have protective effects on TFC, which, like all nucleated cells, are resistant to complement-mediated cell lysis, through the expression of protective proteins, including CD46, CD55, CD59 and membrane attack complex inhibiting protein/homologous restriction factor. TFC expression of these molecules is upregulated by IL-1, TNF and IFNγ (52,53). IFNγ treatment of human TFC *in vitro* renders these cells resistant to cell-mediated cytotoxicity by mechanisms which are unclear (54). TGFβ₁ may also have a protective effect as it inhibits peripheral and thyroid-derived T cell proliferation in response to nonspecific stimuli. In addition, TFC recognition by thyroid autoantigen-specific T cell clones is reduced by TGFβ₁ treatment *in vitro* (55). The potentially protective effects of cytokines in GD are summarized in Table 2.

Table 2. Potentially protective immunological effects of cytokines on TFC.

Cytokine	Effect on TFC	Potential protective role
IFNγ, TNFα	induction of class II expression	induction of anergy in B-7 dependent T cells
IFNγ	resistance to cell-mediated cytotoxicity	protection against TFC destruction
IL-1, IFNγ, TNFα	increased expression of CD46, CD55 and CD59	protection against complement-mediated cell lysis
TGFβ	reduced recognition by autoantigen-specific T cells	dampening of the inflammatory response
IL-4, IFNα, TGFβ	inhibition of NO production	anti-inflammatory effects

IFN = interferon; TNF = tumor necrosis factor
TGF = transforming growth factor; NO = nitric oxide

Functional effects of cytokines on TFC

In addition to the effects of intrathyroidal cytokines on the inflammatory response itself, the cytokines generated may have autocrine or paracrine effects on TFC which could contribute to disordered thyroid function. IL-1 has a positive effect on the growth of primary TFC *in vitro*, but it also exerts indirect inhibitory effects on TFC proliferation through stimulation of PGE₂ synthesis (56). IL-6 also has a positive effect on TFC growth in the presence of TSH (57), whereas IFNγ inhibits human thyroid cell line growth, an effect that is further potentiated by TNF (58).

Iodine uptake in human TFC cultures is decreased by IL-1, TNFα and IFNγ (59), which is due, at least partly, to downregulation of sodium iodide symporter (NIS) gene expression (60). Accumulation of cAMP in primary TFC is decreased in response to IL-1 treatment *in vitro* (59), whereas results for IL-6, TNFα and IFNγ have been conflicting (61,62). IL-1 (at high concentration), TNFα and IFNγ all decrease TG production and TPO gene expression (which may affect iodine organification) in primary TFC cultures (62,63). IL-6 also decreases TPO expression whereas it has no effect on TG production (64). IFNγ suppresses TSHR gene expression (65) and IL-1, IFNγ and TNF all downregulate TSH-stimulated NIS gene expression in primary TFC cultures (60). It is worth noting that IL-1, IL-2 and TNF exert little, if any, effect on TFC viability (66); the effects of these cytokines on TFC function are not simply due to cytotoxicity. Together these data indicate that cytokines can affect all steps of thyroid hormone synthesis by regulating TSHR, NIS, TPO and TG gene expression and protein production, potentially resulting in modulation of thyroid function *in vivo*. A major caveat with these studies is the lack of information on intrathyroidal cytokine concentrations in GD tissue, and the concentration of cytokines used may not reflect the actual *in vivo* levels of these molecules. In addition, *in vitro* work analyses the behavior of TFC after exposure to a limited number of agents which certainly does not mirror the complex *in vivo* environment. An example of this is that cytokines can downregulate TSH-stimulated NIS mRNA expression in GD-derived TFC cultures yet NIS mRNA is upregulated in GD compared with MNG tissue samples (60). This observation suggests that the levels of cytokines in tissue samples are too low to result in NIS gene inhibition. Alternatively, it is possible that this discrepancy is due to the effects of TSAb (that have been shown to increase NIS mRNA expression) counteracting any inhibitory effects exerted by cytokines. The effects of cytokines on TFC growth and function are summarized in Table 3.

Table 3. Functional effects of cytokines on cultured human thyroid follicular cells.

	Growth	Iodide uptake	cAMP accumulation	TG production	TPO expression	TSHR expression
IL-1	↑, ↓	↓	↓	↓	↓	NS
IL-6	↑	NS	↓, →	→	↓	NS
IFNγ	↓	↓	↓, →	↓	↓	↓
TNF	↓, →	↓	↑, ↓, →	↓	↓	NS

NS = not studied; ↑ = increased; ↓ = decreased; → = no effect
IFN = interferon; TNF = tumor necrosis factor
TG = thyroglobulin; TPO = thyroid peroxidase

CYTOKINES IN ORBITAL TISSUE

The autoimmune process in TAO involves mainly the extraocular muscles (EOM), although the orbital fat and connective tissue are also affected. A patchy infiltration of activated lymphocytes can be identified in EOM from patients with TAO, with deposition of glycosaminoglycans (GAG) produced by activated fibroblasts, causing edema and muscle swelling, in turn leading to proptosis.

Cytokine production in orbital tissue and orbital-derived lymphocytes

The inflammatory infiltrate in TAO consists of T cells (mainly CD4$^+$), macrophages and B cells (67, 68). All these cells have the capability to produce cytokines. In addition, human orbital fibroblasts also appear to contribute to the local cytokine pool in TAO (69). Studies of *in vivo* cytokine expression in TAO tissue have been limited due mainly to the technical difficulties related to small sample size and the infrequency with which biopsy material is available. Using immunohistochemistry, IFNγ, IL-1α and TNFα have been detected in the retrobulbar connective tissue from patients with TAO but not in normal controls (70). The more sensitive RT-PCR has shown both IL-4 and IL-10 expression in 2 of 5 orbital fat specimens and in a single muscle biopsy obtained from TAO patients, but failed to detect IFNγ in any of the samples analyzed, indicating a Th2-like immune response (18). A more recent study on TAO-derived orbital muscle samples has also shown predominance of a Th2 response (71). Moreover, Many *et al.* (72) have elegantly demonstrated the likely importance of the Th2 response in the development of a model of TAO. Immunizing NOD mice with TSHR has been shown to result in destructive thyroiditis with the production of IFNγ in the thyroid, a Th1 response, without any associated orbital pathology. In contrast, immunizing Balb/c mice, under the same conditions, has been associated with a thyroid infiltrate rich in IL-4 and IL-10, which is accompanied, at least in some cases, with the development of orbital changes compatible with TAO. Therefore, it is possible that a thyroid cross-reactive Th2 immune response is necessary for the development of TAO.

Although IFNγ has been infrequently detected in TAO-derived tissue samples, several *in vitro* studies have documented IFNγ production by TAO-derived T cells (71,73,74). This discrepancy may be due to culture conditions that favor the expansion of Th1 cells *in vitro*, in particular after repeated non-specific stimulation. Alternatively, it could be related to the stage of the disease, as it has been suggested that a Th1 response is primarily involved in the initial stages of TAO, whereas the Th2 response takes place in the recovery phase of the disease process (75). However, this remains highly speculative, given the expression of IL-2 in EOM samples (indicating an ongoing inflammatory process) without the detection of IFNγ transcripts (71), suggesting that a Th1 response is not a feature of active disease. The same study has also shown a variability in cytokine mRNA expression between different EOM samples from the same patient. This most probably reflects the patchy inflammatory infiltration associated with TAO, as a result of which biopsies might have been taken from an area which was not infiltrated with inflammatory cells. This finding emphasizes the importance of investigating multiple samples in studies such as this, because analyzing a single sample from each patient would clearly have given misleading results.

Immunological and functional effects of cytokines in orbital tissue

Cytokine effects on orbital fibroblasts have been studied *in vitro* and it has been shown that retrobulbar fibroblast proliferation is stimulated by cytokines, including IL-1α, IL-4 and TGFβ, but not IL-2 or IL-6 (76). Fibroblast function is also modulated by cytokines. IFNγ, TNFα, TGFβ and IL-1 all induce GAG production, whereas IFNα and IL-6 have no effect (77,78). Fibroblast stimulation by these cytokines is further enhanced by hypoxia, which may explain the adverse effects of smoking on thyroid eye disease (77). Cytokines also stimulate fibroblasts to produce metalloproteinase inhibitors (79), suggesting that excessive accumulation of extracellular matrix in orbital tissue in TAO is due not only to increased production but also to impaired degradation.

In addition to these direct effects, cytokines may indirectly affect the inflammatory process through augmenting adhesion molecule, MHC class II and heat shock protein (HSP) expression in the retrobulbar tissue. ICAM-1 is overexpressed in disease-affected tissue and its expression in retrobulbar fibroblasts and vascular endothelial cells is stimulated by IL-1α, TNFα and IFNγ *in vitro* (80,81). Furthermore, these cytokines induce *de novo* expression of endothelial leukocyte adhesion molecule-1 and vascular cell adhesion molecule-1 in vascular endothelial cells from both TAO and normal control patients (81). Increased adhesion molecule expression modulated by cytokines could be a mechanism responsible for orbit-specific lymphocyte recruitment in TAO.

MHC class II expression in cultured fibroblasts, from both TAO and normal control tissue, increases with IFNγ treatment, though this expression is significantly greater in the TAO group. Concomitant treatment with TNFα further enhances class II expression, whereas addition of TNFβ, EGF or IL-6 attenuates IFNγ-induced class II expression. Moreover, enhanced class II expression is more prominent in retrobulbar fibroblasts compared to abdominal fibroblasts taken from the same patient, possibly explaining the selective involvement of the retrobulbar connective tissue in TAO (82).

Heat shock proteins (HSP) are thought to be involved in TAO as their expression is detected, both *in vitro* and *in vivo*, in fibroblasts from TAO but not normal orbital tissue (83, 84). IFNγ and TNFα enhance HSP expression in TAO-derived fibroblasts but not fibroblasts from normal controls, whereas IL-1, IL-6 and TGFβ increase HSP expression in fibroblasts from both normal and TAO tissue (83).

Cytokine-stimulated proliferation of orbital fibroblasts can be inhibited by corticosteroids (76), which could be a mechanism by which corticosteroids exert their therapeutic effects clinically. Antithyroid drugs inhibit H_2O_2- and heat-induced expression of HSP in cultured retrobulbar fibroblasts, which may be related in part to the oxygen radical-scavenging activity of these drugs, but it is unclear whether this is therapeutically important (85). A new therapeutic approach in TAO has been proposed recently by the use of cytokine antagonists such as IL-1 receptor antagonist (IL-1RA) and soluble IL-1 receptor (sIL-1R) which inhibit IL-1-induced GAG production by orbital fibroblasts *in vitro* (86). Clinical trials in other disorders have shown that systemic administration of IL-1RA does not carry significant toxicity (87), but it is currently unknown whether IL-1 blockade alone will be enough to suppress GAG production by orbital fibroblasts *in vivo*. The likely immunological and functional effects of cytokines in orbital tissue are summarized in Table 4.

Table 4. Potential immunological and functional effects of cytokines in TAO.

	IL-1	IL-4	IFNγ	TNFα	TGFβ
GAG synthesis	↑	→	↑	↑	↑
Cell proliferation	↑	↑	→	→	↑
Class II expression	↑	NS	↑	↑	NS
Adhesion molecule	↑	NS	↑	↑	NS
HSP expression	↑	NS	↑	↑	↑
Metalloproteinase	↑	NS	↑	↑	↑

NS = not studied; ↑ = increased; ↓ = decreased; → = no effect
IFN = interferon; TNF = tumor necrosis factor; TGF = transforming growth factor
GAG = glycosaminoglycans; HSP = heat shock proteins

SUMMARY

In conclusion, cytokines are likely to play a major role in the pathogenesis of GD. These molecules can alter the immunological properties of TFC through modulation of adhesion molecule and MHC class I and class II expression, potentially resulting in localization of the inflammatory reaction to the thyroid gland. Furthermore, cytokine production by TFC may further augment the inflammatory reaction and again help in tissue localization of the autoimmune process. In addition to the immunological effects, *in vitro* evidence suggests that cytokines can directly affect the function of TFC. However, it remains unclear whether this results in modulation of thyroid function *in vivo*. Cytokines have also a role in the pathogenesis of extrathyroidal complications of GD. The exact mechanism of TAO remains unclear but it involves the recruitment of T cells to retrobulbar tissue, probably as a result of these cells recognizing an antigen cross reactive with thyroid tissue (and yet to be defined). These T cells are activated, producing cytokines which may lead to perpetuation of the inflammatory process through a number of mechanisms. Cytokines increase class II, HSP and adhesion molecule expression in retrobulbar tissue, resulting in amplification of the inflammatory reaction. Also, cytokines increase fibroblast proliferation locally and help the recruitment of new inflammatory cells, thereby further augmenting the inflammatory activity. In addition to cellular growth, cytokines may increase the accumulation of extracellular matrix in orbital tissue through their stimulatory effects on GAG and metalloproteinase inhibitor production by retrobulbar fibroblasts, consequently resulting in the clinical features of TAO.

REFERENCES

1.   **Mosmann TR, Coffman RL.** 1989 Th1 and Th2 cells. Different patterns of lymphokine secretion lead to different functional properties. Ann Rev Immunol. 7:145-73.

2.   **Firestein GS, Roeder WD, Laxer JA, et al.** 1989 A new murine CD4+ T cell subset with an unrestricted cytokine profile. J Immunol. 143:518-25.

3.   **Mosmann TR, Sad S.** 1996 The expanding universe of T-cell subsets: Th1, Th2 and more. Immunol Today. 17:138-46.

4.   **Kelso A.** 1995 Th1 and Th2 subsets: paradigms lost? Immunol Today. 16:374-379.

5.   **Muraille E, Leo O.** 1998 Revisiting the Th1/Th2 paradigm. Scand J Immunol. 47:1-9.

6.   **Rincon M, Anguita J, Nakamura T, Fikrig E, Flavell RA.** 1997 Interleukin (IL)-6 directs the differentiation of IL-4-producing CD4(+) T cells. J Exp Med. 185:461-469.

7.   **Garside P, Mowat AM.** 1995 Polarization of Th-cell response: a phylogenetic consequence of nonspecific immune defence?. Immunol Today. 16:220-223.

8.   **Desmedt M, Rottiers P, Dooms H, Fiers W, Grooten J.** 1998 Macrophages induce cellular immunity by activating Th1 cell responses and suppressing Th2 cell responses. J Immunol. 160:5300-5308.

9.   **Constant SL, Bottomly K.** 1997 Induction of Th1 and Th2 CD4+ T cell responses: the alternative approaches. Ann Rev Immunol. 15:297-322.

10.   **Ajjan RA, Watson PF, Weetman AP.** 1996 Cytokines and thyroid function. Adv Neuroimmunol. 6:359-386.

11.   **Hamilton F, Black M, Farquharson MA, Stewart C, Foulis AK.** 1991 Spatial correlation between thyroid epithelial cells expressing class II MHC molecules and interferon-gamma containing lymphocytes in human thyroid autoimmune disease. Clin Exp Immunol. 83:64-68.

12.   **Zheng RQH, Abney ER, Chu CG.** 1991 Detection of interleukin-6 and interleukin-1 production in human thyroid epithelial cells by non-radioactive in situ hybridization and immunohistochemical methods. Clin Exp Immunol. 83:314-319.

13.   **Zheng RQH, Abney ER, Chu CQ, et al.** 1992 Detection of *in vivo* production of tumour necrosis factor-alpha by human thyroid epithelial cells. Immunology. 75:456-462.

14.   **Kayser L, Broholm H, Francis D, et al.** 1996 Immunocytochemical localisation of tumor necrosis factor α in thyroid tissues from patients with neoplastic or autoimmune thyroid disorders. Autoimmunity. 23:91-97.

15.   **Grubeck-Loebenstein B, Buchan G, Chantry D, et al.** 1989 Analysis of intrathyroidal cytokine production in thyroid autoimmune disease: thyroid follicular cells produce interleukin-1α and interleukin-6. Clin Exp Immunol. 77:324-330.

16.   **Rutenfranz I, Kruse A, Rink L, Wenzel B, Arnholdt H, Kirchner H.** 1992 In situ hybridization of the messenger mRNA for interferon-γ, interferon-α, interferon-β, interleukin-1β and interleukin-6 and characterization of infiltrating cells in thyroid tissues. J Immunol Method. 148:233-242.

17.   **Kimoto Y.** 1998 A single human cell expresses all messenger ribonucleic acids: the arrow of time in a cell. Mol Gen Genet. 258:233-239.

18.   **McLachlan SM, Prummel MF, Rapoport B.** 1994 Cell-mediated or humoral immunity in GravesÕ ophthalmopathy? Profiles of T-cell cytokines amplified by polymerase chain reaction from orbital tissue. J Clin Endocrinol Metab. 78:1070-1074.

19. **Watson PF, Pickerill AP, Davies R, Weetman AP.** 1994 Analysis of cytokine gene expression in Graves' disease and multinodular goiter. J Clin Endocrinol Metab. 79:355-360.

20. **Paschke R, Schuppert F, Taton M, Velu T.** 1994 Intrathyroidal cytokine gene expression profiles in autoimmune thyroiditis. J Endocrinol. 141:309-315.

21. **Paschke R, Kist A, Jännicke R, Eck T, Velu T, Usadel KH.** 1993 Lack of intrathyroidal tumour necrosis factor alpha in Graves' disease. J Clin Endocrinol Metab. 76:97-102.

22. **Aust G, Heuer S, Laue I, et al.** 1996 Expression of tumour necrosis factor-alpha mRNA and protein in pathological thyroid tissue and carcinoma cell lines. Clin Exp Immunol. 105:148-154.

23. **Heuer M, Aust G, Ode-Hakim S, Scherbaum WA.** 1996 Different cytokine mRNA profile in Graves' disease, Hashimoto's thyroiditis, and non autoimmune thyroid disorders determined by quantitative reverse transcriptase polymerase chain reaction (RT-PCR). Thyroid. 6:97-105.

24. **Ajjan RA, Watson PF, Weetman AP.** 1997 Detection of IL-12, IL-13 and IL-15 in the thyroid of patients with autoimmune thyroid disease. J Clin Endocrinol Metab. 82:666-669.

25. **Ajjan RA, Watson PF, McIntosh RS, Weetman AP.** 1996 Intrathyroidal cytokine gene expression in Hashimoto's thyroiditis. Clin Exp Immunol. 105:523-528.

26. **McKenzie GJ, Bancroft A, Grencis RK, McKenzie ANJ.** 1998 A distinct role for interleukin-13 in Th2-cell-mediated immune responses. Curr Biol. 8:339-342.

27. **Del Prete GF, Tiri A, De Carli M, et al.** 1989 High potential to tumour necrosis factor-α production of thyroid infiltrating lymphocytes in Hashimoto's thyroiditis: A peculiar feature of thyroid autoimmunity. Autoimmunity. 4:267-276.

28. **Bagnasco M, Venuti D, Prigione I, Torre GC, Ferini S, Canonica GW.** 1988 Graves' disease: Phenotypic and functional analysis at the clonal level of the T cell repertoire in peripheral blood and in thyroid. Clin Immunol Immunopathol. 47:230-239.

29. **Del Prete GF, Tiri A, Mariotti S, Pinchera A, Ricci M, Romagnani S.** 1987 Enhanced production of γ-interferon by thyroid-derived T cell clones from patients with Hashimoto's thyroiditis. Clin Exp Immunol. 69:323-331.

30. **Mullins RJ, Chernajovsky Y, Dayan C, Londei M, Feldmann M.** 1994 Transfection of thyroid autoantigens into EBV-transformed B cell lines: Recognition by Graves' disease thyroid T cells. J Immunol. 152:5572-5580.

31. **Mullins RJ, Cohen SBA, Webb LMC, et al.** 1995 Identification of thyroid-stimulating hormone receptor-specific T cells in Graves' disease thyroid using autoantigen-transfected Epstein-Barr virus-transformed B cell lines. J Clin Invest. 96:30-37.

32. **Fisfalen ME, Palmer EM, Van Seventer GA, et al.** 1997 Thyrotropin-receptor and thyroid peroxidase-specific T cell clones and their cytokine profile in autoimmune thyroid disease. J Clin Endocrinol Metab. 82:3655-3663.

33. **Roura-Mir C, Catalfamo M, Sospedra M, Alcalde L, Pujol-Borrell R, Jaraquemada D.** 1997 Single-cell analysis of intrathyroidal lymphocytes shows differential cytokine expression in Hashimoto's and Graves' disease. Eur J Endocrinol. 27:3290-3302.

34. **Kallmann BA, Huther M, Tubes M, et al.** 1997 Systemic bias of cytokine production toward cell-mediated immune regulation in IDDM and toward humoral immunity in Graves' disease. Diabetes. 46:237-243.

35. **Hidaka Y, Okumura M, Shimaoka Y, Takeoka K, Tada H, Amino N.** 1998 Increased serum concentration of interleukin-5 in patients with Graves' disease and Hashimoto's thyroiditis. Thyroid. 8:235-239.

36. **Okumura M, Hidaka Y, Matsuzuka F, et al.** 1999 CD30 expression and interleukin-4 and interferon-γ production of intrathyroidal lymphocytes in Graves' disease. Thyroid. 9:333-339.

37.   **Hidaka Y, Okumura M, Fukata S, Shimaoka Y, Takeoka K, Tada H, Amino N.** 1999 Increased serum concentration of interleukin-12 in patients with silent thyroiditis and Graves' disease. Thyroid. 9:149-153.

38.   **Weetman AP, Bennett GL, Wong WLT.** 1992 Thyroid follicular cells produce interleukin-8. J Clin Endocrinol Metab 75:328-330.

39.   **Cowin AJ, Bidey SP.** 1994 Transforming growth factor-β_1 synthesis in human thyroid follicular cells. J Endocrinol. 141:183-190.

40.   **Watson PF, Pickerill AP, Davies R, Weetman AP.** 1995 Semi-quantitative analysis of interleukin-1-α, interleukin-6 and interleukin-8 mRNA expression by human thyrocytes. J Mol Endocrinol. 15:11-21.

41.   **Mandrup-Poulsen T, Nerup J, Rimers JI, et al.** 1996 Cytokine and the endocrine system. II. Roles in substrate metabolism, modulation of thyroidal and pancreatic endocrine cell functions and autoimmune endocrine disease. Eur J Endocrinol. 134:21-30.

42.   **Bottazzo GF, Pujol-Borrell R, Hanafusa T, Feldmann M.** 1983 Role of aberrant HLA-DR expression and antigen presentation in induction of endocrine autoimmunity. Lancet. 2:1115-1119.

43.   **Sospedra M, Obiols G, Babi LFS, et al.** 1995 Hyperinducibility of MHC class-II expression of thyroid follicular cells from Graves' disease - a primary defect. J Immunol. 154:4213-4222.

44.   **Chiovato L, Lapi P, Mariotti S, Del Prete G, De Carli M, Pinchera A.** 1994 Simultaneous expression of thyroid peroxidase and human-leukocyte antigen-DR by human thyroid cells. Modulation by thyrotropin, thyroid-stimulating antibody, and interferon-γ. J Clin Endocrinol Metab. 79:653-56.

45.   **Londei M, Bottazzo GF, Feldmann M.** 1985 Human T cell clones from autoimmune thyroid glands: specific recognition of autologous thyroid cells. Science. 228:85-89.

46.   **Marelli-Berg FM, Weetman A, Frasca L, et al.** 1997 Antigen presentation by epithelial cells induces anergic immunoregulatory CD45RO$^+$ T cells and deletion of CD45RA$^+$ T cells. J Immunol. 159:5853-5861.

47.   **Kasai K, Hattori Y, Nakanishi N, et al.** 1995 Regulation of inducible nitric oxide production by cytokines in human thyrocytes in culture. Endocrinology. 136:4261-4270.

48.   **Vladutiu AO.** 1995 Role of nitric-oxide in autoimmunity. Clin Immunol Immunopathol. 76:1-11.

49.   **Giordano C, Stassi G, De Maria R, et al.** 1997 Potential involvement of Fas and its ligand in the pathogenesis of Hashimoto's thyroiditis. Science. 275:960-963.

50.   **Mitsiades N, Poulaki V, Kotoula V, et al.** 1998 Fas/Fas ligand up-regulation and bcl-2 down-regulation may be significant in the pathogenesis of Hashimoto's thyroiditis. J Clin Endocrinol Metab. 83:2199-2203.

51.   **Kawakami A, Eguchi K, Matsuoka N, et al.** 1996 Thyroid-stimulating hormone inhibits Fas antigen-mediated apoptosis of human thyrocytes *in vitro*. Endocrinology. 137:3163-3169.

52.   **Tandon N, Morgan BP, Weetman AP.** 1992 Expression and function of membrane attack complex inhibitory proteins on thyroid follicular cells. Immunology. 75:372-377.

53.   **Tandon N, Yan SL, Morgan BP, Weetman AP.** 1994 Expression and function of multiple regulators of complement activation in autoimmune thyroid disease. Immunology. 81:643-647.

54.   **Bogner U, Sigle B, Schleusener H.** 1988 Interferon-γ protects human thyroid epithelial cells against cell-mediated cytotoxicity. Immunobiology. 176:423-431.

55.   **Widder J, Dorfinger K, Wilfing A, et al.** 1991 The immunoregulatory influence of transforming growth factor-β (TGFβ) in thyroid autoimmunity: TGFβ inhibits autoreactivity in Graves' disease. J Autoimmunity. 4:689-701.

56.   **Kawabe Y, Eguchi K, Shimomura L, et al.** 1989 Interleukin-1 production and action in thyroid tissue. J Clin Endocrinol Metab. 68:1174-83.

57.   **Nishiyama S, Takada K, Tada H, Takano T, Amino N.** 1993 Effect of interleukin-6 on cell proliferation of FRTL-5 cells. Biochem Biophys Res Commun. 192:319-323.

58.   **Huber GK, Davies TF.** 1990 Human fetal thyroid cell growth *in vitro:* System characterization and cytokine inhibition. Endocrinology. 126:869-875.

59.   **Sato K, Satoh T, Shizume K, et al.** 1990 Inhibition of I^{125} organification and thyroid-hormone release by interleukin-1, tumor necrosis factor-alpha, and interferon-gamma in human thyrocytes in suspension-culture. J Clin Endocrinol Metab. 70:1735-1743.

60.   **Ajjan RA, Kamaruddin NA, Crisp M, Watson PF, Ludgate M, Weetman AP** 1998 Regulation and tissue distribution of the human sodium iodide symporter gene. Clin Endocrinol. 49:517-523.

61.   **Deuss U, Buscema M, Schumacher H, Winkelmann W.** 1992 *In vitro* effects of tumor-necrosis-factor-alpha on human thyroid follicular cells. Acta Endocrinol. 127:220-25.

62.   **Rasmussen AK, Kayser L, Rasmussen UF, Bendtzen K.** 1994 Influence of tumour necrosis factor-β and interferon-γ, separately and added together with interleukin-1β, on the function of cultured human thyroid cells. J Endocrinol. 143:359-365.

63.   **Ashizawa K, Yamashita S, Tobinaga T, et al.** 1989 Inhibition of human thyroid peroxidase gene expression by IL-1. Acta Endocrinol. 121:465-69.

64.   **Tominaga T, Yamashita S, Nagayama Y, et al.** 1991 Interleukin-6 inhibits human thyroid peroxidase gene expression. Acta Endocrinol. 124:290-96.

65.   **Nishikawa T, Yamashita S, Namba H, et al.** 1993 Interferon-γ inhibition of human thyrotropin receptor gene expression. J Clin Endocrinol Metab. 77:1084-1089.

66.   **McLachlan SM, Taverne J, Atherton MC, Middleton SL, Young ET, Smith R.** 1990 Cytokine, thyroid autoantibody synthesis and thyroid cell survival in culture. Clin Exp Immunol. 79:175-181.

67.   **Weetman AP, Cohen S, Gatter KS, Fells P, Shine B.** 1989 Immunohistochemical analysis of the retrobulbar tissues in Graves' ophthalmopathy. Clin Exp Immunol. 75:222-227.

68.   **Kahaly G, Hansen C, Felke B, Dienes HP.** 1994 Immunohistochemical staining of retrobulbar adipose tissue in Graves' ophthalmopathy. Clin Immunol Immunopathol. 73:53-62.

69.   **Sempowski GD, Rozenblit J, Smith TJ, Phipps RP.** 1998 Human orbital fibroblasts are activated through CD40 to induce proinflammatory cytokine production. Am J Cell Physiol. 43:C707-C714.

70.   **Heufelder AE, Bahn RS.** 1993 Detection and localization of cytokine immunoreactivity in retro-ocular connective tissue in Graves' ophthalmopathy. Eur J Clin Invest. 23:10-17.

71.   **Pappa A, Calder V, Ajjan R, et al.** 1997 Analysis of extraocular muscle-infiltrating T cells in thyroid-associated ophthalmopathy (TAO). Clin Exp Immunol. 109:362-369.

72.   **Many MC, Costagliola S, Detrait M, Denef JF, Vassart G, Ludgate M.** 1999 Development of an animal model of autoimmune thyroid eye disease. J Immunol. 162:4966-4974.

73.   **Forster G, Otto E, Hansen C, Ochs K, Kahaly G.** 1998 Analysis of orbital T cells in thyroid-associated ophthalmopathy. Clin Exp Immunol. 112:427-434.

74.   **Yang DM, Hiromatsu Y, Hoshino T, Inoue Y, Itoh K, Nonaka K.** 1999 Dominant infiltration of T(H)-1-type $CD4^+$ T cells at the retrobulbar space of patients with thyroid-associated ophthalmopathy. Thyroid. 9:305-310

75.   **Natt N, Bahn RS.** 1997 Cytokines in the evolution of Graves' ophthalmopathy. Autoimmunity. 26:129-136.

76.   **Heufelder AE, Bahn RS.** 1994 Modulation of Graves' orbital fibroblast proliferation by cytokines and glucocorticoid receptor agonists. Invest Ophthalmol Vis Sci. 35:120-127.

77. **Metcalfe RA, Weetman AP.** 1994 Stimulation of extraocular muscle fibroblasts by cytokines and hypoxia: possible role in thyroid-associated ophthalmopathy. Clin Endocrinol. 40:67-72.

78. **Imai Y, Ibaraki K, Odajima R, Shishiba Y.** 1994 Analysis of proteoglycan synthesis by retro-ocular tissue fibroblasts under the influence of interleukin-1β and transforming growth factor-β_1. Eur J Endocrinol. 131:630-638.

79. **Seibold M, Spitzweg C, Joba W, Heufelder A.E.** 1997 Detection and regulation of tissue inhibitor of metalloproteinase-1 (TIMP-1) and matrix metalloproteinase-1 (MMP-1) in Graves' and normal orbital fibroblasts. Exp Clin Endocrinol Diab. 105 (supp. 1): 38-39.

80. **Heufelder AE, Bahn RS.** 1992 Graves' immunoglobulins and cytokines stimulate the expression of intercellular-adhesion molecule-1 (ICAM-1) in cultured Graves' orbital fibroblasts. Eur J Clin Invest. 22:529-537.

81. **Heufelder AE, Scriba PC.** 1996 Characterization of adhesion receptors on cultured microvascular endothelial cells derived from the retroorbital connective tissue of patients with Graves' ophthalmopathy. Eur J Endocrinol. 134:51-60.

82. **Heufelder AE, Smith TJ, Gorman CA, Bahn RS.** 1991 Increased induction of HLA-DR by interferon-γ in cultured fibroblasts derived from patients with Graves' ophthalmopathy and pretibial dermopathy. J Clin Endocrinol Metab. 73:307-313.

83. **Heufelder AE, Wenzel BE, Gorman CA, Bahn RS.** 1991 Detection, cellular localization, and modulation of heat shock proteins in cultured fibroblasts from patients with extrathyroidal manifestations of Graves' disease. J Clin Endocrinol Metab. 73:739-745.

84. **Heufelder AE, Wenzel BE, Bahn RS.** 1992 Cell surface localization of a 72 kilodalton heat shock protein in retroocular fibroblasts from patients with Graves' ophthalmopathy. J Clin Endocrinol Metab. 74:732-735.

85. **Heufelder AE, Wenzel BE, Bahn RS.** 1992 Methimazole and propylthiouracil inhibit the oxygen free radical-induced expression of a 72 kilodalton heat shock protein in Graves' retroocular fibroblasts. J Clin Endocrinol Metab. 74:737-742.

86. **Tan GH, Dutton CM, Bahn RS.** 1996 Interleukin-1 (IL-1) receptor antagonist and soluble IL-1 receptor inhibit IL-1-induced glycosaminoglycan production in cultured human orbital fibroblasts from patients with Graves' ophthalmopathy. J Clin Endocrinol Metab. 81:449-452.

87. **Van Zee K, Coyle S, Calvano S, et al.** 1995 Influence of IL-1 receptor blockade on the human response to endotoxemia. J Immunol. 154:1499-507.

7

CO-STIMULATORY MOLECULES IN GRAVES' DISEASE

Francesca Paolieri, Giampaola Pesce, Claudia Salmaso, Paola Montagna and Marcello Bagnasco

INTRODUCTION

Most immune responses depend on the activation of T cells. This class of lymphocytes consists of functionally and phenotypically distinct populations, the best characterized of which are helper and cytotoxic T cells. CD4+ helper T cells can be divided into two subtypes. Type 1 helper T cells (Th1) mainly synthesize interferon-γ and interleukin (IL)-2; type 2 helper T cells (Th2) principally secrete IL-1, IL-5, and IL-10 (1). The pathogenesis and outcome of certain diseases appears to be strongly influenced by the type of helper T cells involved. For example in leishmaniasis the development of a response polarized toward Th1 is important for a successful immune defence, but a response polarized toward Th2 is detrimental as demonstrated in an animal model (2).

There is agreement that several human organ-specific autoimmune diseases, using Hashimoto's thyroiditis (HT) as a prototype, are characterized by the presence at the level of the target organ of Th1 and/or cytotoxic (Tc1) T cells (3,4,5). Infiltrating Th1 cells are believed to induce tissue lesions through activation of cytolytic effector cells and secretion of lymphokines.

At least two signals for proliferation and cytokine secretion by T cells are required (6). The first signal is delivered through the interaction of the T cell receptor (TCR) with antigen (Ag)-major histocompatibility complex (MHC) expressed on the surface of Ag-presenting cells (APC). The second or costimulatory signal, neither Ag-specific nor MHC-restricted, is delivered by cell surface molecules expressed by APC (7). In the absence of such costimulatory signal, cognate antigen recognition will result in inhibitory events, such as anergy or unresponsiveness to further stimulation, or apoptosis.

At least seven distinct molecular combinations, including intercellular adhesion molecule (ICAM)-1/ICAM-2 with lymphocyte function associated antigen (LFA)-1, LFA-3 with CD2, vascular cell adhesion molecule (VCAM-1) with very late antigen-4 (VLA-4), CD40 antigen with its ligand CD40L and B7.1 (CD80)/B7.2(CD86) with CD28/ Cytolytic T lymphocyte associated antigen-4 (CTLA-4), are involved in T cell activation. Among these interactions, the combination of B7.1/B7.2 with CD28/CTLA-4 provide the most potent costimulatory signal for T cell activation (8,9,10). CD40 antigen and its ligand (CD40L; also called CD154 and gp39) have been shown to play a major role in regulating both humoral and cellular immune responses (11).

B7: CD28/CTLA-4 COSTIMULATORY PATHWAY

This pathway consists of two costimulatory ligands on APC, B7.1 and B7.2, each of which binds to two receptors on T cells, called CD28 and CTLA-4 (Table 1). The CD28 and CTLA-4 proteins share amino acid sequences and have a similar overall structure, but are differently expressed and display different functions. CD28 is expressed by both resting and activated T cells. CTLA-4 is expressed only by activated T cells (12). Different from CD28, which is able to deliver potent activation signals, CTLA-4 signaling displays an inhibitory effect (13).

Table 1. B7.1 and B7.2 Costimulation.

B7.1 (CD80)		**B7.2 (CD86)**
Glycoprotein 55-60 kDa		Glycoprotein 70 kDa
	Immunoglobulin Superfamily	
Expression:		Expression:
Resting dendritic cells		Resting dendritic cells
Activated T, B, NK cells		Monocytes
Macrophages	Ligands: CD28 and CTLA-4	Activated T, B, NK cells
CD28		**CTLA-4**
	Immunoglobulin Superfamily	
Expression:		Expression:
Resting T cells		Activated T cells
	Function on T cell activation	
Costimulation (positive regulator)		Inhibition (negative regulator)
	Ligands: B7.1 and B7.2	

B7.1 (CD80) and B7.2 (CD86) belong to the immunoglobulin supergene family and sharing about 25% structural homologies. Both B7 molecules are expressed on professional APC: dendritic cells, activated macrophages and activated B cells. On the other hand B7.1 has not been found on resting T, B, NK cells or monocytes (14). Although the stimuli able to induce B7.1 and B7.2 expression on B cells and monocytes are similar (15), B7.2 is induced more rapidly than B7.1 and is usually expressed at higher levels (16).

Several cytokines modulate the expression of B7.1 and B7.2. IL-2 and IL-4 enhance the induction of B7.1 expression on mitogen-stimulated tonsillar B cells (17). IL-7 treatment of T cells results in the induction of B7.1 expression (18). The interaction of CD40 with its ligand and of TCR with MHC class II have both been shown to induce B7.1 expression on B cells (19,20). We have demonstrated that IL-1β is able to induce B7.1 expression on cultured thyroid follicular cells (TFC); bacterial lipopolysaccharide (LPS) stimulation has the same effect (21).

THE B7:CD28/CTLA-4 PATHWAY IN AUTOIMMUNITY

The expression and function of B7.1 and B7.2 have been studied in mice with systemic lupus erythematosus, insulin-dependent diabetes mellitus, and experiment-ally induced allergic encephalomyelitis. Systemic lupus erythematosus occurs spontaneously in several strains of inbred or cross-bred mice. To examine the individual roles of B7.1 and B7.2, mice were injected with specific antibodies anti-B7.1 and B7.2 (22). Injection of anti-B7.1 alone had little effect; by contrast, the injection of anti-B7.2 antibodies inhibited the production of anti-DNA antibodies. B7 antagonists inhibit the development of insulitis and diabetes mellitus in nonobese diabetic mice (23). Anti-B7.2 antibodies blocked the development of diabetes when administered in mice two to four weeks of age, whereas anti-B7.1 antibodies had no protective effect (23). These results suggest that B7.2 is more important than B7.1 in the pathogenesis of autoimmune disorders. By contrast, in experimentally induced murine allergic encephalomyelitis, where B.7.1 is preferentially expressed on APC, B7.1 seems more important than B7.2. In fact injections with anti-B7.1 antibodies, but not with anti-B7.2 antibodies, reduced the severity of disease (24,25).

We have demonstrated in Hashimoto's thyroiditis (HT) the expression of B7.1 (and not B7.2) on TFC (21). This molecule could provide a local costimulatory signal for T-lymphocyte differentiation toward the type 1 cytokine secretion pattern and maintenance of a sustained Th1 response (21). The differential expression of the two B7 antigens in thyroid tissue of HT is reminiscent of a report concerning human multiple sclerosis, another Th1-cell-mediated autoimmune disease. In specific lesions of the central nervous systems, the expression of B7.1, but not B7.2, was observed on different cell structures, whereas in nonspecific (vascular) lesions, B7.2 predominated (26).

The effect of anti-B7 antibodies on autoimmune disorders may be explained in two ways. In one model, the interaction of B7.1 and B7.2 with the same receptors on a precursor helper T cell results in the generation of different subsets of Th. According to this model, B7.1 preferentially acts as a costimulator for Th1 and B7.2 induces the production of Th2 (24). The difficulty with this explanation is that the development of diabetes in the nonobese diabetic mouse (mediated by Th1 and CD8) is inhibited by the administration of anti-B7.2 antibodies but not anti-B.1 (23).

In a second model, B7.1 and B7.2 induce similar signals in precursor helper T cells but can have distinct roles in immune responses because of their different expression kinetics; B7.2 expression occurs earlier and at higher levels than B7.1. Thus it is possible that anti-B7.2 antibodies inhibit the production of both Th1 and Th2 cytokines while B7.1 antibodies inhibit only Th1 lymphokine pattern secretion. Some experimental data support this latter hyphothesis (22).

The role of the CTLA-4 receptor in the pathogenesis of autoimmunity is not known. A lethal lymphoproliferative disease develops in CTLA-4 deficient mice that is characterized by T infiltration of multiple organs and destruction of tissue (27,28). This phenotype is evidence of a suppressive role for the CTLA-4 receptor and raises the possibility that mutations in the CTLA-4 gene can lead to autoimmune disease in humans. Studies of the association between a polymorphism in the CTLA-4 gene and autoimmune thyroid disease, using polymorphic microsatellite markers located within this gene, indicated a lack of linkage to date (29).

B7: CD28/CTLA-4 COSTIMULATORY PATHWAY IN GRAVES'DISEASE

There is considerable evidence that in autoimmune thyroid diseases thyroid follicular cells cross-talk with locally recruited immunocompetent cells via different surface molecules (Table 2). More than 15 years ago, constitutive follicular

Table 2. Constitutive expression of surface molecules on thyroid follicular cells involved in "cross-talking" with lymphocytes in autoimmune thyroid diseases.

	Graves' disease	Hashimoto's Thyroiditis
MHC Class II	+	+
ICAM-1	+/-	+
LFA-3	+	+
B7.1	-	+
B7.2	-	-
CD40	+	+
Fas	-	+
Fas Ligand	+	+

Data are summarized from references 30, 32, 33, 34, 35, 36, 37, 39, 40, 49, 56, 58.

expression of MHC class II antigens in Graves' Disease (GD) and HT (together with upregulation of Class I antigens) was reported (30,31). A functional role of Class II antigens has been suggested on the basis of the observed capability of Class II-bearing thyroid epithelial cells to present antigenic peptides (31). Follicular expression of ICAM-1 (CD54) was observed by us and others in HT, whereas conflicting and in most part negative results have been reported in GD (32-37). These findings suggest that TFC expressing MHC Class II antigens can serve as APC. It has been demonstrated that thyrocytes from patients with GD induce proliferation of autologous peripheral blood T cells in response to soluble antigens (38). The antigen-specific T cell response induced by TFC is blocked completely by anti-human leukocyte antigen-DR monoclonal antibody and partially by anti-ICAM-1. Furthermore, the synergistic augmentation of the T cell response, induced by the addition of suboptimal number of monocytes, is suppressed completely by combining anti B7.1 and B7.2, to a level equivalent to that observed when TFC are used alone as APC (39). These data suggest that the delivery of costimulatory signals on bystander professional APC enhances T cell activation by TFC.

The question of whether thyroid follicular cells express costimulatory molecules has been raised in different studies (39,40,41). Using specific anti-B7.1and anti B7.2 antibodies these studies failed to show any follicular staining in a series of GD patients, whereas positive infiltrating cells were observed. We recently reported that B7.1 (and not B7.2) may be expressed on the surface of TFC in HT but not in GD. Moreover co-cultures of infiltrating T cells with TFC have proved that the molecule is functional (21).

The major histological differences between HT and GD are the infiltrate amount and the damage to follicular structure. The expression of B7.1 on TFC in HT could provide a local costimulatory signal for T-lymphocyte differentiation toward the type 1 cytokine secretion pattern and maintenace of a sustained Th1 response. A role has been demonstrated for B7 antigen interaction with their T cell ligands in preventing T-cell apoptosis (42). Follicular B7.1 expression in HT may contribute to main-tenance of large lymphocyte infiltrates by increasing their survival, whereas in GD interaction of infiltrating T-cells with MHC Class II-positive, B7-negative follicular cells may results in inactivation or apoptosis. Matsuoka et al. (39) demonstrated low expression of CD28 on intrathyroidal versus peripheral blood CD8 bright+ cells indicating the possibility of an anergic state in these populations.

The most important source of intrathyroidal costimulatory molecules in GD appears to be activated B cells, although many intrathyroidal dendritic cells are B7+ (8). In GD, TFC are unable to provide a costimulatory signal via B7.1 and antigen presentation by Class II + TFC may, therefore, induce peripheral tolerance. This may be an important protective mechanism against the development of tissue damage.

CD40L/CD40 COSTIMULATION

CD40L/CD40 costimulation has been show to play a major role in regulating both humoral and cellular immune responses (11) (Table 3). The role for CD40L/CD40 stimulation in regulating Th1 responses could involve at least two mechanisms; first, direct induction of IL-12 production by APCs and, second, augmentation of expression of costimulatory molecules such as B7.1 and B7.2 on APCs, leading to increased T cell stimulation and IFN-γ production (44).

Table 3. CD40/CD40L costimulation.

CD40	CD40L
Glycoprotein 45-50kDa	Glycoprotein 39 kDa
Cell surface molecule of the TNF receptor/nerve growth factor receptor family	TNF gene family
Expression: B cells, dendritic cells, epithelial cells , endothelial cells	Expression: activated T, mast cells
Counter-receptor: CD40L	Counter-receptor: CD40

As already mentioned, Th1 responses are important in mediating protective immunity against certain intracellular infections, as well as in initiating or exacerbating specific autoimmune diseases (2,24). Recently it has been shown that IFN-γ production involves a complex interaction between two interdependent, yet distinct, costimulatory pathways and there is evidence that CD40L/CD40 interaction may be crucial in regulating IFN-γ production by peripheral blood mononuclear cells (11). In fact, in vivo experiments demonstrated that CD40-/- mice are highly susceptible to Leishmania major infection as a result of impaired production of IFN-γ (45). In contrast, CD28-/- mice infected with L. major exhibit normal Th1 responses and are able to control infection (46). In addition, there is evidence that CD40L/CD40 stimulation has a central role in regulating T cell-dependent antibody production. These data prompted investigation of the possible involvement of the CD40L/ CD40 signaling pathway in the pathogenesis of infectious and autoimmune disease.

CD40L/CD40 PATHWAY IN THYROID AUTOIMMUNITY

There is considerable evidence that the CD40L/CD40 pathway is involved in the pathogenesis and outcome of autoimmune diseases (47). The role of this pathway has been showed in an animal model of GD: treatment with anti-CD40L monoclonal antibodies of severe combined immunodeficient (SCID) mice with GD thyroid explants reduced levels of thyroid-reactive antibodies and thyroid lymphocytic infiltration (48). Recently, detection of CD40 on TFC has been reported in both autoimmune and non-autoimmune glands (49); CD40 expression was up-regulated by IL-1 β and IFN-γ (49).

CD40L/CD40 signaling enhances cytokine production (50) and induces expression of other costimulatory molecules on APC (51-53). CD40 stimulation of TFC increases IL-6 synthesis (49). In addition to IL-6, TFC have been implicated in the production of a number of other cytokines: for example IL-1α, IL-8, IL-12, TNF-α (54).

In thyroid autoimmunity, ligation of CD40 on TFC may result in increased synthesis of proinflammatory cytokines, with stimulation of T cell maturation and alteration of cytokine synthesis patterns (55). In HT, expression of CD40, B7.1 together with MHC Class II antigens and ICAM-1 on TFC could provide a local costimulatory signal for T-lymphocyte differentiation toward the type 1 cytokine secretion pattern and maintenance of the autoimmune process. Infiltrating Th1 are believed to induce tissue lesions through activation of cytolytic effector cells and secretion of lymphokines.

It is conceivable that, at least in part and/or in some phases of the natural history of HT, TFC may effectively act as autoantigen-presenting cells. The finding of colocalization of Class II and B7.1 antigens on the same follicular structure is consistent with such hypothesis (21). We observed that B7.1 can be induced on TFC by LPS and IL-1β, and that large amounts of IL-1β are present within HT thyroid tissue (56). IL-1β secretion may be promoted by products of Th1 infiltrating cells, far more abundant in HT than in GD.

In TFC of GD, where expression of MHC Class II and CD40 but not B7.1 has been observed, interaction of infiltrating T cells with TFC may result in T cell inactivation or anergy more easily than in HT because TFC are unable to provide a costimulatory signal. This mechanism may be important in protecting against the development of tissue damage in GD as opposed to HT. In GD, however, the expression of CD40 together with MHC Class II on TFC suggests the additional possibility of T cell-TFC interactions, with possible implications both for TFC synthesis of immunological mediators and for the biasing of T cell behaviour (IFN-γ secretion).

CONCLUSIONS

GD differs from chronic lymphocytic thyroiditis in two main respects: the crucial role of the autoimmune reaction against the TSH receptor and, on the other hand, the far less pronounced mononuclear cell infiltration and the lack of follicular structural damage. The role of costimulatory phenomena is probably different in the two diseases and this may, at least in part, account for the aforementioned differences. In GD, effective autoantigen presentation is possibly mainly via professional B7-positive APC (39). No expression of B7 antigens is detectable on TFC, therefore their interaction with infiltrating T-cells will result more easily in anergy, or apoptosis (6,7). The CD40 molecule, on the other hand, has been reported to be widely expressed on both non-autoimmune and autoimmune TFC (including GD) (49). Its presence in association with MHC class II antigens may facilitate TFC/T cell interactions resulting in proinflammatory cytokine release. This mechanism may be consistent with the inflammatory pattern (though limited; zones of mononuclear cell infiltrates) observed in some GD thyroid specimens. However the lack of B7 expression on TFC in GD may prevent the perpetuation and expansion of the autoimmune reaction resulting in tissue damage.

We demonstrated that IL1β promotes B7.1 expression on TFC. Of note, the same cytokine promotes expression of the Fas (CD95) molecule on TFC. The interaction of Fas molecule with its ligand (FasL) is able to transduce apoptotic signals. We also demonstrated (56,57) constitutive FasL expression on TFC from different sources, whereas Fas expression is far higher in HT than in GD (56 and our unpublished results). Thus, TFC FasL expression in GD may be effective mainly in inducing apoptosis of infiltrating lymphocytes that are in an activated state and may readily express Fas (58). The lack of B7.1 on TFC would prevent rescue from apoptosis of such lymphocytes. This mechanism is at variance with that occuring in HT, where TFC damage may occur via a "fratricidal" interaction between TFC mediated by Fas/FasL (56).

In summary, in GD costimulatory mechanisms (mainly B7-dependent) are likely to favor autoantigen presentation via professional APC. TFC are less efficient in delivering costimulatory signals in comparison with HT, and their interaction with infiltrating T-cells will more likely result in limited clonal expansion of the latter and, consequently, less tissue damage.

REFERENCES

1. **Seder RA, Paul WE.** 1994 Acquisition of lymphokine-producing phenotype by CD4+ T cells. Annu Rev Immunol. 12:635-673.
2. **Corry DB, Reiner SL, Linsley PS, Locksley RM.** 1994 Differential effects of blockade of CD28-B7 on the development of Th1 or Th2 effector cells in experimental leishmaniasis. J Immunol.153:4142-4148.
3. **Del Prete GF, Tiri A, Mariotti S, Pinchera A, Ricci M, Romagnani S.** 1987 Enhanced production of γ-interferon by thyroid-derived T cell clones from patients with Hashimoto's Thyroiditis. Clin Exp Immunol. 69:323-331.
4. **Del Prete GF, Tiri A, De Carli M et al.** 1989 High potential to tumor necrosis factor alpha production of thyroid infiltrating T lymphocytes in Hashimoto's thyroiditis: a peculiar feature of destructive thyroid autoimmunity. Autoimmunity. 4:267-270.
5. **Bagnasco M, Ferrini S, Venuti D et al.** 1987 Clonal analysis of T lymphocytes infiltrating the thyroid gland in Hashimoto's thyroiditis. Int Arch. Allergy Appl Immunol. 82:141-146.
6. **Guerder S, Meyerhoff J, Flavell R.** 1994 The role of the T cell costimulator B7.1 in autoimmunity and in the induction and maintenance of tolerance to peripheral antigen. Immunity. 1:155-163.
7. **Lanier LL, O'Fallon S, Somoza C et al.** 1995 CD80 (B7) and CD86 (B70) provide similar costimulatory signals for T cell proliferation, cytokine production and generation of CTL. J Immunol. 154:97-105.
8. **June CH, Bluestone JA, Nadler LM, Thompson CB.** 1994 The B7 and CD28 receptor families. Immunol Today. 15:321-330.
9. **Olive D, Pages F, Klasen S et al.** 1994 Stimulation via the CD28 molecule: regulation of signalling, cytokine production and cytokine receptor expression. Fundam. Clin. Immunol. 2:185-196.
10. **Reiser H, Stadecker MJ.** 1996 Costimulatory B7 molecules in the pathogenesis of infectious and autoimmune disease. New Engl J Med. 335:1369-1377.
11. **McDyder J, Goletz JT, Thomas E, June HC, Seder AR.** 1998. CD40 Ligand/CD40 stimulation regulates the production of IFN-γ from human peripheral blood mononuclear

cells in an IL-12 and/or CD28-dependent manner. J Immunol. 160:1704-1707.

12. **Linsley PS, Greene JL, Brady W, Bajorath J, Ledbetter JA, Peach R.** 1995 Human B7.1 (CD80) and B7.2 (CD86) bind with similar avidities but distinct kinetics to CD28 and CTLA-4 receptors. Immunity. 1:793-801.

13. **Krummel MF, Allison JP.** 1995 CD28 and CTLA-4 have opposing effect on the response of T cells to stimulation. J Exp Med. 182:459-465.

14. **Azuma M, Ito D, Yagita H et al.** 1993 B70 antigen is a second ligand for CTLA-4 and CD28. Nature. 366:76-78.

15. **Creery WD, Diaz-Mitoma F, Filion L, Kumar A.** 1996 Differential modulation of B7.1 and B7.2 isoform expression on human monocytes by cytokines which influence the development of T helper cell phenotype. Eur J Immunol. 26:1273-1277.

16. **Hathcock KS, Laszlo G, Pucillo C, Linsley P, Hodes RJ.** 1994 Comparative analysis of B7.1 and B7.2 costimulatory ligands: expression and function. J Exp Med. 180:631-637.

17. **Valle A, Aubry JP, Durand I, Bancherau J.** 1991 IL-4 and IL-2 upregulate the expression of antigen B7, the B cell counterstructure to T cell CD28: an amplification mechanism for T-B cell interactions. Int Immunol. 3:229-235

18. **Yssel H, Schneider PV, Lanier LL** 1993 Interleukin-7 specifically induces the B7/BB1 antigen onhuman cord blood and peripheral blood T cells and T cell clones. Int Immunol. 5:753-759

19. **Ranheim EA, Kipps TJ** 1993 Activated T cells induce expression of B7/BB1 on normal or leukemic B cells through a CD40-dependent signal. J Exp Med. 177:925-935

20. **Nabavi N, Freeman GJ, Gault A et al.** 1992 Signalling through the MHC class II cytoplasmatic domain is reqiured for antigen presentation and induces B7 expression. Nature 360:266-268.

21. **Battifora M, Pesce G, Paolieri F, Fiorino N, Giordano C, Riccio A, Toree G, Olive D, Bagnasco M.** 1998 B7.1 costimulatory molecule is expressed on thyroid follucular cells in Hashimoto's thyroiditis, but not in Graves'disease. J Clin Endocrinol Metab. 83:4130-4139.

22. **Nakajima A, Azuma M, Kodera S et al.** 1995 Preferential dependence of autoantibody production in murine lupus on CD86 costimulatory molecule. Eur J Immunol. 25:3060-3069.

23. **Lenschow DJ, Ho SC, Sattar H et al.** 1995 Differential effects of anti B7.1 and anti B7.2 monoclonal antibody treatment on the development of diabetes in the nonobese diabetic mouse. J Exp Med. 181: 1145-1155.

24. **Kuchroo VK, Das MP, Brown JA, et al.** 1995 B7.1 and B7.2 costimulatory molecules differentially activate the Th1/Th2 developmental pathways: application to autoimmune disease therapy. Cell 80:707-718.

25. **Miller SD, Vanderlugt CL, Lenschow DJ et al.** 1995 Blockage of CD28/B7.1 interaction prevents epitope spreading and clinical relapses of murine EAE. Immunity 3:739-745.

26. **Windhagen BA, Newcombe J, Dangond F et al.** 1995 Expression of costimulatory molecules B7.1 (CD80), B7.2 (CD86) and IL-12 cytokine in multiple sclerosis lesions. J Exp Med. 182:1985-1991.

27. **Waterhouse P, Penninger JM Timms E et al.** 1995 Lymphoproliferative dis-orders with early lethality in mice deficient in CTLA-4. Science 270: 985-988.

28. **Tivol EA, Boriello F, Schweitzer AN, Lynch WP, Bluestone JA Sharpe AH.** 1995 Loss of CTLA-4 leads to massive lymphoproliferation and fatal multiorgan tissue destruction, revealing a critical negative regulatory role of CTLA-4. Immunity 3:541-547.

29. **Barbesino G, Tomer Y, Concepcion E, Davies TF, Greenberg DA.** 1998 Linkage

analysis of candidate genes in autoimmune thyroid disease: 1. Selected immunoregolatory genes. International Consortium for the Genetics of Autoimmune Thyroid Disease. J Clin Endocrinol Metab. 83(5): 1580-1584.

30. **Hanafusa T, Pujol-Borrell R, Chiovato L, Bottazzo GF.** 1983 Aberrant expression of HLA-DR antigen on thyrocytes in Graves' disease. Lancet 2:1111-1115.

31. **Londei M, Lamb JR, Bottazzo GF, Feldmann M.** 1984 Epithelial cells expressing aberrant MHC class II determinants can present antigen to cloned human T cells. Nature 312:639-641.

32. **Bagnasco M, Caretto A, Olive D, Pedini B, Canonica GW, Betterle C.** 1991 Expression of intercellular adhesion molecule-1 (ICAM-1) on thyroid epithelial cells in Hashimoto's thyroiditis but not in Graves' disease or papillary thyroid cancer. Clin Exp Immunol. 83:309-313.

33. **Weetman AP, Cohen SB, Makgoba MW, Borysiewicz LK.** 1989 Expression of an intercellular adhesion molecule, ICAM-1, by human thyroid cells. J Endocrinol. 122:185-191.

34. **Zheng RQH, Abney ER, Grubeck-Loebenstein B, Dayan C, Maini RN, Feldmann M.** 1990 Expression of intercellular adhesion molecule-1 and lymphocyte function-associated antigen-3 on human thyroid epithelial cells in Graves' and Hashimoto's disease. J Autoimmunity 3:727-732.

35. **Tolosa E, Roura C, Catalfamo M, et al.** 1992 Expression of intercellular adhesion molecule-1 in thyroid follicular cells in autoimmune, non-autoimmune and neoplastic diseases of the thyroid gland: discordance with HLA. J. Autoimmunity 5:107-118.

36. **Miyazaki A, Mirakian R, Bottazzo GF.** 1992 Adhesion molecule expression in Graves' thyroid glands; potential relevance of granule membrane protein (GMP-140) and intercellular adhesion molecule-1 (ICAM-1) in the homing and antigen presentation process. Clin Exp Immunol. 89:52-57.

37. **Nakashima M, Eguchi K, Ida H, et al.** 1994 The expression of adhesion molecules in thyroid glands from patients with Graves' disease. Thyroid 4:19-25.

38. **Eguchi K, Otbubo T, Kawabe Y et al.** 1988 Synergy in antigen presentation by thyroid epithelial cells and monocytes from patients with Graves'disease. Clin Exp Immunol. 72:84-90.

39. **Matsuoka N, Eguchi K, Kawakami A, Tsuboi M, Nakamara H, Kimura H, Ishikawa N, Ito K, Nagataki S**. 1996 Lack of B7.1/BB1 and B7.2/B70 expression on thyrocytes of patients with Graves'disease. Delivery of costimulatory signals from bystander professional antigen-presenting cells. J Clin Endocrinol Metab. 81:41374143.

40. **Tandon N, Metcalfe RA, Barnett D, Weetman AP.** 1994 Expression of the costimulatory molecule B7/BB1 in autoimmune thyroid disease. Q J Med. 87:231-236.

41. **Lombardi G, Arnold K, Uren J, et al.** 1997 Antigen presentation by IFN-γ treated thyroid follicular cells inhibits IL2 and support IL4 production by B7-dependent human T cells. Eur J Immunol. 27:62-71.

42. **Wagner DH, Hagman J, Linsley PS, Hodsdon W, Freed JII, Newell MK.** 1996 Rescue of thymocytes from glucocorticoid-induced cell death mediated by CD28/CTLA-4 costimulatory interactions with B7.1/B7.2. J Exp Med. 184:1631-1638.

43. **Cella M, Scheidegger D, Palmer-Lehmann K, Lane P, Lanzavecchia A, Alber G.** 1996 Ligation of CD40 on dendritic cells triggers production of high levels of IL-12 and enhances T cell stimulatory capacity: T-T help via APC activation. J Exp Med. 18:747-753.

44. **Kiener P, Moran-Davis P, Rankin BM, Wahl AF, Aruffo A Hollenbaugh D.** 1995 Stimulation of CD40 with purified soluble gp39 induces proinflammatory responses in human monocytes. J Immunol. 155:4917-4923.

45. **Campbell KA, Ovendale PJ, Kennedy MK, Fanslow WC, Reed GS, Maliszewski**

CR. 1996 CD40 ligand is required for protective cell-mediated immunity to Leishmania major. Immunity 4:283-289.

46. **Brown DR, Green MJ, Moskowitz NH, Davis M, Thompson BC, Reiner SL.** 1996 Limited role of CD28-mediated signals in T helper subset differentiation. J Exp Med. 184:803-808.

47. **Buhlmann JE, Noelle RJ.** 1996 Therapeutic potential for blockade of the CD40 ligand, gp39. J Clin immunol. 16:83-89.

48. **Resetkova E, Kawai K, Enomoto T et al.** 1996. Antibody to gp39, the ligand for CD40 significantly inhibits the humoral response from Graves' thyroid tissue xenografted into severe combined immunodeficient (scid) mice. Thyroid 6:267-273.

49. **Metcalfe RA, McIntosh SR, Marelli-Berg F, Lombardi G, Lechler R, Weetman AP.** 1998. Detection of CD40 on human thyroid follicular cells: analysis of expression and function. J Clin Endocrinol Metab. 83:1268-1274.

50. **Heloisa Blotta M, Marshall JD, DeKruyff RH, Umetsu DT.** 1996 Cross-linking of the CD40 ligand on human CD4+ T lymphocytes generates a costimulatory signal that up-regulates IL-4 synthesis. J Immunol. 156:3133-3140.

51. **Clark LB, Foy TM, Noelle RJ.** 1996 CD40 and its ligand. Adv Immunol. 63:43-78.

52. **Yang YP, Wilson JM.** 1996 CD40 ligand-dependent T cell activation: requirement of B7-CD28 signaling through CD40. Science. 273: 1862-1864.

53. **Scinde S, Wu Y, Guo Y et al.** 1996 CD40L is important for induction of, but not response to, costimulatory activity: ICAM-1 as the second costimulatory molecule rapidly up-regulated by CD40L. J Immunol. 157: 2764-2769.

54. **Ajjan RA, Watson PF, Weetman AP.** 1997 Cytokines and cytokine function. Adv Neuroimmunol. 36: 359-386.

55. **Lombardi G, Arnold K, Uren J, et al.** 1997 Antigen presentation by interferon-gamma-treated thyroid follicular cells inhibits interleukin-2 (IL-2) and support IL-4 production by B7-dependent human T cells. Eur J Immunol. 27:62-71.

56. **Giordano C, Stassi G, De Maria R, et al.** 1997 Potential involvement of Fas and its ligand in the pathogenesis of Hashimoto's thyroiditis. Science 275:960-963.

57. **Griffith TS, Ferguson TA.** 1997. The role of FasL-induced apoptosis in immune privilege. Immunol Today 18: 240-244.

58. **Papoff G, Stassi G, De Maria R et al.** 1998. Technical Comment: Constitutive expression of FasL in thyrocytes. Science 279: 2015a.

8

APOPTOSIS IN AUTOIMMUNE THYROID DISEASE

Peiqing Wu and James R. Baker, Jr

INTRODUCTION

Autoimmune thyroid disease

The thyroid is the most common target for organ-specific autoimmune destruction in humans. In 1912, Hashimoto described 4 cases of goiter with diffuse lymphocyte infiltration, eosinophilic changes of follicular cells, and various degrees of atrophy and fibrosis (1). Autoantibodies were found in the patients with this disorder nearly half a century later (2), establishing Hashimoto's thyroiditis (HT) as an organ-specific autoimmune disease. It is the most common thyroid disorder, with a female to male ratio of 20:1, affecting up to 2% of the female population (3). Besides HT, which can also present clinically as 'silent thyroiditis' or as atrophic thyroiditis, the other major autoimmune thyroid disease (AITD) is Graves' disease (GD).

Mode of thyroid destruction in autoimmune thyroid disease

A major clinical manifestation of HT is hypothyroidism resulting from the immune destruction of thyroid follicular cells. Histologically, HT is characterized by extensive lymphoid infiltration with germinal center formation, loss of thyroid epithelial cells, atrophy of thyroid follicles, and diffuse fibrosis of the thyroid. In its late stage there is total disruption of normal thyroid architecture and few, if any, thyrocytes are present (4,5). Thyroid follicular cells in close proximity to infiltrating lymphocytes are apoptotic (6,7). The mechanism(s) of thyroid destruction in AITD are not yet fully understood. Some possible destructive pathways are discussed below.

Complement-mediated Cytolysis

Thyroid epithelial cells can be damaged by thyroid-specific antibodies and ensuing complement fixation. Anti-thyroglobulin antibodies (2,8,9) and antithyroperoxidase (TPO) antibodies (previously known as anti-microsomal antibodies) (8-11) are present in the majority of HT and GD patients. Anti-TPO antibodies can fix complement *in vitro* and are toxic to human thyrocytes (3,10).

Tandon *et al.*, however, argued that thyrocytes from GD and HT were not vulnerable to complement-mediated lysis due to the expression of CD59 and inhibitory proteins of membrane attack complexes (MACs) (12). These molecules prevent the insertion of MACs into the cell membrane and are upregulated by IL-1, TNF, and IFN-γ (12). In AITD, infiltrating lymphocytes and macrophages provide a local source for these cytokines, which render thyrocytes more resistant to complement-mediated attack. Although GD patients have an anti-TPO response similar to that in HT patients (11), there is no evidence for thyroid destruction. Therefore, this process does not seem to be the major mechanism of thyrocyte destruction in AITD.

Antibody-dependent cellular cytotoxicity

In antibody-dependent cell-mediated cytotoxicity (ADCC), antibodies recognize antigens on the cell surface. Subsequently macrophages, monocytes, nature killer cells (NK cells) and cytotoxic T lymphocytes (CTLs), which have IgG Fc receptors (FcγR) on their surface, bind the Fc portion of the bound antibodies and phagocytose or kill the IgG-coated cells. Thyroid antibodies mediate ADCC *in vitro* (13). Using normal lymphocytes as effectors and thyrocytes as targets, HT sera, unlike GD sera, were twice as potent as normal sera in killing thyrocytes (14). NK cell number was reported to be increased in thyroids of HT patients (15), but to be decreased in those of GD patients (15,16). However, there is no evidence that ADCC plays a primary role in thyroid destruction in AITD.

Apoptosis triggered by cytotoxic T lymphocytes and nature killer cells

Apoptosis is believed to be a major factor in the destruction of the thyroid in AITD. Thyrocyte killing by CTLs and NK cells has been shown in HT and GD (14,17). The majority of T cell clones isolated from infiltrating T lymphocytes (ITLs) of the thyroid glands of AITD were CTLs and cytotoxic against thyrocytes (18-20). CTLs and NK cells execute killing by inducing apoptosis in their target cells (21-23) primarily in the following two ways. CD8$^+$ CTLs and NK cells mainly utilize the granule-exocytosis pathway that relies on the release of perforin and granzyme B. The latter cleaves and activates caspase-3, which is a component in the apoptotic cascade (24). CD4$^+$ CTLs elicit programmed cell death in target cells by the Fas-mediated apoptotic pathway.

AN OVERVIEW OF APOPTOSIS

Characteristics of apoptosis

There are two major morphologically and biochemically distinct categories of cell death in a living body. *Accidental cell death* is a pathological death that occurs in response to environmental or traumatic stimuli, for instance, severe hypoxia, hyperthermia, toxins or poisons, complement attack, and viral lysis (25). The term *necrosis* (Greek for deadness) refers to this form of cell death, featured morphologically by (a) organelle swelling and rupture, (b) cell autolysis, © focal cell death, and (d) local inflammation. It is characterized biochemically by (a) metabolic collapse and ATP depletion, (b) release of lysosomal enzymes, © generation of toxic oxygen radicals, and (d) activation of Ca^{2+}-dependent phospholipases (25).

The other category is *programmed cell death*. In 1972, Kerr *et al.* (26) proposed the term *apoptosis* (Greek for falling of leaves off trees in the autumn) to describe a distinct mode of cell death, in which cells die from an inherent program, as opposed to mitosis, in the regulation of animal cell populations. Apoptosis is a physiological death and an active suicidal event depending upon active metabolism, including (a) activation of caspases (cyteine aspases), (b) activation of Ca^{2+}/Mg^{2+}-dependent endonucleases, and © energy supply. Apoptosis is featured morphologically by (a) nuclear condensation, (b) DNA fragmentation into multiples of 180 base pairs (the length of one nucleosome), © membrane blebbing, (d) single cell death surrounded by viable neighbors, (e) shrunken apoptotic cells and/or apoptotic bodies (multiple membrane-enclosed vesicles resulting from breaking down of apoptotic cells) phagocytosed by macrophages and neighboring cells without eliciting a local inflammation, and (f) fast progression (usually 30 to 60 minute) (27-32).

Apoptosis is a vital mechanism in the development and homeostasis of multicellular organisms. It is part of an organized tissue reaction, such as embryogenesis and morphogenesis, tissue atrophy following hormone withdrawal, the controlled normal tissue turnover, and tumors in regression. One of the critical functions of apoptosis is to eliminate autoreactive B and T cells. In the negative selection during T cell maturation in the thymus, for instance, the deletion of 95% of immature T cells is a result of programmed cell death through apoptosis. Another important function of apoptosis is to dispose of cells with non-repairable damage in their genome (for example, DNA breakage by ionizing irradiation) to avoid passing the abnormal genome to their progeny. Dysregulation of apoptosis may result in a variety of clinical situations, including autoimmunity, neoplasm, and the deletion of uninfected $CD4^+$ T cell in AIDS (27-32).

Pathways and regulation of apoptosis

In mammalian cells two apoptotic pathways are being extensively studied. One is the caspase-8 apoptotic pathway (Figure 1A), which can be initiated by binding of Fas ligand (FasL), tumor necrosis factor (TNF), and TRAIL (TNF-related apoptosis-inducing ligand) to their receptors Fas, TNFR1, and DR4 and DR5, respectively. The other is the caspase-9 apoptotic pathway (Figure 1B), which may be triggered by γ-irradiation and glucocorticoids. Caspases are a group of cyteine aspases that play a pivotal role in the activating cascade of apoptosis (33).

Fas-mediated apoptotic pathway

Fas (CD95/Apo-1) is a type I transmembrane protein with a cysteine-rich extra-cellular domain belonging to the tumor necrosis factor (TNF) receptor family (34, 35). It contains an 80 amino acid cytoplasmic sequence known as the death domain (36,37). Fas is reported to be constitutively expressed on lymphocytes and to be detected on some nonhematopoeitic cells (35,38).

Fas ligand (FasL) is a type II transmembrane protein and a member of the TNF superfamily (39). A matrix metalloprotease releases the membrane-bound FasL into

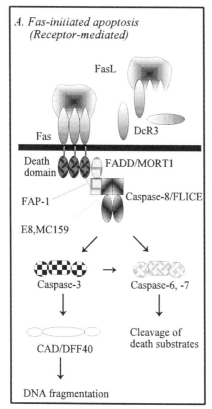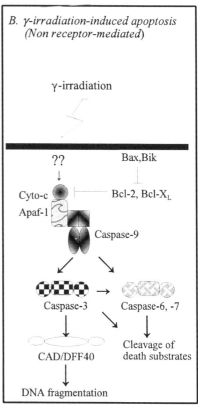

Figure 1. Apoptotic signal transduction pathways. *(A) Caspase-8 pathway.* This pathway can be mediated by Fas. Upon ligation by FasL, Fas trimerizes and, via its death domain, binds an adaptor FADD. Caspase-8 is subsequently recruited to FADD through their death effector domains. The bound caspase-8 then oligomerizes and self-cleaves to become an active form. It in turn activates effector caspases (caspase-3, -6, -7, -x) that digest death substrates (PARP, lamin, gho-GDI, *etc.*). Caspase-3 is also responsible for activating CAD/DFF40 that executes DNA fragmentation. FAP-1 binds to the C-terminus of Fas and prevents Fas-FADD association. Viral inhibitors E8 and MC159 interfere with FADD-caspase-8 binding. Viral protein CrmA inhibits activities of several caspases (not shown in the figure). Soluble decoy receptor DcR3 neutralizes FasL and prevents the triggering of Fas apoptosis pathway. *(B) Caspase-9 pathway.* The immediate early events following γ-irradiation are not clear. The first confirmed event is the release of cytochrome c from mitochondria. It then binds to and activates Apaf-1. This process is dATP-dependent. The activated Apaf-1 recruits and activates caspase-9. The active caspase-9 then activates effector caspases. Bcl-2 and Bcl-x_L inhibit the release of cytochrome c and block this apoptotic pathway. Bax and Bik relieve this inhibition by forming heterodimers with Bcl-2.

intercellular space, where it exists as a homotrimer (40). FasL is expressed on activated CTLs and NK cells (39,40). It is believed to be a major tool for CTLs and NK cells in killing virally infected cells and tumor cells (21,35).

A cascade of intracellular events leading to apoptosis is initiated following binding of cell surface Fas (24,35, 41-44). This apoptotic signal transduction pathway is highly complicated and yet to be fully understood. A brief picture of it is illustrated below and in Figure 1A.

Upon ligation by FasL, Fas trimerizes and, via its death domain, recruits an adaptor known as FADD (Fas-associated protein with death domain) (45) or MORT1 (mediator of receptor-induced toxicity) (46). FADD/MORT1 has a death effector domain (DED). Through its own DED, FADD then attracts the DED of FLICE (a FADD-like interleukin-1β-converting enzyme) (47). This complex is now called a DISC (death-inducing signal complex) or an apoptosome (24). The members of interleukin-1β-converting enzyme (ICE) family have been designated caspases (cyteine aspases) (33). In this nomenclature, FLICE is referred to as caspase-8. The formation of the DISC causes caspase-8 to oligomerize and self-cleave into its active form, which in turn activates a number of downstream effector caspases (caspase-3, -6, -7, *etc.*). Active form of caspase-3 then activates a DNA fragmentation factor (DFF) (48). DFF is a 40 kDa nuclease (DFF40), also known as caspase-activated DNase (CAD). In non-apoptotic cells, DFF40/CAD is complexed with a 45 kDa inhibitor (DFF45 or ICAD, inhibitor of CAD), so that the cleavage of chromosomal DNA is prevented. Caspase-3 elicits the nuclease activity of DFF40 by cutting DFF45/ICAD at two sites and setting DFF40/CAD free from its inhibitor DFF45/ICAD (48-51). The nuclease activity of DFF40/CAD is further boosted by histone 1 (but not core histones). This explains why chromosomal DNA is cut at internucleosomal locations (50). Other caspase activities are also observed. For instance, a 116 kDa death substrate poly (ADP-ribose) polymerase (PARP) is cleaved into a 102 kDa fragment by caspase-3 and caspase-6 (52, 53). Lamin is digested by caspase-6 (53). The proteolysis of gho-GDI and actin is also reported (54,55).

Although DNA fragmentation is a hallmark of apoptosis, it has recently been considered dispensable. The virtue of DNA degradation during apoptosis its that it seems to facilitate efficient disposal of the genome of the dead cell, to minimize gene transfer to the phagocytosing cells, and to prevent the formation of anti-DNA antibodies and the ensuing autoimmunity (44,56).

γ-irradiation-induced apoptotic pathway

Apoptosis triggered by γ-irradiation and glucocorticoids proceeds through Apaf-1-caspase-9 signal transduction pathway without a specific membrane receptor (Figure 1B). Apaf-1 stands for apoptotic protease-activating factor 1 (57). The receptor(s) and the immediate early events following γ-irradiation and exposure to dexamethasone are currently unknown. The first confirmed step in this signal transduction series is the release of cytochrome c from mitochondria. The released cytochrome c then binds and activates Apaf-1. This process requires dATP (32,57). Through its CARD (caspase recruitment domain), Apaf-1 binds the prodomain of caspase-9, which leads to aggregation and self-cleavage of caspase-9 and the activation of caspase-9. The active caspase-9 in turn cleaves and activates caspase-3 and other downstream effector caspases (procaspase-6, –7, *etc.*). The rest of the signal transduction events are similar to those in Fas-mediated apoptosis. In knockout mouse models, caspase-9 was shown to be required for cytochrome c-mediated activation of caspase-3. Thymocytes and splenocytes from caspase-9$^{-/-}$ mice were resistant to apoptosis induced by γ-irradiation and dexamethasone. However, apoptosis induced by Fas and TNF-α in these mice remained intact (58,59).

Other death pathways

Currently known death pathways cannot account for the negative selection in the thymus, where autoreactive T cells are sentenced to death (60-62). Mutations in the *fas* gene did not inhibit clonal deletion of autoreactive T cells in the thymus (63-65). Also, *bcl-2* transgene expression did not block apoptosis during negative selection in the thymus (66-68). The combination of Fas deficiency and Bcl-2 excess did not completely suppress negative selection (69). Furthermore, there is recent evidence that in the presence of caspase inhibitors, apoptosis proceeded when induced by appropriate agents and conditions (70). In fact, Kuida *et al.* reported that caspase-9 was not essential for negative selection in the thymus (58). Therefore, additional death pathways may exist.

Other death receptors

At the present time there are 5 known death receptors (DRs) belonging to the TNF receptor family. They are Fas (34), TNFR1 (71), DR3 (72), DR4 (73), and DR5 (74). Their ligands FasL, TNF and Apo3L bind to Fas, TNFR1, and DR3, respectively. Apo2L or TRAIL (TNF-related apoptosis-inducing ligand) (75) recognizes DR4 and DR5. These death receptors have an intracellular death domain and trigger similar pathways, which merge at some point down the signal transduction cascade. A detailed discussion of these pathways is beyond the scope of this chapter.

Inhibitors of apoptosis

Inhibitors of apoptosis exist in nature through evolution. The CTL-induced apoptosis serves to kill cells with intracellular organisms (viruses, protozoa, *etc.*). Viruses have found ways to keep their host cells alive to support viral replication. Viral inhibitors of apoptosis can be functionally classified into two groups. One group of such inhibitors, exemplified by viral inhibitors E8 (a herpesvirus protein) and MC159 (a poxvirus protein), binds to the molecules in the apoptotic pathway and block the signal transduction. Both E8 and MC159 contain a DED that binds to FLICE/caspase-8 and FADD, respectively (76,77). The binding interferes with the formation of the DISC, whereby blocking apoptosis. The other group acts by inhibiting the enzymatic activity of caspases (32). They include CrmA, p35, and a family of IAP (inhibitors of apoptosis). The cowpox virus protein CrmA inhibits caspase-1 and caspase-3 (78).

In mammals, cellular inhibitors of apoptosis include the products of the protooncogene *bcl-2* family Bcl-2, Bcl-x$_L$, Bcl-w. The relatives of Bcl-2 family Bax, Bik, Bak, Bad and Bcl-x$_S$, on the other hand, facilitate apoptosis. Bcl-2 and its homologs bind to mitochondria and prevent the release of cytochrome c. This in turn blocks activation of Apaf-1 and the caspase-9 apoptotic pathway, which can be induced by γ-irradiation and glucocorticoids (44). However, most studies demonstrated that Bcl-2 failed to block Fas-induced apoptosis (69,79,80), which is a caspase-8 apoptotic pathway. In the periphery, apoptosis induced by antigen stimulation depends upon Fas death pathway (81-84). Bcl-2 has been shown to be unable to inhibit this process (69). Bax and Bik act by forming heterodimers with Bcl-2 and resolving the inhibition of cytochrome-c release. Therefore, the apoptotic cascade proceeds (44).

EVIDENCE FOR APOPTOSIS IN AUTOIMMUNE THYROID DISEASE

In the thyroid there is a basal level of apoptosis serving to regulate glandular formation and cell turnover (6,7,85,86). In animal experiments, the deprivation of thyroid stimulating hormone (TSH) led to apoptosis in canine thyrocytes (87). In patients with idiopathic myxedema, thyroid stimulation blocking antibodies (TSBAb) caused thyroid atrophy and hypothyroidism in a situation similar to TSH withdrawal (88). In GD patients, on the other hand, thyroid-stimulating antibodies (TSAb) caused goiter and hyperthyroidism, presumably due to decreased apoptosis (88).

There is a growing body of evidence supporting the idea that apoptosis is a major contributing factor in AITD (reviewed in ref. 89 and 90). Morphological changes characteristic of apoptosis have been observed in AITD (6,7,91). In HT, the numbers of apoptotic follicular cells are increased in areas in close proximity to infiltrating lymphocytes (6,7,85,86), whereas they are decreased in intact follicles further away from germinal centers (6,85). In GD, where the lymphocyte infiltration is milder, the number of apoptotic cells is decreased, but apoptosis that is noted is also associated with areas of infiltrates (7,85).

FAS-MEDIATED APOPTOSIS IN AUTOIMMUNE THYROID DISEASE

Animal models have provided valuable insight into the functions of Fas and FasL. Mice carrying mutations in *fas* gene have a lymphoproliferative phenotype (*lpr* mice) and manifest systemic autoimmune reactivities mimicking human systemic lupus erythematosus (SLE)(92,93). Mice with generalized lymphoproliferative disease (*gld* mice) have mutations in the *fasl* gene (94,95). Both *lpr* and *gld* mice develop lymphadenopathy and splenomegaly due to accumulation of CD3$^+$CD4$^-$CD8$^-$ T cells in peripheral lymphoid tissues. Subsequently, autoimmune diseases develop in some strains of these mice. In the periphery, the Fas death pathway is involved in activation-induced suicide of T cells (81-84), which serves to hold the immune response at a certain magnitude, and to terminate the immune response after the offending pathogen is cleared. In *lpr* and *gld* mice, however, mature T cells do not die after activation and accumulate in the spleen and lymph nodes.

In humans, mutations in the *fas* gene have been reported in autoimmune lymphoproliferative syndrome (ALPS) (96), lymphoproliferative syndrome (97) and Canale-Smith syndrome (98), which may, in fact, be a single disorder. Mutation in the *fasl* gene was also reported in a patient with SLE and lymphoproliferative disease (99).

Evidence for Fas-mediated apoptosis in autoimmune thyroid disease

Monoclonal antibodies against Fas induce apoptosis in cell lines *in vitro* (34,100). A number of reports have shown a correlation between the number of Fas-positive cells in the thyroid and the number of apoptotic cells detected by flow cytometry, electron microscopy, and terminal deoxy-UTP nick end labeling (TUNEL)(85,91,101,102). HT is most clearly associated with apoptosis, compared with GD and multinodular goiter (85). By combining FACS and *in situ* immunofluorecence, they found that apoptosis tended to be more concentrated in areas where lymphocytes infiltrated. Kawakami *et al.* reported that, upon up-regulation of Fas expression by IFN-γ and IL-1β, apoptosis was induced by anti-Fas antibody (103). When Fas expression was down-regulated by TSH, apoptosis was inhibited (103). It is also believed that there is a correlation between the level of Fas expression and the degree of apoptosis in the thyroid.

Expression of Fas and FasL on thyrocytes

Fas expression in the thyroid

Various levels of Fas expression on thyroid epithelial cells have been demonstrated by a number of laboratories using immunohistochemistry (7,85,101,102,104), reverse transcription-polymerase chain reaction (RT-PCR) (104,105), ribonuclease protection assay (104,105), Western blot (104), and flow cytometry (101,103,106). In contrast, others have found no Fas expression on normal thyrocytes (85,101,107). However, Hammond *et al.* examined normal thyroid tissue from only one patient (85). Hammond's and Leithauser's groups detected Fas expression by immunohistochemistry only (85,107). Using thyrocytes from nontoxic goiter patients as their normal tissue, Giordano *et al.* found no Fas expression unless IL-1β was added (101)

Although thyrocytes are capable of expressing Fas, it is not yet fully understood how this expression is regulated in these cells. Kawakami *et al.* reported that Fas was constitutively expressed on thyroid cells, but it did not induce apoptosis unless these cells were exposed to IFN-γ or IL-1β (103). Arscott *et al.* showed that Fas was constitutively expressed on thyroid follicular cells and that its expression on these cells did not vary regardless of culture conditions, and not affected by IFN-γ or IL-1β (104). There are several studies regarding Fas expression on thyrocytes from HT patients. Using immunohistochemistry, Hammond *et al.* (85) reported a slight increase in Fas expression, and Mitsiades *et al.* found the increased expression of Fas was localized to follicles in close proximity to lymphocyte infiltration (102). In contrast, Tanimoto *et al.* found reduced Fas expression on HT thyrocytes as compared with that on thyrocytes from GD and tumor patients and normal subjects (7). Using immunohistochemistry and flow cytometry, Giordano's group showed a high level of Fas expression upon induction by IL-1β (101). They also reported that normal and HT thyrocytes constitutively express FasL. They believe that in HT, the upregulation of Fas results in apoptosis, implicating that thyrocytes kill their neighboring thyrocytes.

One of the possible regulatory elements for Fas expression is TSH, which has an anti-apoptotic effect upon thyroid epithelial cells. Kawakami *et al.* reported that Fas expression on thyrocytes was down-regulated by TSH (103,106). Likewise, thyroid stimulating antibodies to the TSH receptor that are found in GD patients, had a similar effect. Kawakami's group found that in GD, these antibodies significantly down-regulated Fas expression on thyrocytes *in vitro* (106). In their studies, Fas expression was down-regulated by TSH and IgG from GD patients, but not by IgG from patients with idiopathic myxedema. Furthermore, the upregulation of Fas by IL-1β and IFN-γ was suppressed by TSH and Graves' IgG. Also, anti-Fas antibody-induced apoptosis was inhibited by TSH and Graves' IgG (106).

FasL expression in the thyroid

Reports of FasL expression on thyroid epithelial cells have resulted in an ongoing debate. Xerri *et al.* detected no FasL expression by thyrocytes using Southern blot, RT-PCR, and Western blot analysis (108). In contrast, Giordano *et al.* (101) showed that normal and HT thyrocytes constitutively expressed FasL using immunohistochemistry, RT-PCR, and flow cytometry. However, Stokes *et al.* (105) found no FasL mRNA by RT-PCR and ribonuclease protection assay, and suspected that the FasL mRNA detected by Giordano's group might come from contaminating lymphocytes in their samples, or from their use of "goiter" cells as normal thyrocytes. Stokes' and Fiedler's groups (105) and Smith *et al.* (109) also questioned the specificity of the commercial antibodies used in the Giordano's study.

More recently Mitsiades *et al.* also found high levels of FasL expression on HT thyrocytes but virtually none on normal thyrocytes and infiltrating lymphocytes (102). Another study by the Giordano's group, without using the questioned antibodies, again argued for the expression of FasL on thyrocytes from HT patients (110). Using their own antibodies in Western blot and immunohistochemistry, Tamura *et al.* detected a high level of FasL expression on rat thyrocytes (91).

Overall, the issue regarding the expression of FasL in normal and autoimmune thyroid glands remains unsettled. Further studies are needed to clarify the controversy.

Cytokines in the regulation of Fas and FasL expression

Infiltrating lymphocytes and macrophages in AITD provide a local source for cytokines (111). Intrathyroid $CD4^+$ T cell clones from HT and GD produced IFN-γ, IL-2, IL-6, TGF-β, TNF-α, and lymphotoxin (TNF-β)(112). IFN-γ was up-regulated in thyroid-derived T cell clones from HT (113), and TNF-α was up-regulated in thyroid infiltrating T lymphocytes (114). IL-1 was shown to be produced by macrophages, thyrocytes, and endothelial cells in the autoimmune thyroid gland (115).

There is evidence that apoptosis in thyrocytes is induced by anti-Fas monoclonal antibodies only when these cells are pre-incubated with inflammatory cytokines, presumably due to the up-regulation of Fas (22,101). In the HT thyroid, where infiltrating T cells are predominately Th1 that produce IL-1 and IFN-γ, Kotani *et al.* believe that the up-regulation of Fas might be a result of cytokine stimulation (6). A number of other studies also showed that Fas expression was up-regulated by cytokines IFN-γ, IL-1β, and TNF-α (85,101,102,103,116), whereas others found no such an effect (104,105). Kawakami *et al.* reported that the up-regulation of Fas by IL-1β and IFN-γ is suppressed by TSH and IgG from GD patients (103,106).

Infiltrating T lymphocytes in autoimmune thyroid disease

The Fas apoptotic pathway has been recognized as an important mechanism used by CTLs and NK cells to kill their targets (22,35). Up-regulation of FasL expression on activated killer cells is an efficient way to induce apoptosis in Fas positive target cells (117). First, CTLs were found in areas in the thyroid where apoptosis occurred (6,7). Second, CTLs were shown to induce apoptosis in target cells (21,22,118-120). Infiltrating T lymphocytes (ITLs) found in the thyroid from HT patients were mostly autoreactive cytotoxic T cells, leading to the suspicion that these ITLs might be inducing apoptosis in thyrocytes (121,122).

However, Stassi *et al.* (110) found that ITLs from HT did not express high levels of FasL. In their tissue cultures, 24-36% of ITLs died by apoptosis within 36 hours. *In situ* TUNEL showed that virtually all ITLs near FasL-expressing thyrocytes were pre-apoptotic, as measured by expression of high levels of GD3 ganglioside, a glycolipid responsible for the generation of apoptotic signals following Fas ligation. About 10-15% of these ITLs were apoptotic. They concluded that, in HT, ITLs were not directly involved in the killing of thyrocytes, rather, Fas-FasL interaction among thyrocytes was responsible for the destruction of thyrocytes. This conclusion was instead in agreement with Giordano *et al.* (101) in that thyrocyte destruction is due to suicide or fratricide by thyrocytes that simultaneously express Fas and FasL. Again, this issue is not yet settled due to the controversy over whether thyrocytes express FasL.

Regulation of Fas-mediated apoptosis in autoimmune thyroid disease

Although increased apoptosis may account for the pathogenesis of HT, decreased apoptosis may be a contributing factor in GD. As a result, GD presents with hyperthyroidism and thyrotoxicosis from thyroid hyperplasia. The modulation of programmed cell death pathways in the thyroid by modifying the susceptibility of thyrocytes to immune-mediated apoptosis will change the landscape of our under-standing of autoimmune thyroid disease.

Thyroid stimulating hormone

Apoptosis in the canine thyroid has been observed following withdrawal of TSH (87). TSH also inhibits Fas-induced apoptosis in the human thyroid (103). While Kawakami *et al.* reported that TSH down-regulate Fas expression (103,106), Arscott *et al.* found no such an effect (104). They instead observed an increased apoptosis associated with IFNγ or IL-1β only in the presence of cycloheximide (104). This implies that a protein inhibitor may override the effect of TSH on apoptosis in thyrocytes.

Bcl-2 and its homologs

Earlier studies on the inhibition of Fas-mediated apoptosis by Bcl-2 provided confusing results. While some reported that Bcl-2 inhibited this process (123,124), others did not agree (69,125-127). Scaffidi *et al.* proposed two Fas death pathways

(128). In their model, Fas triggering in type I cells results in strong caspase-8 activation at the DISC that bypasses mitochondria and directly leads to activation of other caspases. This process, therefore, is not inhibitable by Bcl-2. In type II cells, on the other hand, only a little DISC is formed leading to activation of mitochondria and the caspases downstream of mitochondria, which can be inhibited by Bcl-2 and Bcl-x_L.

Tanimoto *et al.* found various levels of Bcl-2 in HT thyrocytes, but much higher levels in GD thyrocytes (7). Hammond *et al.* and Mitsiades *et al.* found decreased expression of Bcl-2 in HT thyroids (85,102). Bcl-2 expression was shown unchanged by TSH and Graves' IgG, idiopathic myxedema IgG, or IL-1β and IFN-γ (106).

Although in most cases Bcl-2 and its homologs cannot block Fas-mediated apoptotic pathway, they may play an important role in inhibiting apoptosis induced by ionizing irradiation and steroids, and in promoting survival of Fas-negative cells.

Other inhibitors of apoptosis

Studies have suggested that the expression of certain apoptosis inhibitors might be increased in thyroid glands from GD patients (7,106). As mentioned above, Arscott *et al.* found that thyroid epithelial cells were resistant to Fas-mediated apoptosis, even in the presence of IFN-γ or IL-1β. In spite of high levels of Fas expression, thyrocytes did not undergo apoptosis unless cycloheximide was added. This indicates that there exists a labile protein inhibitor of the Fas-mediated apoptosis cascade (104). Sato's group had found a protein tyrosine phosphatase FAP-1 (Fas-associated phosphatase-1) (129). It interacts with the carboxyl terminus of Fas, whereby prevents the recruitment of FADD and blocks apoptotic signal transduction pathway (130). Preliminary studies by Myc *et al.* suggest that FAP-1 is present in the thyroid (131).

Recently two more cellular inhibitors of apoptosis have been characterized. I-FLICE (inhibitor of FLICE) binds to FLICE/caspase-8 but not FADD, and prevents FLICE/caspase-8 from being associated with FADD (132). FLIPs (FLICE-inhibitory proteins) associate strongly with FADD to form a stable Fas-FADD-FLIP complex that is not capable of recruiting FLICE/caspase-8 (133). They are highly expressed in tumors. Their involvement in AITD is yet to be determined.

Decoy receptors for FasL

Decoy receptors do not have an intracellular death domain, or have a defective DD. Recently Pitti *et al.* described such a decoy receptor, DcR3, for FasL (134). The soluble DcR3 inhibits apoptosis by binding to FasL. It has been found in a number of cancers, implying a potential mechanism in the pathogenesis of neoplasm. However, the role that DcR3 plays in autoimmune thyroid disease such as GD remains to be demonstrated.

OTHER APOPTOSIS PATHWAYS IN AUTOIMMUNE THYROID DISEASE

Very little is known about the involvement of other death pathways in AITD. In addition to Fas, the caspase-8 pathway of apoptosis can also be triggered by TNF and TRAIL. They recognize their own receptors and utilize additional adaptors for the formation of DISC. The caspase-9 pathway of apoptosis can be elicited by a variety of factors, including γ-irradiation, glucocorticoids, genotoxic damage, cytotoxic stress, and growth factor deprivation. The role(s) that these factors play in the induction of apoptosis in AITD are currently unknown. It is also possible that perforin and granzyme B, which are released by CD8[+] CTLs and NK cells, may also play a role in triggering apoptosis of thyrocytes in AITD.

Le[Y], an apoptosis-associated antigen, has been related to early apoptotic changes (135). It was reported that the Le[Y] positivity correlates with ISEL (immunohisto-chemical and *in situ* end-labeling of fragmented DNA) positivity. Using ISEL, Tanimoto *et al.* (7) noted Le[Y] expression and DNA fragmentation in thyrocytes from Hashimoto's thyroiditis and thyroid cancer. While in Graves' disease, bcl-2 and Le[Y] are expressed without DNA fragmentation. Normal thyrocytes were not stained with either Le[Y] or ISEL. The apoptotic pathway(s) that Le[Y] may be related to are not yet discovered.

PATHOGENESIS OF AUTOIMMUNE THYROID DISEASE

To date the pathogenesis of AITD remains unresolved. Initially, it was believed that the autoreactive CD4[+] T cells, which have escaped negative selection, might be responsible for the development of AITD. This would have led to a mainly antibody-mediated destruction of the thyroid. As previously mentioned, however, more recent studies have presented a body of evidence supporting that cell-mediated killing of thyrocytes via apoptosis is most likely the major mechanism of AITD. The question now comes down to how the immune privilege of the thyroid is negated, in other words, how autoimmune responses against the thyroid get started in the first place.

Immune privilege

There are a number of sites in the human body, such as the epithelial cells of the cornea, the anterior chamber of the eyes, Sertoli cells of the testis, and neurons, where inflammatory reactions and immune responses are prevented. An earlier hypothesis was that relative restriction of T cell access might account for the protection of these tissues. It has recently been proposed that constitutive expression of FasL on Fas-negative cells, for instance, the stroma cells of the eyes and testis, may induce apoptosis in invading CTLs and contribute to the establishment of these immune privileged sites (136-139). Tumor cells seem to use the same strategy to counterattack NK cells by up-regulating FasL expression, and/or to escape immune-mediated killing by down-regulating Fas expression (140). In the normal thyroid gland, there may be a similar mechanism that keeps thyrocytes from attack by the immune system.

The Bottazzo-Feldmann hypothesis

How self-destruction of the thyroid is initiated has been a puzzle for decades. To account for the pathogenesis of organ-specific autoimmune endocrine disease, Bottazzo and Feldmann proposed a hypothesis in 1983 (141). In their model, local aberrant expression of MHC class II molecules on thyroid epithelial cells and subsequent presentation of autoantigens to T cells might initiate the destructive cascade of thyrocytes. Cytokines secreted by Th1 cells were blamed for the aberrant expression of MHC class II on thyrocytes (142). According to this model, the following may be operating: viral infection of the thyroid results in production of IFNγ by infiltrating T cells (142) leading to up-regulation of MHC class II expression on thyrocytes, presentation by thyrocytes of thyroid autoantigen in the context of MHC class II to T cells and, finally, killing of thyrocytes by activated T cells. In support of this hypothesis, they were able to demonstrate that in Graves' disease thyroid autoantigens were MHC class II-restricted (143,144) and that thyroid follicular cells were strongly positive for MHC class II (145).

This model is noteworthy for two reasons. Firstly, CD4$^+$ CTLs are MHC class II-restricted. And secondly, CD4$^+$ CTLs utilize Fas death pathway in killing their targets. On the other hand, we know that co-stimulatory molecules CD80 and CD86 are needed for the activation of T cells. However, thyrocytes have not been shown to express these molecules (146).

More recently Dayan *et al.* (147) suggested that co-expression of MHC class II and FasL on thyrocytes might protect these cells against attack by infiltrating T cells through induction of apoptosis in those T cells that express Fas. They put forward this modification in light of the report by Giordano *et al.* (101) that thyrocytes constitutively expressed FasL. In this scenario, IFN-γ produced by ITLs up-regulate the expression of MHC class II on thyrocytes. Then thyroid antigens are presented to CD4$^+$ T cells in the context of MHC class II in the presence of FasL, without the requirement for other co-stimulation signals. As a result, autoreactive T cells are activated and the expression of Fas on these T cells is up-regulated. Subsequently, cross-linking of FasL on thyrocytes and Fas on T cells induces T cell apoptosis. However, more studies are required to clear the controversy over the issue of FasL expression on thyrocytes.

Once this protective system fails, as it might be the case in AITD, the balance between Fas-FasL might be altered so that the protection mechanism against attack by ITLs is damaged. Hammond *et al.* found that, in contrast to GD and multinodular goiter glands, thyroid follicular cells in HT showed a decreased level of FasL, and that ITLs in HT were clearly positive for FasL (148). Therefore ITLs killed thyrocytes whose Fas expression had been up-regulated by IFN-γ secreted by these ITLs. Normal thyroid epithelial cells do express low levels of MHC class I but no class II (149). It is possible that in AITD, the expression of MHC class II may be up-regulated by IFN-γ. This effect can be enhanced by TNF-α (115). Although it may not be true that up-regulation of MHC class II on thyrocytes initiates AITD, it may contribute to the maintenance and amplification of AITD.

CONCLUSIONS

Apoptosis in normal thyroid follicular cells is complicated and under tight control. The Fas-mediated apoptotic pathway is well characterized and present in the thyroid. The expression of FasL on thyroid epithelial cells is currently under debate. While Fas-mediated apoptosis contributes to the destruction of thyrocytes in autoimmune thyroid disease, other apoptotic pathways may be operating as well. More research is necessary to understand how immune destruction of the thyroid is initiated, how it progresses, how inhibitory mechanism(s) of apoptosis fail under these circumstances, and how apoptosis can be modulated. The outcome of these studies will shed light on our search for a cure for autoimmune thyroid disease, and for autoimmune disease in general.

REFERENCES

1.   **Hashimoto H**. 1912 Zur Kenntniss der lymphomatosen Veranderung der Schilddruse (Struma lymphomatosa). Arch Klin Chir. 97:219-248.
2.   **Roitt IM, Doniach D, Campbell PN, Hudson RV.** 1956 Auto-antibodies in Hashimoto's disease (lymphadenoid goitre). Lancet ii:820-821.
3.   **Levine SN.** 1983 Current concepts of thyroiditis. Arch Intern Med. 143:1952-1956.
4.   **Baker JR Jr.** 1997 Endocrine diseases. In: Stites DP, Terr AI, Parslow TG, eds. Medical Immunology, 9th ed. Stamford: Appleton & Lange; 480-492.
5.   **Nagataki S.** 1993 The concept of Hashimoto disease. In: Nagataki S, Mori T, Torizuka K, eds. Eighty years of Hashimoto disease. Amsterdam: Elsevier Science Publishers B.V.; 539-545.
6.   **Kotani T, Aratake Y, Hirai K, et al.** 1995 Apoptosis in thyroid tissue from patients with Hashimoto's thyroiditis. Autoimmunity. 20:231-236.
7.   **Tanimoto C, Hirakawa S, Kawasaki H, et al.** 1995 Apoptosis in thyroid diseases: a histochemical study. Endocr J. 42:193-201.
8.   **McLachlan SM, Pegg CA, Atherton MC, et al.** 1986 Subpopulations of thyroid autoantibody secreting lymphocytes in Graves' and Hashimoto thyroid glands. Clin Exp Immunol. 65:319-328.
9.   **Baker JR Jr., Saunders NB, Wartofsky L, et al.** 1988 Seronegative Hashimoto's thyroiditis with thyroid autoantibody production localized to the thyroid. Ann Intern Med. 108:26-30.
10.   **Forbes IJ, Roitt IM, Doniach D, Solomon IL.** 1962 The thyroid cytotoxic autoantibody. J Clin Invest. 41:996-1006.
11.   **Bermann M, Magee M, Koenig RJ, et al.** 1993 Differential autoantibody responses to thyroid peroxidase in patients with Graves' disease and Hashimoto's thyroiditis. J Clin Endocr Metab. 77:1098-1101.
12.   **Tandon N, Morgan BP, Weetman AP.** 1992 Expression and function of membrane attack complex inhibitory proteins on thyroid follicular cells. Immunology 75:372-377.
13.   **Weetman AP, Black CM, Cohen SB, et al.** 1989 Affinity purification of IgG subclasses and the distribution of thyroid auto-antibody reactivity in Hashimoto's thyroiditis. Scand J Immunol. 30:73-82.
14.   **Bogner U, Schleusener H, Wall Jr.** 1984 Antibody-dependent cell mediated cytotoxicity against human thyroid cells in Hashimoto's thyroiditis but not Graves' disease. J Clin Endocr Metab. 59:734-738.
15.   **Amino N, Mori H, Iwatani Y, et al.** 1982 Peripheral K lymphocytes in autoimmune thyroid disease: decrease in Graves' disease and increase in Hashimoto's disease. J Clin Endocr Metab. 54:587-591.
16.   **Iwatani Y, Amino N, Kabutomori O, et al.** 1984 Decrease of peripheral large granular lymphocytes in Graves' disease. Clin Exp Immunol. 55:239-244.
17.   **Iwatani Y, Amino N, Mori H, et al.** 1982 A microcytotoxicity assay for thyroid-specific cytotoxic antibody, antibody-dependent cell-mediated cytotoxicity and direct lymphocyte cytotoxicity using human thyroid cells. J Immunol Methods. 48:241-250.

18. **Del Prete GF, Maggi E, Mariotti S, et al.** 1986 Cytolytic T lymphocytes with natural killer activity in thyroid infiltrate of patients with Hashimoto's thyroiditis: analysis at clonal level. J Clin Endocr Metab. 62:52-57.
19. **DeGroot LJ, Quintans J.** 1989 The causes of autoimmune thyroid disease. Endocr Rev. 10:537-562.
20. **Weetman AP, McGregor AM.** 1994 Autoimmune thyroid disease: further developments in our understanding. Endocr Rev. 15:788-830.
21. **Kagi D, Vignaux F, Ledermann B, et al.** 1994 Fas and perforin pathways as major mechanisms of T cell-mediated cytotoxicity. Science. 265:528-530.
22. **Lowin B, Hahne M, Mattmann C, Tschopp J.** 1994 Cytolytic T-cell cyto-toxicity is mediated through perforin and Fas lytic pathways. Nature 370:650-652.
23. **Shresta S, Pham CTN, Thomas DA, et al.** 1998 How do cytotoxic lymphocytes kill their targets? Curr Opin Immunol. 10:581-587.
24. **Green DR.** 1998 Apoptotic pathways: the roads to ruin. Cell. 94:695-698.
25. **Duvall E, Wyllie AH.** 1986 Death and the cell. Immunol Today. 7:115-119.
26. **Kerr JFR, Wyllie AH, Currie AR.** 1972 Apoptosis: a basic biological phenomenon with wide ranging implications in tissue kinetics. Brit J Cancer. 26:239-257.
27. **Wyllie AH, Kerr JFR, Currie AR.** 1980 Cell death: the significance of apoptosis. Int Rev Cytol. 68:251-306.
28. **Arends MJ, Morris AG, Wyllie AH.** 1990 Apoptosis: the role of the endonuclease. Am J Pathol .136:593-608.
29. **Arends MJ, Wyllie AH.** 1991 Apoptosis: mechanisms and roles in pathology. Int Rev Exp Pathol. 32:223-254.
30. **Fesus L, Davies PJA, Piacentini M.** 1991 Apoptosis: molecular mechanisms in programmed cell death. Eur J Cell Biol. 56:170-177.
31. **Thompson CB.** 1995 Apoptosis in the pathogenesis and treatment of disease. Science 267:1456-1462.
32. **Thornberry NA, Lazebnik Y.** 1998 Caspases: enemies within. Science 281:1312-1316.
33. **Salvesen GS, Dixit VM.** 1997 Caspases: intracellular signaling by proteolysis. Cell 91:443-446.
34. **Itoh N, Yonehara S, Ishii A, et al.** 1991 The polypeptide encoded by the cDNA for human cell surface antigen Fas can mediate apoptosis. Cell. 66:233-243.
35. **Nagata S, Golstein P.** 1995 The Fas death factor. Science. 267:1449-1456.
36. **Itoh N, Nagata S.** 1993 A novel protein domain required for apoptosis. Mutational analysis of human Fas antigen. J Biol Chem. 268:10932-10937.
37. **Tartaglia LA, Ayres TM, Wong GH, Goeddel DV.** 1993 A novel domain within the 55 kd TNF receptor signals cell death. Cell. 74:845-853.
38. **Owen-Schaub LB, Yonehara S, Crump WL 3d, Grimm EA.** 1992 DNA fragmentation and cell death is selectively triggered in activated human lymphocytes by Fas antigen engagement. Cell Immunol. 140:197-205.
39. **Suda T, Takahashi T, Golstein P, Nagata S.** 1993 Molecular cloning and expression of the Fas ligand, a novel member of the tumor necrosis factor family. Cell. 75:1169-1178.
40. **Tanaka M, Suda T, Haze K. et al.** 1996 Fas ligand in human serum. Nature Med. 2:317-322.
41. **Peter ME, Krammer PH.** 1998 Mechanisms of CD95 (APO-1/Fas)-mediated apoptosis. Curr Opin Immunol. 10:545-551.
42. **Singh A, Ni J, Aggarwal BB.** 1998 Death domain receptors and their role in cell demise. J Interferon Cytokine Res. 18:439-450.
43. **Nagata S.** 1997 Apoptosis by death factor. Cell. 88:355-365.
44. **Cory S.** 1998 Cell death throes. Proc Natl Acad Sci USA. 95:12077-12079.

45. **Chinnaiyan AM, O'Rourke K, Tewari M, Dixit VM.** 1995 FADD, a novel death domain-containing protein, interacts with the death domain of Fas and initiates apoptosis. Cell. 81:505-512.

46. **Boldin MP, Varfolomeev EE, Pancer Z, et al.** 1995 A novel protein that interacts with the death domain of Fas/APO1 contains a sequence motif related to the death domain. J Biol Chem. 270:7795-7798.

47. **Muzio M, Chinnaiyan AM, Kischkel FC, et al.** 1996 FLICE, a novel FADD-homologous ICE/CED-3-like protease, is recruited to the CD95 (Fas/APO-1) death--inducing signaling complex. Cell. 85:817-827.

48. **Liu X, Zou H, Slaughter C, Wang X.** 1997 DFF, a heterodimeric protein that functions downstream of caspase-3 to trigger DNA fragmentation during apoptosis. Cell. 89:175-184.

49. **Enari M, Sakahira H, Yokoyama H. et al.** 1998 A caspase-activated DNase that degrades DNA during apoptosis, and its inhibitor ICAD. Nature. 391:43-50.

50. **Liu X, Li P, Widlak P, et al.** 1998 The 40-kDa subunit of DNA fragmentation factor induces DNA fragmentation and chromatin condensation during apoptosis. Proc Natl Acad Sci USA. 95:8461-8466.

51. **Sakahira H, Enari M, Nagata S.** 1998 Cleavage of CAD inhibitor in CAD activation and DNA degradation during apoptosis. Nature. 391:96-99.

52. **Tewari M, Quan LT, O'Rourke K, et al.** 1995 Yama/CPP32 beta, a mammalian homolog of CED-3, is a CrmA-inhibitable protease that cleaves the death substrate poly(ADP-ribose) polymerase. Cell. 81:801-809.

53. **Takahashi A, Alnemri ES, Lazebnik YA, et al.** 1996 Cleavage of lamin A by Mch2 alpha but not CPP32: multiple interleukin 1 beta-converting enzyme-related proteases with distinct substrate recognition properties are active in apoptosis. Proc Natl Acad Sci USA. 93:8395-8400.

54. **Enari M, Talanian RV, Wong WW, Nagata S.** 1996 Sequential activation of ICE-like and CPP32-like proteases during Fas-mediated apoptosis. Nature. 380:723-726.

55. **Nagata S.** 1998 Fas-induced apoptosis. Int Med. 37:179-181.

56. **Zhang J, Liu X, Scherer DC, et al.** 1998 Resistance to DNA fragmentation and chromatin condensation in mice lacking the DNA fragmentation factor 45. Proc Natl Acad Sci USA. 95:12480-12485.

57. **Liu X, Kim CN, Yang J, et al.** 1996 Induction of apoptotic program in cell-free extracts: requirement for dATP and cytochrome c. Cell. 86:147-157.

58. **Kuida K, Haydar TF, Kuan CY, et al.** 1998 Reduced apoptosis and cytochrome c-mediated caspase activation in mice lacking caspase 9. Cell. 94:325-337.

59. **Hakem R, Hakem A, Duncan GS, et al.** 1998 Differential requirement for caspase 9 in apoptotic pathways in vivo. Cell. 94:339-352.

60. **Kappler JW, Roehm N, Marrack P.** 1987 T cell tolerance by clonal elimination in the thymus. Cell. 49:273-280.

61. **Murphy KM, Heimberger AB, Loh DY.** 1990 Induction by antigen of intrathymic apoptosis of CD4+CD8+TCRlo thymocytes in vivo. Science. 250:1720-1723.

62. **Nossal GJ.** 1994 Negative selection of lymphocytes. Cell. 76:229-239.

63. **Sidman CL, Marshall JD, Von Boehmer H.** 1992 Transgenic T cell receptor interactions in the lymphoproliferative and autoimmune syndromes of lpr and gld mutant mice. Eur J Immunol. 22:499-504.

64. **Herron LR, Eisenberg RA, Roper E, et al.** 1993 Selection of the T cell receptor repertoire in Lpr mice. J Immunol. 151:3450-3459.

65. **Singer GG, Abbas AK.** 1994 The fas antigen is involved in peripheral but not thymic deletion of T lymphocytes in T cell receptor transgenic mice. Immunity. 1:365-371.

66. **Sentman CL, Shutter JR, Hockenbery D, et al.** 1991 bcl-2 inhibits multiple forms of apoptosis but not negative selection in thymocytes. Cell. 67:879-888.
67. **Strasser A, Harris AW, Cory S.** 1991 bcl-2 transgene inhibits T cell death and perturbs thymic self-censorship. Cell. 67:889-899.
68. **Strasser A, Harris AW, von Boehmer H, Cory S.** 1994 Positive and negative selection of T cells in T-cell receptor transgenic mice expressing a bcl-2 transgene. Proc Natl Acad Sci USA. 91:1376-1380.
69. **Strasser A, Harris AW, Huang DC, et al.** 1995 Bcl-2 and Fas/APO-1 regulate distinct pathways to lymphocyte apoptosis. EMBO J. 14:6136-6147.
70. **Green DR, Reed JC.** 1998 Mitochondria and apoptosis. Science. 281:1309-1312.
71. **Smith CA, Farrah T, Goodwin RG.** 1994 The TNF receptor superfamily of cellular and viral proteins: activation, costimulation, and death. Cell. 76:959-962.
72. **Chinnaiyan AM, O'Rourke K, Yu GL, et al.** 1996 Signal transduction by DR3, a death domain-containing receptor related to TNFR-1 and CD95. Science. 274:990-992.
73. **Pan G, O'Rourke K, Chinnaiyan AM, et al.** 1997 The receptor for the cytotoxic ligand TRAIL. Science. 276:111-113.
74. **Chaudhary PM, Eby M, Jasmin A, et al.** 1997 Death receptor 5, a new member of the TNFR family, and DR4 induce FADD-dependent apoptosis and activate the NF-kappaB pathway. Immunity. 7:821-830.
75. **Wiley SR, Schooley K, Smolak PJ, et al.** 1995 Identification and characterization of a new member of the TNF family that induces apoptosis. Immunity. 3:673-682.
76. **Bertin J, Armstrong RC, Ottilie S, et al.** 1997 Death effector domain-containing herpesvirus and poxvirus proteins inhibit both Fas- and TNFR1-induced apoptosis. Proc Natl Acad Sci USA. 94:1172-1176.
77. **Hu S, Vincenz C, Buller M, Dixit VM.** 1997 A novel family of viral death effector domain-containing molecules that inhibit both CD-95- and tumor necrosis factor receptor-1-induced apoptosis. J Biol Chem. 272:9621-9624.
78. **Ray CA, Black RA, Kronheim SR, et al.** 1992 Viral inhibition of inflammation: cowpox virus encodes an inhibitor of the interleukin-1 beta converting enzyme. Cell. 69:597-604.
79. **Smith KG, Strasser A, Vaux DL.** 1996 CrmA expression in T lymphocytes of transgenic mice inhibits CD95 (Fas/APO-1)-transduced apoptosis, but does not cause lymphadenopathy or autoimmune disease. EMBO J. 15:5167-5176.
80. **Newton K, Harris AW, Bath ML, et al.** 1998 A dominant interfering mutant of FADD/MORT1 enhances deletion of autoreactive thymocytes and inhibits proliferation of mature T lymphocytes. EMBO J. 17:706-718.
81. **Russell JH, Wang R.** 1993 Autoimmune gld mutation uncouples suicide and cytokine/proliferation pathways in activated, mature T cells. Eur J Immunol. 23:2379-2382.
82. **Dhein J, Walczak H, Baumler C, et al.** 1995 Autocrine T-cell suicide mediated by APO-1/(Fas/CD95). Nature. 373:438-441.
83. **Brunner T, Mogil RJ, LaFace D, et al.** 1995 Cell-autonomous Fas (CD95)/Fas-ligand interaction mediates activation-induced apoptosis in T-cell hybridomas. Nature. 373:441-444.
84. **Ju ST, Panka DJ, Cui H, et al.** 1995 Fas(CD95)/FasL interactions required for programmed cell death after T-cell activation. Nature. 373:444-448.
85. **Hammond LJ, Lowdell MW, Cerrano PG, et al.** 1997 Analysis of apoptosis in relation to tissue destruction associated with Hashimoto's autoimmune thyroiditis. J Pathol. 182:138-144.
86. **Okayasu I, Saegusa M, Fujiwara M, et al.** 1995 Enhanced cellular proliferative activity and cell death in chronic thyroiditis and thyroid papillary carcinoma. J Cancer Res Clin Oncol. 121:746-752.

87. **Dremier S, Golstein J, Mosselmans R, et al.** 1994 Apoptosis in dog thyroid cells. Biochem Biophy Res Comm. 200:52-58.

88. **Fenzi GF, Vitti P, Marcocci C, et al.** 1987 TSH receptor autoantibodies affecting thyroid function. In: Pinchera A, Ingber SH, Mckenzie JM, Fenzi GF, eds. Thyroid autoimmunity. New York: Plenum Press; 83-90.

89. **Arscott PL, Baker JR Jr.** 1998 Apoptosis and thyroiditis. Clin Immunol Immunopathol. 87:207-217.

90. **Borgerson KL, Bretz JD, Baker JR Jr.** 1999 The role of Fas-mediated apoptosis in thyroid autoimmune disease. Autoimmunity. In press.

91. **Tamura M, Kimura H, Koji T, et al.** 1998 Role of apoptosis of thyrocytes in a rat model of goiter. A possible involvement of Fas system. Endocrinology. 139:3646-3653.

92. **Watanabe-Fukunaga R, Brannan CI, Copeland NG, et al.** 1992 Lympho-proliferation disorder in mice explained by defects in Fas antigen that mediates apoptosis. Nature. 356:314-317.

93. **Adachi M, Suematsu S, Kondo T, et al.** 1995 Targeted mutation in the Fas gene causes hyperplasia in peripheral lymphoid organs and liver. Nature Genet. 11:294-300.

94. **Lynch DH, Watson ML, Alderson MR, et al.** 1994 The mouse Fas-ligand gene is mutated in gld mice and is part of a TNF family gene cluster. Immunity. 1:131-136.

95. **Takahashi T, Tanaka M, Brannan CI, et al.** 1994 Generalized lympho-proliferative disease in mice, caused by a point mutation in the Fas ligand. Cell. 76:969-976.

96. **Fisher GH, Rosenberg FJ, Straus SE, et al.** 1995 Dominant interfering Fas gene mutations impair apoptosis in a human autoimmune lymphoproliferative syndrome. Cell. 81:935-946.

97. **Rieux-Laucat F, Le Deist F, Hivroz C, et al.** 1995 Mutations in Fas associated with human lymphoproliferative syndrome and autoimmunity. Science. 268:1347-1349.

98. **Drappa J, Vaishnaw AK, Sullivan KE, et al.** 1996 Fas gene mutations in the Canale-Smith syndrome, an inherited lymphoproliferative disorder associated with autoimmunity. New Engl J Med. 335:1643-1649.

99. **Wu J, Wilson J, He J, et al.** 1996 Fas ligand mutation in a patient with systemic lupus erythematosus and lymphoproliferative disease. J Clin Invest. 98:1107-1113.

100. **Yonehara S, Ishii A, Yonehara M.** 1989 A cell-killing monoclonal antibody (anti-Fas) to a cell surface antigen co-downregulated with the receptor of tumor necrosis factor. J Exp Med. 169:1747-1756.

101. **Giordano C, Stassi G, De Maria R, et al.** 1997 Potential involvement of Fas and its ligand in the pathogenesis of Hashimoto's thyroiditis. Science. 275:960-963.

102. **Mitsiades N, Poulaki V, Kotoula V, et al.** 1998 Fas/Fas ligand up-regulation and Bcl-2 down-regulation may be significant in the pathogenesis of Hashimoto's thyroiditis. J Clin Endocr Metab. 83:2199-2203.

103. **Kawakami A, Eguchi K, Matsuoka N, et al.** 1996 Thyroid-stimulating hormone inhibits Fas antigen-mediated apoptosis of human thyrocytes in vitro. Endocrinology. 137:3163-3169.

104. **Arscott PL, Knapp J, Rymaszewski M, et al.** 1997 Fas (APO-1, CD95)-mediated apoptosis in thyroid cells is regulated by a labile protein inhibitor. Endocrinology. 138:5019-5027.

105. **Stokes TA, Rymaszewski M, Arscott PL, et al. and Fiedler P, Schaetzlein CE, Eibel H.** 1998. Constitutive expression of FasL in thyrocytes. Science. 279:2015a-2015a.

106. **Kawakami A, Eguchi K, Matsuoka N, et al.** 1997 Modulation of Fas-mediated apoptosis of human thyroid epithelial cells by IgG from patients with Graves' disease (GD) and idiopathic myxoedema. Clin Exp Immunol. 110:434-439.

107. **Leithauser F, Dhein J, Mechtersheimer G, et al.** 1993 Constitutive and induced expression of APO-1, a new member of the nerve growth factor/tumor necrosis factor receptor superfamily, in normal and neoplastic cells. Lab Invest. 69:415-429.

108. **Xerri L, Devilard E, Hassoun J, et al.** 1997 Fas ligand is not only expressed in immune privileged human organs but is also coexpressed with Fas in various epithelial tissues. Mol Pathol. 50:87-91.

109. **Smith D, Sieg S, Kaplan D.** 1998 Technical note: Aberrant detection of cell surface Fas ligand with anti-peptide antibodies. J Immunol. 160:4159-4160.

110. **Stassi G, Todaro M, Bucchieri F, et al.** 1999 Fas/Fas ligand-driven T cell apoptosis as a consequence of ineffective thyroid immunoprivilege in Hashimoto's thyroiditis. J Immunol. 162:263-267.

111. **Watson PF, Pickerill AP, Davies R, Weetman AP.** 1994 Analysis of cytokine gene expression in Graves' disease and multinodular goiter. J Clin Endocr Metab. 79:355-360.

112. **Grubeck-Loebenstein B, Turner M, Pirich K, et al.** 1990 CD4+ T-cell clones from autoimmune thyroid tissue cannot be classified according to their lymphokine production. Scand J Immunol. 32:433-440.

113. **Del Prete GF, Tiri A, Mariotti S, et al.** 1987 Enhanced production of gamma-interferon by thyroid-derived T cell clones from patients with Hashimoto's thyroiditis. Clin Exp Immunol. 69:323-331.

114. **Del Prete GF, Tiri A, De Carli M, et al.** 1989 High potential to tumor necrosis factor alpha (TNF-alpha) production of thyroid infiltrating T lymphocytes in Hashimoto's thyroiditis: a peculiar feature of destructive thyroid autoimmunity. Autoimmunity. 4:267-276.

115. **Nagataki S, Eguchi K.** 1992 Cytokines and immune regulation in thyroid autoimmunity. Autoimmunity 13:27-34.

116. **Yamashita S.** 1998 Endocrine disease and apoptosis. Int Med. 37:194-196.

117. **Ridgway WM, Weiner HL, Fathman CG.** 1994 Regulation of autoimmune response. Curr Opin Immunol. 6:946-955.

118. **Duke RC, Cohen JJ, Chervenak R.** 1986 Differences in target cell DNA fragmentation induced by mouse cytotoxic T lymphocytes and natural killer cells. J Immunol. 137:1442-1447.

119. **Ucker DS.** 1987 Cytotoxic T lymphocytes and glucocorticoids activate an endogenous suicide process in target cells. Nature. 327:62-64.

120. **Sellins KS, Cohen JJ.** 1991 Cytotoxic T lymphocytes induce different types of DNA damage in target cells of different origins. J Immunol. 147:795-803.

121. **Del Prete GF, Vercelli D, Tiri A, et al.** 1986 In vivo activated cytotoxic T cells in the thyroid infiltrate of patients with Hashimoto's thyroiditis. Clin Exp Immunol. 65:140-147.

122. **MacKenzie WA, Schwartz AE, Friedman EW, Davies TF.** 1987 Intrathyroidal T cell clones from patients with autoimmune thyroid disease. J Clin Endocr Metab. 64:818-824.

123. Itoh N, Tsujimoto Y, Nagata S. 1993 Effect of bcl-2 on Fas antigen-mediated cell death. J Immunol. 151:621-627.

124. **Kawahara A, Kobayashi T, Nagata S.** 1998 Inhibition of Fas-induced apoptosis by Bcl-2. Oncogene. 17:2549-2554.

125. **Chiu VK, Walsh CM, Liu CC, et al.** 1995 Bcl-2 blocks degranulation but not fas-based cell-mediated cytotoxicity. J Immunol. 154:2023-2032.

126. **Van Parijs L, Biuckians A, Abbas AK.** 1998 Functional roles of Fas and Bcl-2-regulated apoptosis of T lymphocytes. J Immunol. 160:2065-2071.

127. **Owen-Schaub LB, Radinsky R, Kruzel E, et al.** 1994 Anti-Fas on nonhemato-poietic tumors: levels of Fas/APO-1 and bcl-2 are not predictive of biological responsiveness. Cancer Res. 54:1580-1586.

128. **Scaffidi C, Fulda S, Srinivasan A, et al.** 1998 Two CD95 (APO-1/Fas) signaling pathways. EMBO J. 17:1675-1687.

129. **Sato T, Irie S, Kitada S, Reed JC.** 1995 FAP-1: a protein tyrosine phosphatase that associates with Fas. Science. 268:411-415.

130. **Yanagisawa J, Takahashi M, Kanki H, et al.** 1997 The molecular interaction of Fas and FAP-1. A tripeptide blocker of human Fas interaction with FAP-1 promotes Fas-induced apoptosis. J Biol Chem. 272:8539-8545.

131. **Myc A, Arscott PL, Baker JR Jr.** 1998 FAP-1 is present in human thyroid follicular cells and functions as an inhibitor of Fas-mediated signaling of programmed cell death. 71st Annual Meeting of the American Thyroid Association. Portland, Oregon, September, 1998. Program and Abstract Book, #148, p74.

132. **Hu S, Vincenz C, Ni J, et al.** 1997 I-FLICE, a novel inhibitor of tumor necrosis factor receptor-1- and CD-95-induced apoptosis. J Biol Chem. 272:17255-17257.

133. **Irmler M, Thome M, Hahne M, et al.** 1997 Inhibition of death receptor signals by cellular FLIP. Nature. 388:190-195.

134. **Pitti RM, Marsters SA, Lawrence DA, et al.** 1998 Genomic amplification of a decoy receptor for Fas ligand in lung and colon cancer. Nature. 396:699-703.

135. **Hiraishi K, Suzuki K, Hakomori S, Adachi M.** 1993 Le[Y] antigen expression is correlated with apoptosis (programmed cell death). Glycobiology. 3:381-390.

136. **French LE, Hahne M, Viard I, et al.** 1996 Fas and Fas ligand in embryos and adult mice: ligand expression in several immune-privileged tissues and coexpression in adult tissues characterized by apoptotic cell turnover. J Cell Biol. 133:335-343.

137. **Griffith TS, Yu X, Herndon JM, et al.** 1996 CD95-induced apoptosis of lymphocytes in an immune privileged site induces immunological tolerance. Immunity. 5:7-16.

138. **Griffith TS, Brunner T, Fletcher SM, et al.** 1995 Fas ligand-induced apoptosis as a mechanism of immune privilege. Science. 270:1189-1192.

139. **Bellgrau D, Gold D, Selawry H, et al.** 1995 A role for CD95 ligand in preventing graft rejection. Nature. 377:630-632.

140. **Hahne M, Rimoldi D, Schroter M, et al.** 1996 Melanoma cell expression of Fas(Apo-1/CD95) ligand: implications for tumor immune escape. Science. 274:1363-1366.

141. **Bottazzo GF, Pujol-Borrell R, Hanafusa T, Feldmann M**. 1983 Role of aberrant HLA-DR expression and antigen presentation in induction of endocrine autoimmunity. Lancet. ii:1115-1119.

142. **Todd I, Pujol-Borrell R, Hammond LJ, et al.** 1985 Interferon-gamma induces HLA-DR expression by thyroid epithelium. Clin Exp Immunol. 61:265-273.

143. **Dayan CM, Londei M, Corcoran AE, et al.** 1991 Autoantigen recognition by thyroid-infiltrating T cells in Graves disease. Proc Natl Acad Sci USA. 88:7415-7419.

144. **Londei M, Bottazzo GF, Feldmann M.** 1985 Human T-cell clones from autoimmune thyroid glands: specific recognition of autologous thyroid cells. Science. 228:85-89.

145. **Hanafusa T, Pujol-Borrell R, Chiovato L, et al.** 1983 Aberrant expression of HLA-DR antigen on thyrocytes in Graves' disease: relevance for autoimmunity. Lancet. ii:1111-1115.

146. **Tandon N, Metcalfe RA, Barnett D, Weetman AP.** 1994 Expression of the co-stimulatory molecule B7/BB1 in autoimmune thyroid disease. Q J Med. 87:231-236.

147. **Dayan CM, Elsegood KA, Maile R.** 1997 FasL expression on epithelial cells: the Bottazzo-Feldman hypothesis revisited. Immunol Today. 18:203-203.

148. **Hammond LJ, Cerrano PG, Torre GC, et al.** 1997 Apoptosis in thyroid disease. Immunology 92 (Suppl.) OP76.

149. **Lucas-Martin A, Foz-Sala M, Todd I, et al.** 1988 Occurrence of thyrocyte HLA class II expression in a wide variety of thyroid diseases: relationship with lymphocytic infiltration and thyroid autoantibodies. J Clin Endocr Metab. 66:367-375.

9

ANIMAL MODELS OF GRAVES' DISEASE

Marian Ludgate, Sabine Costagliola and Gilbert Vassart

INTRODUCTION

It will be evident to the reader, from other chapters in this book, that Graves' Disease (GD) is polygenic and multifactorial, a combination which makes unravelling relevant pathogenic mechanisms exceedingly difficult. GD is very common but patients present when disease has advanced to the extent of causing clinical signs and symptoms, which is likely to be temporally removed from the initiating immune events. Thus it has long been recognized that fundamental progress in our understanding of GD would benefit from an appropriate animal model.

What is meant by 'appropriate'? Obviously a model should mimic, as closely as possible, human GD with some or all of the animals demonstrating:-

1. elevated thyroxine and/or reduced thyrotropin levels;
2. antibodies to the thyrotropin receptor (TSHR), preferably thyroid stimulating antibodies (TSAb);
3. changes in thyroid architecture;
4. lymphocytic thyroiditis;
5. clinical signs of hyperthyroidism such as weight loss, and
6. orbital changes akin to those of thyroid eye disease (TED)

Ideally the GD model should be spontaneous and not rely on administration of antigen preparations and immunological adjuvants. However there are very few spontaneous models of autoimmunity and the best examples for autoimmune thyroid disease are the obese strain chicken (1), the BB rat (2) and some colonies of NOD mice (3) which develop destructive thyroiditis with antibodies directed to thyroglobulin in the chicken and rat and thyroid peroxidase in the mouse. In the absence of spontaneity, we would expect induced models to depend on a relevant autoantigen, which in the case of GD is the TSHR.

This chapter will review the differing approaches taken and attempt to evaluate how close we are to an appropriate model of GD but will begin with a brief reflection on the properties of the TSHR which may contribute to its autoantigenicity.

THE THYROTROPIN RECEPTOR AS AN AUTOANTIGEN

The TSHR is a G protein-coupled receptor, with the characteristic seven membrane spanning regions. It is a member of the glycoprotein hormone subfamily and, along with the receptors for luteinizing hormone (LH) and follicle stimulating hormone (FSH), has a large extracellular domain (ECD) which confers ligand binding specificity (reviewed in 4). Unlike the receptors for LH and FSH, the TSHR undergoes a post-translational cleavage with a metalloprotease (5) such that a proportion of surface receptors are in the form of two subunits, with the ECD linked to the membrane spanning region via (a) disulfide bridge(s).

Relative to the other glycoprotein hormone receptors, the TSHR ECD has a unique 'insertion' of some 50 amino acids, which comprises the probable sites of cleavage and is highly immunogenic, as determined from hydropathy profiles and borne out by the development of monoclonal antibodies which bind linear sequences in this region (6-8). The immunogenicity may simply be the result of a free carboxyl terminus created in the ECD following cleavage of the receptor; in most proteins the N and C termini are immunogenic (reviewed in 9) and indeed in the TSHR a second 'hot-spot' for generated monoclonals is the amino terminus (10,11). An alternative explanation to the immunogenicity of the TSHR is that a portion of the ECD or even the entire ECD may be released into the circulation, either following maturation or upon ligand mediated receptor activation, and there is some evidence for a circulating TSH binding protein (12,13). Whether receptor fragments in the circulation might have a role in breaking peripheral tolerance remains conjectural but there is evidence for widespread autoimmunity to the TSHR, defined as T cell epitopes (14) or in assays measuring direct antibody binding to the receptor (15), in normal individuals without GD.

RECEPTOR INDUCED ANIMAL MODELS

The TSHR has a low level of expression in the thyroid, precluding the preparation of autoantigen for injection from animal or human tissues as had been achieved for thyroglobulin. With few exceptions, most models depend on the provision of recombinant receptor which in turn required its cloning. The problem of low receptor expression was circumvented by detergent extraction and TSH affinity purification of receptor from a human thyroid cell line, GEJ (16). When five different H-2 strains received repeated immunizations with the receptor preparation, H-2^s developed low levels of TBII and mild thyroiditis was observed in H-2^s, H-2^b and H-2^q mice. The disadvantage of this model is that even with a cell line, limited quantities of antigen can be obtained and with considerable effort, the advantage is its use of TSHR in a conformation able to bind TSH, a problem that was to trouble many of the earliest attempts using recombinant TSHR.

Recombinant strategies have varied with improvements in technology and fall into the following categories:-

1. Injection of synthetic receptor peptides.
2. Injection of receptor protein produced in procaryotic cells.
3. Injection of receptor protein produced in eukaryotic cells.
4. Genetic immunization.
5. Injection of receptor transfected cells.
6. Transfer of receptor with in vivo primed T cells (priming via either strategy 1,2,4 or 5).

Synthetic Peptides

There was an initial rush of papers claiming induction of TSAb, TSH blocking antibodies (TBAb), TSH binding inhibitory antibodies (TBII) and increased thyroxine levels in several species treated with synthetic peptides based on the TSHR sequence (17-20). To our knowledge lymphocytic thyroiditis was not reported in any of these studies and in some cases the antibody and hormone changes have subsequently become more questionable for the reasons described in more detail below. In retrospect it would have been surprising if this approach had been successful in generating an animal model but it remains a useful route for producing antibodies for validating receptor protein produced in vitro (21).

Recombinant Receptor from Procaryotic Cells

Several groups, including ourselves, have produced recombinant receptor fusion proteins in bacteria. We employed the ECD (21) coupled to maltose binding protein (MBP), enabling us to hyperimmunize male and female BALBc mice with 50 or 100 μg doses of a purified receptor preparation. Our protocol uses the intra-peritoneal route and an adjuvant of alum and pertussis toxin and always involves the study of test animals receiving ECD-MBP and control mice treated with the fusion partner, MBP, alone. In our initial experiments (22), in which individual sera from male mice receiving ECD-MBP or MBP were pooled, we reported the induction of TBII in both groups early on in the immunization schedule but which persisted only in the ECD-MBP group. When testing immunoglobulins (IgGs), the TBII were confirmed only in the receptor treated mice indicating that false positive TBII can be demonstrated using unfractionated sera. Similarly we noted reduced T4 levels in both groups early on but the MBP mice recovered, unlike the ECD-MBP whose thyroids also displayed increased vascularity and focal lymphocytic thyroiditis.

Subsequently we extended the study to examine individual male and female BALBc mice (H-2^d) hyperimmunized with ECD-MBP or MBP alone (23). We confirmed the induction by the receptor antigen, but not MBP, of TBII and TBAb (measured in IgG) in both males and females. These antibodies were often accompanied by reduced circulating T4. Thyroiditis was induced in 50% of male and 100% of surviving female mice.

When testing mice of differing genetic background (24), particularly in the MHC, H-2^b (C57) and H-2^k (CBA) animals did not develop thyroiditis although antibodies to the receptor, measured by ELISA on a different ECD fusion protein, were present at similar levels to those in the H-2^d (BALBc) mice. In the same series of experiments, NOD mice, which have a unique H-2^g haplotype, developed antibodies to the receptor, destructive thyroiditis and reduced T4 levels, when treated with the ECD-MBP antigen. When comparing the phenotype of the lymphocytic infiltrate, in the BALBc mice B cells and immunoreactivity for IL-4 and IL-10 were found, indicating a Th2 immune response. In contrast, in the NOD mice there were very few B cells and immunoreactivity for INFγ was detected, indicating the Th1 nature of the induced disease.

Similar attempts by other groups, even using the same hyperimmunization protocol and strain of BALBc, failed to induce thyroiditis. Does this suggest that environmental factors could be important as in the case of transgenic mice expressing a myelin basic protein specific T cell receptor (25), which develop spontaneous allergic encephelomyelitis only when housed in a non-sterile facility? More recently it has been possible to induce thyroiditis, in a similar protocol to ours but using an ECD truncated in the C terminus (26). The authors have interpreted this finding as being due to the removal of immunodominant non-thyroiditis epitopes, unmasking cryptic disease-inducing T cell epitopes. This seems plausible, especially as our ECD-MBP fusion protein could be truncated in the C terminus either due to incomplete synthesis or degradation during purification, problems associated with proteins in which the fusion partner, which provides the selection for purification, is at the amino terminus.

Recombinant Receptor from Eukaryotic Cells

A major draw back using receptor produced in bacteria was the lack of correct folding and glycosylation and it was hoped that eukaryotic expression in insect cells, using baculovirus vectors, might offer a solution to this problem. Certainly the human ECD produced using this system is superior to the antigen from bacteria in terms of absorbing out TBII activity from GD patients sera (27) but there have been no convincing demonstrations of direct TSH binding to a receptor protein expressed using baculovirus. Nevertheless, useful information has been obtained, with both the human and murine ECD, when injected into animals in combination with various adjuvants. Prabhakar and colleagues (28) studied four different strains of mice treated with the human ECD and observed that antibodies to the receptor, having no biological activity, were induced in all of the mice. In contrast, moderately increased thyroxine levels were present only in the BALBc mice and, despite the absence of thyroiditis, there were changes in the gland, such as budding, indicative of hyperactivity. The same antigen, used by the same group but this time injected into rabbits (29), induced TBII. Perhaps reasoning that an induced immune response to a heterologous antigen is not sufficient to claim autoimmunity, Davies' group have expressed the murine ECD in insect cells and obtained monoclonal antibodies, some of which had TBII and TBAb activities, when measured in vitro on CHO cells expressing the human TSHR (30). Furthermore, when BALBc mice were treated with the same murine antigen and an adjuvant comprised of alum and pertussis toxin (31), TBII and TBAb were induced and mice had reduced levels of T3 accompanied by increased TSH but no signs of thyroiditis or thyroid destruction.

Genetic Immunization

A novel departure from using protein antigens to initiate an immune response is provided by genetic immunization. It was shown that an intramuscular injection, with the cDNA for the coding region of a protein in a eukaryotic expression vector, induced an antibody response in mice (32). It is assumed that the myocytes at the site of injection take up the cDNA and express the encoded protein at the surface of the cell, perhaps in the context of MHC-class I. The resulting inflammation brings dendritic and other professional antigen presenting cells (APC) to the scene, which phagocytose either cDNA or its translated protein released from the muscle cells. This allows, not only antigen presentation with MHC-class II but also the second signals provided by accessory molecules on professional APC, required for inducing an immune response.

This method was applied to groups of female BALBc mice which received three injections of 100 μg TSHR in pcDNAIII, or the empty vector alone, at 3 week intervals (33). The cDNA was administered either in PBS or 25% sucrose, or following pretreatment of the muscle with cardiotoxin. Fourteen of 15 mice treated with receptor cDNA developed antibodies to the TSHR as measured by flow cytometry and the majority contained TBII and TBAb activities. One serum contained TSAb resulting in an 800% increase in cAMP production and which persisted for 18 weeks. Thyroid hormone levels remained normal throughout the experiment. All mice displayed severe thyroiditis with many infiltrating B cells but no thyroid destruction, quite the opposite with signs of epithelial thickening and budding.

Induced animal models traditionally use inbred mouse strains. Reasoning that the failure to develop hyperthyroidism in BALBc mice receiving genetic immunization, might relate to inadequate genetic background, the method was applied to NMRI outbred mice. All mice responded by producing antibodies capable of recognizing the recombinant receptor expressed at the surface of stably transfected CHO cells. The antibodies in the sera of most of the immunized mice scored positive when tested for their ability to block stimulation of cAMP accumulation by TSH in cells expressing the TSHR. Five out of 29 female mice showed biological evidence of hyperthyroidism with elevated total T4 (8.6 ± 0.9 μg/dl vs 4.3 ± 0.4 μg/dl in controls; $p < 0.001$) and suppressed TSH levels (< 0.02 vs > 0.1 ng/ml in controls). The serum of these mice contained thyroid stimulating activity, as measured in a classical assay using CHO cells expressing recombinant TSHR. In contrast, only one male out of thirty had moderately elevated serum total T4 with undetectable TSH values. In addition, the hyperthyroid animals had goiters (thyroid weight: 18.6 ± 5.7 mg vs 5.6 ± 0.4 mg in controls; $p < 0.001$) with extensive lymphocytic infiltration characteristic of a Th2 immune response and displayed edema of their extraocular muscles (34 and manuscript submitted).

Injection of Receptor Transfected Cells

One very promising approach has involved treating mice with fibroblasts which express an MHC-class II molecule and the full length, functional human TSHR (35). The mouse strain used was the AKR/N which is H-2^k, homologous to the RT4.15HP murine fibroblast cell line. Recipient mice and cells used as immunogen are MHC-class I identical. The TSHR was introduced by transfection into the RT4.15HP cells or the parent line lacking the MHC-class II, and surface expression of MHC molecules confirmed by flow cytometry. Furthermore the transfected TSHR was shown to be functional in terms of TSH mediated cAMP production.

Female mice were injected intraperitoneally with 10^7 fibroblasts, a total of six times at intervals of two weeks and examined two weeks following the final injection. The fibroblasts either expressed MHC-class II, or human TSHR or both. A variety of investigations were performed including determination of TBII and circulating thyroid hormone levels in individual mouse sera, TSAb and TBAb activities in protein A-purified IgG samples pooled from pairs of mice, and the gross and microscopic morphology of the thyroid glands. The majority of mice receiving cells expressing MHC-class II and receptor developed TBII. About 20% had increased thyroxine levels and this was shown to be accompanied by TSAb activity. In contrast, TBII positive sera in animals with normal thyroid hormone levels displayed TBAb activity. The precise incidence and magnitude of the TSAb and TBAb are difficult to assess because of the use of paired sera, which was imposed by the practical limitation of blood volumes available for study, and the undefined basal levels for calculating percentage changes, respectively. No TBII, TSAb, TBAb or changes in circulating thyroid hormone were induced in AKR/N mice receiving cells expressing either TSHR or MHC-class II alone and the thyroids of these animals appeared normal.

In contrast, the thyroids of the animals receiving TSHR and MHC-class II expressing fibroblasts were macroscopically enlarged and microscopically displayed changes in architecture, for example hypertrophy and hypercellularity with follicular cells protruding into the lumen, which are similar to those seen in hyperthyroidism. However, there was no lymphocytic infiltration. Of interest, the induction of TBII and TBAb might be expected to reduce circulating thyroid hormone levels. The authors have not commented on the fact that the five mice having the lowest thyroxine levels are in this category, although the induction of increased and reduced T4 levels using this protocol has been noted more recently (see below).

In a second series of experiments, the non-MHC genetic control of the induced disease was investigated (36). As mentioned above, the RT4.15HP fibroblast cell line express murine H-2^k, unfortunately fibroblast cell lines expressing other MHC molecules are apparently not available and the authors have instead examined five different strains of mice, all H-2^k. When treated with fibroblasts expressing MHC-class II and the TSHR, the majority of animals developed TBII, irrespective of the strain. Furthermore, the CBA and C3H strains had circulating TBII even when the fibroblasts expressed only receptor and not MHC-class II. When a larger series of AKR/N and C3H animals were compared, elevated T4 levels, which were said to be associated with detectable TSAb (no data were reported), were found only in C3H mice receiving fibroblasts expressing both receptor and MHC-class II.

From these experiments, in which TBII and increased T4 levels were induced in mice receiving cells co-expressing the TSHR and MHC-class II, it was concluded that aberrant class II expression in human thyrocytes is necessary for the development of GD. Non-MHC genes would play a more limited role.

Subsequently the same authors, using this protocol in the original AKR/N mice (37), investigated whether certain regions of the TSHR might be necessary or sufficient to induce disease. In previous chimera studies, in which portions of the TSHR were substituted with the equivalent part of the LH receptor, the amino terminal of the protein was found to be required for binding and specific recognition by TSAb. A range of such chimeras lacking residues 9-165 (mc 1+2); 90-165 (mc 1) and 261-370 (mc 4) were transfected into the RT4.15Hp and parent cell lines and characterized by FACS analysis as described above for the wild type (WT) receptor. Demonstration of chimeric receptors compared with WT receptors at the cell surface might have been a useful analysis to confirm comparable expression, although all types of receptor expressing cells induced in vitro proliferation of splenocytes which had been primed in vivo with the same receptor, showing that all constructs contain T cell epitopes. TBII were induced in mice receiving MHC-class II expressing fibroblasts transfected with the WT and mc 4 receptors but not the mc 1 or mc 1+2 constructs. Elevated T4 levels, associated with TSAb were present in 2/9 WT and MHC-class II recipients but not in any of the other treated or control groups.

Based on the TBII results, it was concluded that the N terminal segment of the receptor is critical, not only as an epitope for human TSAb but also in the induction of TSHR antibodies in a murine model of GD. However, considering the lack of TSAb in animals receiving the mc 4 construct, the participation of the carboxyl end of the ECD should not be overlooked.

This model has recently been confirmed and extended (38) using the same AKR/N mouse strain, receiving the RT4.15HP cell line transfected with the human TSHR (in a slightly different expression vector) and administered intraperitoneally a total of 8 times with mice being examined 6, 12 and 18 weeks after the first injection. In the basic protocol, most animals developed TBII, and elevated T4 levels (defined as being > 5 μg/dl) were induced in 5/20 recipients of fibroblasts expressing receptor and MHC-class II. A further two mice died prior to levels being measured. One mouse had elevated TSH and reduced T4 but the thyroid was normal, as in the euthyroid and control animals. The five animals with increased serum T4 levels had enlarged thyroids with signs of hypertrophy and colloid droplet formation but no lymphocytic infiltration. When the protocol was modified by including alum, a Th2 adjuvant, increased T4 levels and goiters were found in a greater proportion (9/19) of mice and the onset was earlier (9 compared with 11 weeks). Two mice had increased TSH indicative of hypothyroid-ism. In contrast to alum, the inclusion of Complete Freund's, a Th1 adjuvant, resulted in a slower onset of hyperthyroidism with 10/31 mice having increased serum T4 levels by 14 weeks. This last group comprised male and female animals and no difference was observed in the incidence or severity of induced disease. Epitope mapping by ELISA revealed that 9/13 sera from mice receiving fibroblasts expressing TSHR and MHC-class II, recognized a peptide for amino acid residues 97-116 in the amino terminal region of the ECD, but peptides for residues 322-371 in the carboxyl part of the ECD also showed high absorption by experimental but not control sera.

Transfer of Receptor with In Vivo Primed T Cells

The earliest reported transfer of TSHR primed T cells used synthetic peptides shown to be T cell epitopes for GD patients in the in vivo priming step of DBA mice (23). Treatment with 3/4 T cell epitope peptides elicited weak TSAb activity and T cell lines were developed from one TSAb positive and one TSAb negative mouse. When these lines were transferred to naive syngeneic mice, following a period of in vitro priming with receptor peptides, weak TSAb activity were present in 2/4 mice receiving the line from the TSAb positive donor but no TSAb could be detected in the four mice receiving the line from the TSAb negative donor.

We have used unfractionated T cells and a CD4+ enriched population to transfer disease to syngeneic BALBc and NOD recipients. The in vivo priming step could be performed using the TSHR produced in bacteria (ECD-MBP) or by genetic immunization, but in both cases was followed by an in vitro priming period using ECD-MBP. In our first study (39), BALBc and NOD recipients were examined 16 days after transfer of syngeneic receptor primed T cells and both strains of mice displayed thyroiditis similar in phenotype to that induced in the donors using ECD-MBP, that is Th2 in the BALBc and Th1 with thyroid destruction in the NOD. Neither strain of recipient animals had developed antibodies to the TSHR at this early stage although these antibodies were present in the donor mice.

In more recent experiments (40), we examined the kinetics of disease induction, again using unfractionated T cells and a CD4+ enriched population, at 4, 8 and 12 weeks after transfer. In addition, since we had found evidence for TSHR transcripts and protein in orbital tissue from TED patients (41,42), the mouse orbits were examined. In both BALBc and NOD recipients the Th2 and Th1 nature of induced thyroiditis respectively was confirmed and found to persist for the 12 week duration of the experiment.

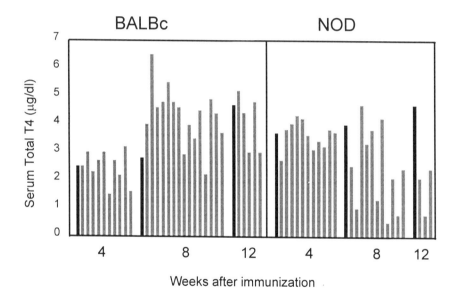

Figure 1. Serum total T4 levels in recipient mice. Black bars, recipients of non-primed T cells. Gray bars, recipients of TSHR primed T cells.

At 4 weeks, TSHR antibodies, including TBII, had been induced in both strains and these too persisted throughout the experiment. Changes in thyroid hormone levels were more difficult to evaluate, especially in the BALBc (Fig. 1). In NOD recipients of TSHR primed T cells, thyroid hormone levels were reduced, as might be expected from the destructive thyroiditis induced in this strain. Four weeks after transfer, BALBc recipients of TSHR primed *and* control non-primed T cells had reduced serum T4 levels which slowly recovered in the latter. At 8 and 12 weeks, some BALBc recipients of receptor primed T cells had increased T4, relative to the control non-primed recipients.

When examining the orbits, all NOD recipients of primed and non-primed cells, displayed normal histology with intact, well organized muscle fibre architecture. BALBc orbits of primed (but not non-primed) T cells appeared strikingly different. The muscle fibres were disorganized and separated by periodic acid Schiff positive edema. There was accumulation of adipose tissue and infiltration by immune cells, especially mast cells. These changes were observed in 17/25 BALBc recipients of receptor primed cells and did not correlate with TBII or T4 levels. However, orbital changes were observed only in mice having the most severe thyroiditis with 25-30% of the gland occupied by interstitium, which also correlated with the most skewed Th2 response, B:T cell ratio of 1.6-1.9 and IL-4:INFγ ratio of >2.5.

Finally, passive transfer to naive recipients was performed using either spleen or intraperitoneal cells from TSHR+, class II+ fibroblast treated mice (38). The sole criterion for successful transfer was thyroid hormone status. Of a total of 8 animals receiving cells from hyperthyroid donors, only one recipient was transiently hyperthyroid and one hypothyroid. When transferring hypothyroid donor cells, all four recipients became hypothyroid. We have reported that transfer of non-primed control splenocytes can reduce thyroid hormone levels, particularly in some strains of mice. Therefore we consider it unwise to claim transfer of disease on the basis of change in thyroid hormone levels alone, especially when the relevant controls are not included.

CONCLUDING COMMENTS

So what have all these models taught us? It would seem that it is very easy to induce TSHR antibodies lacking biological activity in almost any mouse strain. TBII (and to a lesser extent TBAb) and reduced serum T4 levels are relatively easy to induce, especially in BALBc mice which can also develop hyperthyroxinemia. It should also be noted that false TBII and TSAb can be detected in whole sera, as opposed to the IgG fraction, and serum T4 levels can be reduced by antigens and T cells completely unrelated to the TSHR!

In contrast to the above parameters, TSAb and thyroiditis (and consequently orbital pathology akin to TED) are very difficult to induce. Generation of TSAb require administration of TSHR with the correct conformation capable of binding TSH, namely by injection of cDNA or cells transfected with the full-length TSHR. Thyroiditis, the hallmark of an autoimmune response to the endogenous receptor, may require the conjunction of an adequate genetic background and ill-defined environmental factors or immunological challenges. Orbital pathology, at least in the mouse, seems to depend on a Th2 response to the thyroidal TSHR but does not require TSAb.

Both protocols that induce convincing TSAb activity accompanied by increased serum T4 levels also result in the production of TBAb. Many GD patients' sera contain a cocktail of receptor antibodies, TSAb, TBAb and probably antibodies having no biological function with the clinical outcome dictated by the antibody which is most abundant or has the highest affinity. There are reports of patients with hyperthyroid GD developing hypothyroidism and vice versa. All of these observations imply that TBAb and TSAb are very similar immunoglobulins with subtle differences causing their biological effects.

Of all the approaches the most promising is the most recent, that is genetic immunization of outbred mice, which replicates most of the principal signs and symptoms of GD. Hopefully this model will stand the test of time since it offers a unique opportunity for identifying the genes implicated in the loss of tolerance to the TSHR. The use of outbred animals makes the model similar to a human model which was happened on by chance (43). Patients with multiple sclerosis treated in vivo with a monoclonal antibody (Campath-1H) to CD52, resulting in elimination of >95% of circulating lymphocytes, displayed considerable improvement of their disease. Eighteen months after treatment, T cell numbers had returned to 35% and B cells to 180% of pretreatment values, but 12/34 patients had developed GD with hyperthyroidism and antibodies to the TSHR. Campath-1H results in immune deviation away from Th1, hence the improvement in multiple sclerosis, but unfortunately allows the expansion of a Th2 response with production of TSAb leading to GD.

REFERENCES

1. **Wick G, Most J, Schauenstein K**. 1985 Spontaneous autoimmune thyroiditis.A bird's eye view. Immunol Today 6:359-364.
2. **Allen EM, Braverman LE**. 1996 The biobreeding worcester rat - A model of organ-specific autoimmunity. Exp Clin Endocrinol Diab. 104:7-10.
3. **Bernard N F, Ertrug F, Margoleses H**. 1992 High incidence of thyroiditis and anti-thyroid autoantibodies in NOD mice. Diabetes 41:40-46.
4. **Paschke R, Ludgate M**. 1997 The thyrotropin receptor and thyroid disease. N Engl J Med. 337: 1675-1681.
5. **Couet J, Sar S, Jolivet A, Hai MTV, Milgrom E, Misrahi M**. 1996 Shedding of human thyrotropin receptor ectodomain - Involvement of a matrix metallo-protease. J Biol Chem. 271:4545-4552.
6. **Johnstone AJ, Cridland C, DaCosta C, Harfst E, Sheperd P**. 1994 Monoclonal antibodies that recognise native human thyrotropin receptor. Mol Cell Endocrinol. 105:R1-R8.
7. **Nicholson LB, Vlase H, Graves P, Nilsson M, Molne J, Huang GC, Morgenthaler NG, Davies TF, McGregor AM, Banga JP**. 1996 Monoclonal antibodies to the human TSH receptor; epitope mapping and binding to the native receptor on the basolateral plasma memebrane of thyroid follicular cells. J Mol Endocrinol. 16:159-170.
8. **Oda Y, Sanders J, Roberts S, Maruyama M, Kato R, Perez M, Petersen VB, Wedlock N, Furmaniak J, Smith BR**. 1998 Binding characteristics of antibodies to the TSH receptor. J Mol Endocrinol 20:233-244.
9. **Pellequer JL, Westhof E, Vanregenmortel MHV**. 1991 Predicting location of discontinuous epitopes in proteins from their primary structure. Meth Enzymol. 203:176-201.
10. **Chazenbalk GD, Wang Y, Guo J, Hutchison JS, Segal D, Jaume JC, McLachlan SM, Rapoport B**. 1999 A mouse monoclonal antibody to a thyrotropin receptor ectodomain variant provides insight into the exquisite antigenic conformational requirement, epitopes and in vivo concentration of human autoantibodies. J Clin Endocrinol Metab 84:702-710.

11. **Seetharamaiah GS, Wagle NM, Morris JC, Prabhakar B S**. 1995 Generation and characterization of monoclonal antibodies to human thyrotropin receptor: antibodies can bind to discrete conformational or linear epitopes and block TSH binding. Endocrinology 136:2817-2826.

12. **Lee G, Aloj S M, Beguinot F, Kohn L D**. 1977 J Biol Chem 752:7967-7970.

13. **Murakami M, Miyashita K, Yamada M, Iriuchijima T, Mori M**. 1992 Characterization of human thyrotropin receptor related peptide like immunoreactivity in peripheral blood of Graves' Disease. Biochem Biophys Res Comm. 186:1074-1080.

14. **Molteni M, Zulian C, Scrofani S, DellaBella S, Bonara P, Kohn LD, Scorza R**. 1998 High frequency of T cell lines responsive to immunodominant epitopes of thyrotropin receptor in healthy subjects. Thyroid 8:241-247.

15. **Crisp MS, Weetman AP, Ludgate M**. 1997 Evidence for thyrotopin receptor antibodies which are not TSH agonists/antagonists in thyroid associated ophthalmopathy. J Endocr Invest. 20 S5:58.

16. **Marion S, Braun J, Ropars A, Kohn L, Charreire J**. 1994 Induction of autoimmunity by immunization of mice with human thyrotropin receptor. Cell Immunol. 158:329-341.

17. **Ohmori M, Endo T, Onaya T**. 1991 Development of chicken antibodies toward the human thyrotropin receptor and their bioactivities. Biochem Biophys Res Comm. 174 :399-403.

18. **Endo T, Ohmori M, Ikeda M, Onaya T**. 1991 Thyroid stimulating activity of rabbit antibodies towards the human thyrotropin receptor peptide. Biochem Biophys Res Comm. 177:145-150.

19. **Sakata S, Ogawa T, Matsui I, Manshouri T, Atassi MZ**. 1992 Biological activities of rabbit antibodies against synthetic human thyrotropin receptor peptides representing thyrotropin binding regions. Biochem Biophys Res Comm. 182:1369-1375.

20. **Hidaka Y, Guimaraes V, Soliman M, Yanagawa T, Okomoto Y, Quintans J, DeGroot L**. 1995 Production of thyroid stimulating antibodies in mice by immunization with T cell epitopes of human receptor. Endocrinology 136:1642-1647.

21. **Costagliola S, Alcalde L, Ruf J, Vassart G, Ludgate M**. 1994 Overexpression of the extracellular domain of the thyrotropin receptor in bacteria; production of thyrotropin binding inhibiting immunoglobulins. J Mol Endocrinol 13 :11-21.

22. **Costagliola S, Alcalde L, Tonacchera M, Ruf J, Vassart G, Ludgate M**. 1994 Induction of thyrotropin receptor (TSH-R) autoantibodies and thyroiditis in mice immunized with the recombinant TSH-R. Biochem Biophys Res Comm. 199: 1027-1034.

23. **Costagliola S, Many MC, SalmansFalys M, Tonacchera M, Vassart G, Ludgate M**. 1994 Recombinant thyrotropin receptor and the induction of autoimmune thyroid-disease in BALB/c mice - a new animal-model. Endocrinology 135: 2150-2159.

24. **Costagliola S, Many MC, StalmansFalys M, Vassart G, Ludgate M**. 1995 Autoimmune-response induced by immunizing female mice with recombinant human thyrotropin receptor varies with the genetic background. Mol Cell Endocrinol. 115:199-206.

25. **Goverman J, Woods A, Larson L, Weiner LP, Hood L, Zaller DM**. 1993 Transgenic mice that express a myelin basic protein specific T cell receptor develop spontaneous autoimmunity. Cell 72:551-560.

26. **Wang SH, Carayanniotis G, Zhang Y, Gupta M, Mcgregor AM, Banga JP**. 1998 Induction of thyroiditis in mice with thyrotropin receptor lacking serologically dominant regions. Clin Exp Immunol. 113:119-125.

27. **Seetharamaiah GS, Dallas JS, Patibandla SA, Thotakura NR, Prabhakar BS**. 1997 Requirement of glycosylation of the human thyrotropin receptor ectodomain for its reactivity with autoantibodies in patients' sera. J Immunol 158:2798-2804.

28. **Wagle NM, Dallas JS, Seetharamaiah GS, Fan JL, Desai RK, Memar O, Rajaraman S, Prabhakar BS**. 1994 Induction of hyperthyroxinemia in BALB/c but not in several other strains of mice. Autoimmunity 18:103-112.

29. **Seetharamaiah GS, Desai RK, Dallas JS, Tahara K, Kohn LD, Prabhakar BS**. 1993 Induction of TSH binding inhibitory immunoglobulins with the extracellular domain of the human thyrotropin receptor produced using baculovirus expression systems. Autoimmunity 14:315-320.

30. **Davies TF, Bobovnikova Y, Weiss M, Vlase H, Moran T, Graves PN**. 1998 Development and characterisation of monoclonal antibodies specific for the murine thyrotropin receptor. Thyroid 8:693-701.

31. **Vlase H, Weiss M, Graves PN, Davies TF**. 1998 Characterization of the murine immune response to the murine TSH receptor ectodomain: induction of hypothyroidism and TSH receptor antibodies. Clin Exp Immunol. 113:111-118.

32. **Tang D C, DeVit M & Johnston S A**. 1992 Genetic immunization is a simple method for eliciting an immune response. Nature 356:152-155.

33. **Costagliola S, Rodien P, Many MC, Ludgate M, Vassart G**. 1998.Genetic immunization against the human thyrotropin receptor causes thyroiditis and allows production of monoclonal antibodies recognizing the native receptor. J Immunol. 160:1458-1465.

34. **Costagliola S, Pohlenz J, Refetoff S, Vassart G**. 1998 Generation of a murine model of Graves' Disease by genetic immunization of outbred mice with human TSH receptor. J Endocrinol Invest. 21 S4.

35. **Shimojo N, Kohno Y, Yamaguchi K I, Kikuoka S, Hoshioka A, Niimi H, Hirai A, Tamura Y, Saito Y,Kohn LD, Tahara K**. 1996 Induction of Graves'-like disease in mice by immunization with fibroblasts transfected with the thyrotropin receptor and a class II molecule. Proc Natl Acad Sci USA 93:11074-11079.

36. **Yamaguchi K I, Shimojo N, Kikuoka S, Hoshioka A, Hirai A, Tahara K, Kohn L D, Kohno Y, Niimi H.** 1997 Genetic control of anti-thyrotropin receptor antibody genereation in H-2 (K) mice immunized with thyrotropin receptor transfected fibroblasts. J Clin Endocrinol Metab. 82: 4266-4269.

37. **Kikuoka S, Shimojo N, Yamaguchi KI, Watanabe Y, Hoshioka A, Hirai A, Saito Y, Tahara K, Kohn LD, Maruyama N, Kohno Y, Niimi H.** 1998 The formation of thyrotropin receptor (TSHR) antibodies in a Graves' animal model requires the N-terminal segment of the TSHR extracellular domain. Endocrinology 139:1891-1898.

38. **Kita M, Ahmad L, Marians RC, Vlase H, Unger P, Graves PN, Davies TF.** 1999 Regulation and transfer of a murine model of thyrotropin receptor antibody mediated Graves' Disease. Endocrinology 140 : 1392-1398.

39. **Costagliola S, Many MC, StalmansFalys M, Vassart G, Ludgate M**.1996. Transfer of thyroiditis, with syngeneic spleen-cells sensitized with the human thyrotropin receptor, to naive BALB/c and nod mice. Endocrinology 137:4637-4643.

40. **Many MC, Costagliola S, Detrait M, Denef JF, Vassart G, Ludgate M**. 1999 Development of an animal model of autoimmune Thyroid Eye Disease. J Immunol. 162: 4966-4974.

41. **Crisp M, Lane C, Halliwell M, Wynford-Thomas D, Ludgate M**. 1997 Thyrotropin Receptor Transcripts In Human Adipose Tissue. J Clin Endocrinol Metab. 82:2003-2005.

42. **Ludgate M, Crisp M, Lane C, Costagliola S, Vassart G, Weetman A, Daunerie C, Many M-C**. 1998 The Thyrotropin Receptor In Thyroid Eye Disease. Thyroid 8: 411-413.

43. **Coles AJ, Wing MG, Hale G, Waldmann H, Weetman AP, Compston DAS, Chatterjee VKK**. 1998 Anti-lymphocyte monoclonal antibody treatment of multiple sclerosis suppresses disease activity but induced Graves' Disease. J Endocrinol Invest. 21 S5.

10
THIONAMIDE DRUG THERAPY

Michael M. Kaplan and Donald A. Meier

INTRODUCTION

Thionamide antithyroid drug therapy is one of the three standard treatments for hyperthyroidism caused by Graves' disease, along with surgery and radioactive iodine (^{131}I)(1-3). These treatments, all directed at the thyroid gland, are necessarily imperfect, because none stops production of stimulatory TSH receptor autoantibodies. It seems unlikely that therapy to interrupt the underlying process of thyroid autoimmunity will be available any time soon. Therefore, antithyroid drugs will continue to be needed. This chapter reviews their actions, use, side effects, and role in the management of the hyperthyroid patient.

The two thionamides in use in the U..S. and Canada are propylthiouracil (6-n-propyl-2-thiouracil, or PTU) and methimazole (1-methyl-2-mercapto-imidazole, or MMI, brand name Tapazole®). A carbethoxy derivative of MMI, carbimazole, not available in the U.S. or Canada, is used in some other countries. It is rapidly transformed to MMI in serum (4), has no advantage over MMI, and can be considered equivalent to MMI. PTU and MMI were introduced into clinical practice by Astwood and coworkers in the late 1940s (5-7).

PHARMACOLOGY

MMI is available in 5 mg and 10 mg tablets. PTU is available only in 50 mg tablets. The retail cost of 50 mg propylthiouracil tablets in our community in 1999 is approximately $20 for 100 tablets and the cost of 10 mg methimazole tablets is about $80 for 100 tablets. MMI oral bioavailability is greater than 90%, but can be altered by food, while oral bioavailability of PTU is 65-75% (8,9). Both drugs can be administered rectally to a very sick patient who cannot take oral medications. However, rectal preparations are not available commercially, and must be made up extemporaneously (8).

MMI reaches peak blood concentrations in 0.5 - 1 h and PTU reaches its peak in about 1 h (10,11). MMI is minimally bound to serum proteins, while about 75% of PTU in serum is bound to albumin (9-12). PTU has a very low lipid solubility, whereas MMI is quite lipid soluble (9). Therefore, PTU is excreted into milk and transported across the placenta to a much lower extent than MMI. Both drugs are metabolized by the liver. The serum half-life of MMI is 5 - 6 h, and that of PTU is 1 - 2 h (9-11). Thionamides are concentrated by active transport into the thyroid gland (9). The duration of action of the thionamides is determined by thyroid tissue levels, not blood levels. The antithyroid effects of MMI last longer than those of PTU. As a result, MMI is often effective when taken once daily, whereas a higher percentage of patients taking PTU need divided doses (13,14).

The main mechanism of thionamide action is to block synthesis of thyroxine (T4) and triiodothyronine (T3) by thyroid follicular cells. This is accomplished by inhibition of the enzyme thyroid peroxidase, which catalyzes both the iodination of tyrosine residues on the thyroglobulin molecule, and coupling of the iodinated tyrosines to form the thyronines, T4 and T3 (15). Thionamides do not interfere with active transport of iodine into the thyroid gland, release of T4 and T3 by hydrolysis of thyroglobulin, or release of T4 and T3 into the blood.

Outside of the thyroid gland, PTU, but not MMI, inhibits the type I iodothyronine deiodinase, one of the two outer ring deiodinases that can convert T4 to T3 (16,17). By this effect, PTU can cause a more rapid decrease than MMI in serum T3 levels in the initial treatment of hyperthyroid patients who also receive a high dose of stable iodine (18). However, in the ordinary clinical setting no therapeutic benefit has been demonstrated from this extrathyroidal action of PTU.

Whether the thionamides have immunomodulatory effects that are clinically significant in patients with Graves' disease is uncertain (19,20). Actions have been demonstrated in vitro that may or may not be relevant in vivo. Also, because the hyperthyroid state, per se, may perpetuate thyroid autoimmunity, the antithyroid action of the thionamides in vivo may reduce the activity of the autoimmune process indirectly. Thus, an additional, more direct effect of the thionamides on thyroid autoimmunity in the clinical setting is difficult to demonstrate unequivocally.

PATIENT SELECTION

Primary therapy with antithyroid drugs

The main advantage of antithyroid drugs over surgery or radioiodine is that antithyroid drugs do not destroy thyroid tissue and therefore allow for the possibility of a remission of Graves' disease. If remission occurs, the patient may not need life-long thyroid hormone replacement, which is usually required after radioiodine. However, some patients progress spontaneously from hyperthyroidism to hypothyroidism without any treatment (21-23). Presumably, they have a significant element of Hashimoto's thyroiditis. Similarly, in a 20 year follow up study of patients who went into remission from hyperthyroidism after treatment only with antithyroid drugs, more than half had evidence of long term thyroid damage (24). Their spectrum of abnormalities included decreased thyroid functional reserve, increased thyrotropin (TSH) response to thyrotropin-releasing hormone, subclinical hypothyroidism, and overt hypothyroidism. Patients who are treated with antithyroid drugs should be informed of this long term possibility, and the need for systematic follow up, even if they achieve a sustained remission.

Antithyroid drug treatment is less attractive for patients who have a low chance of remission of their hyperthyroidism. Remission of hyperthyroidism in patients with toxic adenomas or toxic multinodular goiters is improbable, because these conditions do not have an autoimmune etiology. Factors that are associated with remission in Graves' disease are listed in Table 1.

Table 1. Factors that may favor antithyroid drug treatment for Graves' disease

---

Greater than average chance of spontaneous remission
 Findings at the time of initial diagnosis
  Mild elevations of serum free T4 and free T3
  Normal thyroid size or minimal enlargement
  Short duration of disease or trend toward improvement
  Possible influences: age>20, female sex, non-smoking status
 Findings in the course of treatment
  Decrease in thyroid size during therapy
  Control of hyperthyroidism with a low maintenance drug dose
  No more than one previous relapse
  Negative thyroid stimulating antibody levels

Hyperthyroidism in pregnancy or during breast feeding

Absence of factors that increase the risk of complicated thyrotoxicosis
 Heart disease
 Neuropsychiatric disease
 No medical insurance
 Demonstrated poor compliance taking antithyroid drugs

Presence of ophthalmopathy
 Possible exacerbation after radioiodine
 Concern about side effects of corticosteroids if used with radioiodine

Patient (or parent/guardian) preference

Physician preference

 At initial presentation, relatively mild elevations of serum free thyroxine (T4) and triiodothyronine (T3) levels and only mild thyroid enlargement increase the chance of remission (25,26). Other favorable factors suggested in some studies are female sex, age over 20 years, and being a non-smoker (25). Findings during antithyroid treatment can help predict the chances of remission of Graves' disease. Favorable factors include a decrease in the size of the thyroid gland during therapy, control of hyperthyroidism with a low antithyroid drug dose (27), no more than one previous relapse (25) and a negative thyroid stimulating antibody test (28), although the latter test is not often used in the U.S. There are geographic differences in remission rates. One hypothesis is that low dietary iodine intake increases the chance of remission (29), but this theory is not proven, and does not explain consistently high remission rates found in Japan (30).

 Reported rates of remission of Graves' disease after antithyroid drug treatment vary between 10 and 98% around the world (25). Because the majority of patients in the U.S. are currently treated with radioiodine (31), and because there have been decreases in dietary iodine intake and smoking rates in the U.S. in recent years, current American remission rates are especially uncertain. In any case, none of the clinical or laboratory variables, alone or in combination, allows a reliable prediction of remission of Graves' disease. Only observation after antithyroid drug withdrawal is conclusive. Long term follow-up is essential after a course of thionamide treatment, because relapses can occur after remissions lasting 5 or more years (32).

Because radioiodine is absolutely contraindicated during pregnancy and breast feeding, and because of possible adverse effects of surgery and general anesthesia during pregnancy on pregnancy outcome, antithyroid drugs are the treatment of choice for hyperthyroidism during pregnancy. This topic is discussed in more detail in Chapter 14. In non-pregnant hyperthyroid women who are planning pregnancy in the future, our preference is for radioiodine therapy, to avoid the potential problems of antithyroid drug treatment during pregnancy. There is no indication that radioiodine treatment adversely affects the outcome of a patient's subsequent pregnancies.

Some clinicians prefer to treat hyperthyroid children and adolescents with antithyroid drugs, because of concern about possible very late side effects of radioiodine treatment, especially malignancy. Recent long term follow up studies of patients treated with radioiodine provide considerable reassurance (33,34). The outcomes of both antithyroid drug and radioiodine treatment for children is satisfactory (35-37). Nevertheless, the number of patients treated with radioiodine in childhood, and followed for many years thereafter, is small. Therefore, antithyroid drug treatment is a reasonable choice for primary treatment of Graves' disease in childhood, but radioiodine is also acceptable, especially for children and adolescents whose thyrotoxicosis is not well controlled by antithyroid medication (except for very young children with substantial thyroid enlargement, for whom the necessary radioiodine dose may deliver an unusually high whole body or gonadal radiation dose).

Sherman and coworkers (38) have identified clinical and psychosocial factors that increase a patient's risk for complicated thyrotoxicosis. As noted in Table 1, they include the presence of heart disease, and factors that decrease the chances of compliance with taking the medication as prescribed. Such patients may be best treated with radioiodine, if the up-front cost of radioiodine can be managed.

A long-standing concern is whether radioiodine therapy might worsen or induce Graves' ophthalmopathy (39). Studies to date have been inconsistent. However, because of this concern, some physicians prefer to treat patients with ophthalmopathy with antithyroid medication initially. An alternative is to employ a course of corticosteroids with radioiodine treatment in patients who have significant eye involvement at the time of diagnosis of hyperthyroidism.

Occasionally, a patient with Graves' disease also has a thyroid nodule. All such nodules should be evaluated by needle biopsy. If the cytology is positive or suspicious for malignancy, surgical management is appropriate for both the hyperthyroidism and the nodule.

In addition to the physiological, clinical, and laboratory variables discussed so far, some patients, or their families or guardians, and physicians have personal or philosophical preferences for or against each of the three available treatments for hyperthyroidism in Graves' disease. We advise a full discussion of the advantages and risks of each of the treatments, with documentation of the discussion. After that, we believe it is appropriate for hyperthyroid patients to be given their choice among the therapies that are not medically contraindicated. Even in patients whose chance of remission after antithyroid drug treatment is better than average, we consider radioiodine therapy an acceptable choice, because of a sustained remission rate well under 50% in our patient population, and the potential aide effects of antithyroid drug therapy.

Preparation with antithyroid drugs before radioiodine or surgery

Radioiodine treatment sometimes produces a radiation thyroiditis, with release of stored thyroid hormone (39). This effect peaks about 10 - 14 days post-therapy, and can cause worsening of hyperthyroidism. In addition, improvement of thyroid function after radioiodine does not occur for several weeks or longer, even if there is no initial worsening. Hyperthyroid patients who are to be treated surgically, such as those with large toxic multinodular goiters, probably have a lower incidence of operative and postoperative complication if they are as close to euthyroid as possible at the time of surgery.

To decrease the chances of these problems, pretreatment of patients with a thionamide is sometimes advisable in preparation for radioiodine, and is routine in preparing patients for surgery. The goal is to deplete intrathyroidal thyroid hormone stores and control thyrotoxicosis before radioiodine, or to control thyrotoxicosis before surgery. The target of pretreatment with antithyroid drugs before ablative therapy is high-normal serum free T4 and T3 (or free T3) levels. Sometimes, free T4 and T3 values slightly above normal are satisfactory, if the extent of clinical improvement is adequate. Normalization of serum TSH levels often lags, because of persistent pituitary thyrotrophic cell suppression; hence the TSH level should not be used as a therapeutic guide in this situation. Beta adrenergic blocker treatment is sometimes added to the thionamide, particularly if tachycardia is prominent or atrial fibrillation is present, provided there are no contraindications.

Opinions vary as to which patients should be pretreated before radioiodine (39). Some authors advise thionamide therapy in most, if not all patients before radioiodine. We and others are selective (39). Our recommendation is to pretreat severely thyrotoxic or elderly patients and patients with pre-existing heart disease, fever, severe systemic illness, or debility.

Thionamide pretreatment before radioiodine appears to cause relative radioresistance, necessitating a larger radioiodine dose than would otherwise be selected (39). One study suggests that this effect may occur only with PTU (40), but in another study, carbimazole pretreatment was associated with an increased failure rate in patients receiving a standard radioiodine dose (41). We and others recommend a 25% higher radioiodine dose in patients pretreated with thionamides (39).

PRACTICAL THIONAMIDE USE

In considering which drug to use initially, MMI has several advantages over PTU. MMI is usually effective in a once daily maintenance dose, and PTU may need to be given in divided doses. Because a 10 mg MMI tablet is about 4 times more potent than a 50 mg PTU tablet, fewer MMI tablets are needed for equivalent antithyroid effects. For both of these reasons, patient compliance in taking MMI as prescribed is easier than for PTU, as long as the physician gives the patient appropriate instructions. PTU has some advantages during pregnancy (see chapter 14), but MMI may be used even then.

The appropriate initial dose of either thionamide depends on the severity of the patient's hyperthyroidism and thyroid size. The advantage of using lower doses, when they are likely to be effective, is a lower incidence of side effects. For patients with mild thyroid hormone elevations and small goiters, we often start with MMI 10 once daily, or PTU 100 mg b.i.d. If the thyroid gland is larger (more than about 25 grams, normal up to about 15 - 18 grams), or thyroid hormone blood levels are twice the upper limit of normal or greater, we use MMI 30 mg daily or PTU 100 - 200 mg t.i.d. For severe hyperthyroidism, MMI 40 - 60 mg daily in divided doses or PTU 800 - 1200 mg daily in divided doses may be needed.

During initial treatment, we sometimes prescribe MMI in divided doses, to maximize the chance of prompt control of the hyperthyroidism, because the duration of action in some patients is not a full day. This decision depends on the severity of the hyperthyroidism and patient compliance considerations, e.g. work schedule, the patient's past experience in trying to take other medication in divided daily doses, forgetfulness, and patient preference. In patients with severe palpitations, tremor, or jittery feelings, and no evidence of impaired cardiac ventricular function or other contraindications, addition of a beta adrenergic blocker to the thionamide in the initial weeks of treatment can provide symptomatic relief faster than a thionamide alone. The beta blocker is discontinued when serum thyroid hormone levels approach normal.

We see patients monthly during the initial phase of therapy. Some patients have significant decreases in serum thyroid hormone levels after 2 - 3 weeks of thionamide therapy (42). We monitor serum free T4 and T3 levels as well as TSH, along with the neutrophil count and transaminase level. TSH measurements alone are insufficient, because there may be suppression of pituitary thyrotroph cell function for several months after an episode of hyperthyroidism. The TSH level may be low in a euthyroid patient, and low or normal even in a patient who becomes hypothyroid from thionamide overtreatment. In an occasional patient, the symptoms and some tissue responses may take longer to improve than the serum free T4 and T3 levels (25). Most patients become euthyroid in 1 - 3 months after initiation of treatment. Some patients seem to be resistant to thionamides. In most cases, the cause of apparent resistance is noncompliance (43).

Once patients become euthyroid, the thionamide dose can usually be reduced substantially. One error that we encounter in the use of antithyroid drugs is continuation of a relatively high initial dose after a patient becomes euthyroid. In that case, hypothyroidism usually develops within 1 - 3 months. Maintenance doses for MMI are typically 2.5 - 10 mg daily, and those for PTU are typically 50 - 150 mg daily in one or two daily doses. After the patient has stabilized, we see them every 3 - 4 months, to ascertain that the thionamide dose remains sufficient without becoming excessive, and to monitor for side effects.

Most patients taking antithyroid medication hope to have a remission of their Graves' disease and to be able to stop antithyroid treatment. Many studies have been performed to determine if the therapeutic program can be optimized to increase the chances of remission. The variables examined have been thionamide dose, duration of thionamide treatment, and combined thionamide-thyroxine ('block and replace') treatment.

The studies of thionamide dose have shown no consistent effect of dose on remission rate. Higher doses achieve control of the hyperthyroidism faster, but also cause a higher incidence of side effects (32,44,45). Regarding duration of treatment, usual practice is to treat for 1 - 2 years, and then attempt to discontinue the thionamide. Some studies suggest that remission rates are higher after 18 months - 2 years of treatment than after 6 months, but other studies show no benefit of the longer treatment durations. The phenomenon of spontaneous hypothyroidism in patients with Graves' disease, discussed earlier, makes it difficult to know whether a longer duration of thionamide treatment changes the natural history of Graves' disease. Some patients are incompletely controlled after 1 year or longer of therapy. Obviously, withdrawing them from thionamide treatment will not be successful. Long term thionamide treatment is safe (46).

A 1991 study from Japan reported a spectacular remission rate in patients with Graves' disease treated with a combination of thionamide and thyroxine (47). Unfortunately, multiple subsequent studies, from many parts of the world including Japan, have not found any benefit from adding thyroxine to thionamide therapy (48-52). Therefore, we do not recommend this combination approach, at least for the purpose of promoting remission of Graves' disease. In the U.S., most endocrinologists favor using only a thionamide, and adjust the dose to be as low as possible. This approach minimizes the incidence of side effects, decreases drug cost for patients who pay for medication, and may improve compliance. In addition, knowledge of the lowest dose needed to control the patient's thyroid function helps guide the decision of whether, and when, to try to stop the medication.

In some countries, a more usual practice is to combine thionamide treatment with thyroxine. The theoretical advantage of this approach is that the relative high thionamide dose blocks thyroid function nearly completely, allowing the thyroxine dose to determine the patient's thyroid status, which is more likely to be stable. In other words, fluctuations in the activity of the Graves' disease and variations in patients' sensitivity to thionamides have less effect on the therapeutic response, and the frequency of office visits may be lower. We find the rationale for thionamide treatment alone to be more persuasive.

SIDE EFFECTS

Side effects of thionamides are relatively common (Table 2). Fortunately, the most frequent side effects are not dangerous and are self limited. Drug reactions appear to be more common at high drug doses, i.e., greater than 40 mg of MMI or 600 mg of PTU daily. The most common reaction is a macular pruritic skin rash. Itching without an eruption and urticaria also occur. It is said that cutaneous reactions to the thionamides may subside without discontinuation of the drugs, but it is our practice to either stop the drug or switch to the other thionamide when itching or a rash occurs.

Table 2. Side effects of PTU and MMI

Mild, relatively common
> Skin rash, itching
> Fever
> Bitter taste of PTU for some patients
> Joint pain without true arthritis
> Hypothyroidism from overdose

Mild, rare
> Loss of sense of taste (MMI)
> Nausea, vomiting, stomach pain
> Mild neutropenia
> Arthritis
> Myalgia with elevated creatine kinase
> Hypoglycemia due to insulin autoantibodies
> Cholestasis with MMI
> Aplasia cutis with MMI

Dangerous, rare
> Agranulocytosis
> Hepatocellular damage
> Vasculitis

Other mild side effects are listed in Table 2. For some patients PTU has a very unpleasant, bitter taste. MMI occasionally causes gastrointestinal discomfort or a loss of taste sensation. Either agent can cause fever or joint pain without frank arthritis. In high doses, mild neutropenia, apparently different from the idiosyncratic agranulocytosis, has been reported. However, because Graves' disease, per se, can also cause mild neutropenia, it is advisable to obtain a baseline complete hemogram with differential, to know whether subsequent neutrophil counts represent a drug-induced change. A recent report described a few patients who developed transient myalgias with elevated creatine kinase levels after rapid correction of hyperthyroidism with MMI or PTU, in the absence of hypothyroidism (53). A small number of babies, whose mothers took MMI during pregnancy, have been born with aplasia cutis, which is a small area of undeveloped skin. If the thionamide dose is too high for too long, hypothyroidism will develop, but the dose-response relationship is quite variable. Hypothyroidism sometimes occurs at low doses, sometimes as a prelude to the development of spontaneous hypothyroidism. In one case of a massive one-time PTU overdose, there were no toxic effects (54).

If a patient has one of the mild side effects while taking one thionamide, changing to the other thionamide may be successful. It is best to let the side effect subside before changing to the alternate antithyroid drug. Otherwise, it is difficult to know whether a persistent symptom is a prolonged reaction to the first drug, a similar reaction to the second drug, or a symptom unrelated to either thionamide. A frequently cited incidence for mild thionamide side effects is 5% or less, but recent studies report 16 - 26% incidences of side effects (45,55), or more (52). The 5% figure may represent the frequency of side effects severe enough to require discontinuation of thionamide treatment. Our experience is closer to the studies suggesting the higher incidences of mild side effects. A patient who has had a hypersensitivity reaction to one of the thionamides has about a 50% chance of having a reaction to the other one.

The dangerous side effects of thionamides are, fortunately, rare (Table 2). They include agranulocytosis, hepatic damage, and vasculitis. In our opinion, patients who have one of these serious reactions to one thionamide should not be treated with the other thionamide.

The incidence of agranulocytosis in a large Japanese study was 55 in 15,398 (0.4%) thionamide-treated patients with Graves' disease (56). From the opposite perspective, a population-based study in the Netherlands found that MMI and carbimazole were associated with 17 of 75 cases of agranulocytosis that developed in non-hospitalized patients, and that the relative risk of agranulocytosis in patients treated with either of these two drugs, compared to the general population, was 114.8 (57).

One study found that agranulocytosis is sometimes preceded by a progressive decrease in the neutrophil count, suggesting that it may be advisable to monitor the neutrophil count regularly in patients taking thionamides (56). However, agranulocytosis can develop precipitously. Agranulocytosis is less common in patients taking less than 30 mg of MMI a day, but can occur at lower MMI doses and at any PTU dose (58,59). Agranulocytosis is most common in the first 4 months of thionamide treatment, but can develop in patients who have been treated for years, or who have had a previous course of treatment without problems, and are retreated because they did not stay in remission (60). Rarely, anemia and thrombocytopenia accompany agranulocytosis. Management of thionamide-induced agranulocytosis includes discontinuation of the drug, blood cultures, patient isolation, and administration of broad spectrum antibiotics. Administration of granulocyte colony-stimulating factor may be effective (60-62).

Both PTU and MMI can cause liver damage, including fulminant drug-induced hepatitis and death from liver failure. Transaminase values rise in 8 - 38% of patients treated with thionamides, but the elevations are usually mild, and may resolve with a reduction in drug dose (63). Liver biopsies in such patients have shown histologic damage. If transaminase levels remain less than twice the upper limit of normal, thionamide treatment may be continued cautiously. Because thyrotoxicosis itself can cause abnormal liver function tests, baseline values are appropriate, and it seems advisable to monitor transaminase levels systematically in patients taking antithyroid drugs. MMI can rarely cause a cholestatic hepatitis (64), but alkaline phosphatase levels must be interpreted cautiously, because hyperthyroidism, per se, can elevate the bone alkaline phosphatase isoenzyme.

Treatment of antithyroid drug-induced liver damage is withdrawal of the drug and supportive measures. If fulminant liver failure occurs, liver transplantation might be a consideration, although we are not aware of a case in which this has been done.

The third rare, but potentially serious, side effect of thionamides is vasculitis. It may present as true arthritis (beyond the more common symptom of arthralgia), or with involvement of the kidneys or lungs. Other manifestations of vasculitis occur, including skin rash, fever, pleuritis, or pericarditis, in a lupus-like picture. The etiology of the vasculitis is thought to be autoimmune. Anti-neutrophil cytoplasmic antibodies and other autoantibodies have been found in affected patients. The incidence of the vasculitic syndromes is not clear. Reports have focused on specific organ involvement with about 15 - 40 cases of various vasculitic syndromes identified by literature reviews (65-70). Undoubtedly, many cases are not published.

Because of the potential for serious, even fatal reactions to thionamides, my colleagues and I give patients who are to be treated with PTU and MMI a printed precaution sheet with the information shown in Table 3. One inconvenience in the use of antithyroid drugs stems from the fact that the symptoms possibly signaling a drug reaction are nonspecific. Most patients taking antithyroid drugs and who develop fever or a sore throat have ordinary viral upper respiratory infections. Patients who develop joint pain can have any of the other causes of this symptom. However, when such symptoms appear, a thionamide reaction must be considered, often necessitating an office visit and/or laboratory tests to distinguish a drug side effect from a false alarm. Also, some patients, when advised of the possibility of various symptoms, interpret any musculoskeletal or gastrointestinal discomfort as a definite antithyroid drug reaction and may require evaluation and much reassurance, or even, on occasion, a change to another form of treatment, even when the symptom proves not to be a drug reaction.

Table 3. Precautions for patients taking antithyroid drugs

The main toxic reactions to antithyroid drugs are:-
1. a skin rash, usually itchy
2. a decrease in the number white blood cells that fight infection, often causing fever, sore throat, or sores in the mouth
3. jaundice (yellow skin or eyes) caused by liver damage
4. arthritis, in which joints, especially of the arms and legs, are swollen, stiff, or painful

If any of these problems develop:-
1. STOP THE ANTITHYROID DRUG AT ONCE.
2. call our office so that we can arrange for you to have the appropriate blood tests right away, and see you in our office as soon as possible.

Keep these instruction posted at home as long as you are taking the antithyroid drug.

SUMMARY

Thionamide treatment, though imperfect, is an appropriate treatment for selected patients with hyperthyroidism caused by Graves' disease. It provides the patient with a chance of remission and the avoidance of long term thyroid hormone replacement. It offers an alternative when physicians or patients wish to avoid exposure to radioiodine or the risks and unpleasantness of general anesthesia and surgery. It is very valuable in the preparation of some patients for radioiodine or surgery. Mild side effects occur with low-to-moderate frequency. Dangerous side effects do occur, but they are rare. Patients considered for thionamide treatment should be informed of the advantages and risks of the three available treatments for hyperthyroidism. Those started on thionamide treatment should be instructed on precautions to take in case of drug reactions.

REFERENCES

1. **Singer PA, Cooper DS, Levy EG, et al.** 1995 Treatment guidelines for patients with hyperthyroidism and hypothyroidism. JAMA. 273:808-812.
2. **Garcia M, Baskin HJ, Feld S, et al.** 1995 AACE clinical practice guidelines for the evaluation and treatment of hyperthyroidism and hypothyroidism. Endocr Pract. 1:54-62.
3. **Torring O, Tallstedt L, Wallin G, et al.** 1996 Outcome of Graves' hyperthyroidism with methimazole, surgery, or radioiodine. J Clin Endocrinol Metab. 81:2986-2993.
4. **Nakashima T, Taurog A.** 1979 Rapid conversion of carbimazole to methimazole in serum: evidence for an enzymatic mechanism. Clin Endocrinol. 10:637-648.
5. **Greep RO, Greer MA.** 1985 Edwin Bennett Astwood. 1909 - 1976. national Academy of Sciences Biographical Memoirs, vol 55. Washington, DC, National Academy Press; 1-42.
6. **Astwood EB, Vanderlaan WP.** 1945 Thiouracil derivatives of greater activity for the treatment of hyperthyroidism. J Clin Endocrinol. 5:424-430.
7. **Stanley MM, Astwood EB.** 1949 1-methyl-2-mercaptoimidazole: an antithyroid compound highly active in man. Endocrinology 44:588-589.
8. **United States Pharmacopeial Convention, Inc**. 1999 Antithyroid agents, systemic. In: USP DI. Vol 1. Drug information for the health care professional. 19th ed. Englewood, CO: Micromedex; 446-451.
9. **Kampmann JP, Hansen JM.** 1981 Clinical pharmacokinetics of antithyroid drugs. Clin Pharmacokinetics. 6:401-428.
10. **Cooper DS, Bode HH, Nath B, Saxe V, Maloof F, Ridgway EC.** 1984 Methimazole pharmacology in man: studies using a newly developed radioimmunoassay for methimazole. J Clin Endocrinol Metab. 58:473-479.
11. **Cooper DS, Saxe VC, Maloof F, Radgway EC.** 1981 Studies of propylthiouracil using a newly developed radioimmunoassay. J Clin Endocrinol Metab. 52:204-213.
12. **Zaton A, Martinez A, DeGandarias JM.** 1988 The binding of thioureylene compounds to human serum albumin. Biochem Pharmacol. 37:3127-3131.
13. **Shiroozu A, Okamura K, Ikenoue H, et al.** 1986 Treatment of hyperthyroidism with a small daily dose of methimazole. J Clin Endocrinol Metab. 63:125-128.
14. **Nicholas WC, Fischer RG, Stevenson RA, Bass JD.** 1995 Single daily dose of methimazole compared to every 8 hours propylthiouracil in the treatment of hyperthyroidism. Southern Med J. 88:973-976.
15. **Taurog A.** 1996 Mechanism of action of antithyroid drugs. In: Braverman LE, Utiger RD (eds). Werner and Ingbar's The Thyroid. A Fundamental and Clinical Text, ed 7. Philadelphia: Lippincott Raven; 66-81.
16. **Saberi M, Sterling FH, Utiger RD.** 1975 Reduction in extrathyroidal triiodothyronine production by propylthiouracil in man. J Clin Invest. 55:218-223.
17. **Geffner DL, Azukizawa M, Hershman JM.** 1975 Propylthiouracil blocks extrathyroidal conversion of thyroxine to triiodothyronine and augments thyrotropin secretion in man. J Clin Invest. 55:224-229.
18. **Abuid J, Larsen PR.** 1974 Triiodothyronine and thyroxine in hyperthyroidism, Comparison of the acute changes during therapy with antithyroid agents. J Clin Invest. 54:201-208.
19. **Weetman A.** 1994 The immunomodulatory effects of antithyroid drugs. Thyroid. 4:145-146.
20. **Wenzel KW, Lente JR.** 1984 Similar effects of thionamide drugs and perchlorate on thyroid-stimulating immunoglobulins in Graves' disease; evidence against an immunosuppressive action of thionamide drugs. J Clin Endocrinol Metab. 58:62-69.
21. **Tamaii H, Kasagi K, Takaichi Y, et al.** 1989 Development of spontaneous hypothyroidism in patients with Graves' disease treated with antithyroid drugs: clinical,

immunological, and histological findings in 26 patients. J Clin Endocrinol Metab. 69:49-53.

22. **Shigemasa C, Mitani Y, Taniguchi S, et al.** 1990 Three patients who spontaneously developed persistent hypothyroidism during or following treatment with antithyroid drugs for Graves' hyperthyroidism. Arch Intern Med. 150: 1105-1109.

23. **Lamberg BA, Salmi J, Wagar G, Makinen T.** 1981 Spontaneous hypothyroidism after antithyroid treatment of hyperthyroid Graves' disease. J Endocrinol Invest. 4:399-402.

24. **Wood LC, Ingbar SH.** 1979 Hypothyroidism as a late sequela in patients with Graves' disease treated with antithyroid drugs. J Clin Invest. 64:1429-1436.

25. **Cooper DS.** 1998 Antithyroid drugs for the treatment of hyperthyroidism caused by Graves' disease. Endocrinol Metab Clin North Am. 27:225-247.

26. **Chowdhury TA, Dyer PH.** 1998 Clinical, biochemical and immunological characteristics of relapsers and non-relapsers of thyrotoxicosis treated with antithyroid drugs. J Intern Med. 224:293-297.

27. **Braverman LE.** 1996 Is there one successful antithyroid regimen for Graves' disease? Lancet. 348:607-698.

28. **Davies TF, Roti E, Braverman LE, DeGroot.** 1998 Thyroid controversy - stimulating antibodies. J Clin Endocrinol Metab. 83:3777-3785.

29. **Solomon BL, Evaul JE, Burman KD, Wartofsky L.** 1987 Remission rates with antithyroid drug therapy: continuing influence of iodine intake? Ann Intern Med. 107:510-512.

30. **Sakata S.** 1988 Remission rates with antithyroid drugs. Ann Intern Med. 108:308.

31. **Solomon B, Glinoer D, Lagasse R, Wartofsky L.** 1990 Current trends in the management of Graves' disease. J Clin Endocrinol Metab. 70:1518-1524.

32. **Benker G, Reinwein D, Kahaly G, et al.** 1998 Is there a methimazole dose effect on remission rate in Graves' disease? Results from a long-term prospective study. Clin Endocrinol. 49:451-457.

33. **Ron E, Doody MM, Becker DV, et al.** 1998 Cancer mortality following treatment for adult hyperthyroidism. JAMA. 280:347-355.

34. **Franklyn JA, Maisonneuve P, Sheppard M, Betteridge J, Boyle P.** 1999 Cancer incidence and mortality after radioiodine treatment for hyperthyroidism: a population-based cohort study. Lancet 353:2111-2115.

35. **Zimmerman D, Lteif AN.** 1998 Thyrotoxicosis in children. Endocrinol Metab Clin North Am. 27:109-126.

36. **Rivkees SA, Sklar C, Freemark.** 1998 The management of Graves' disease in children, with special emphasis of radioiodine treatment. J Clin Endocrinol Metab. 83:3767-3776.

37. **Lippe BM, Landaw EM, Kaplan SA.** 1987 Hyperthyroidism in children treated with long term medical therapy: twenty-five percent remission every two years. J Clin Endocrinol Metab. 64:1241-1245.

38. **Sherman SI, Simonson L, Ladenson PW.** 1996 Clinical and socioeconomic predispositions to complicated thyrotoxicosis: a predictable and preventable syndrome? Am J Med. 101:192-198.

39. **Kaplan MM, Meier DA, Dworkin HJ.** 1998 Treatment of hyperthyroidism with radioactive iodine. Endocrinol Metab Clin North Am. 27:205-221.

40. **Imseis RE, VanMiddlesworth L, Massie JD, Bush AJ, VanMiddlesworth NR.** 1998 Pretreatment with propylthiouracil but not methimazole reduces the therapeutic efficacy of iodine-131 in hyperthyroidism. J Clin Endocrinol Metab. 83:685-687.

41. **Sabri O, Zimny M, Schulz G, et al.** 1999 Success rate of radioiodine therapy in Graves' disease: the influence of thyrostatic medication. J Clin Endocrinol Metab. 83:1229-1233.

42. **Roti E, Gardini E, Minelli R, Salvi M, Robuschi G, Braverman LE.** 1989 Methimazole and serum thyroid hormone concentrations in hyperthyroid patients: effects of single and

multiple daily doses. Ann Intern Med. 111:181-182.

43. **Cooper DS.** 1985 Propylthiouracil levels in hyperthyroid patients unresponsive to large doses. Evidence of poor patient compliance. Ann Intern Med. 102:328-331.

44. **Kallner G, Vitols S, Ljunggren JG.** 1996 Comparison of standardized initial doses of two antithyroid drugs in the treatment of Graves' disease. J Intern Med. 239:525-529.

45. **Grebe SK, Feek CM, Ford HC, et al.** 1998 A randomized trial of short-term treatment of Graves' disease with high-dose carbimazole plus thyroxine versus low-dose carbimazole. Clin Endocrinol. 48:585-92.

46. **Slingerland DW, Burrows BA.** 1979 Long-term antithyroid treatment in hyperthyroidism. JAMA. 242:2408-2410.

47. **Hashizume K, Ichikawa K, Sakurai A, et al.** 1991 Administration of thyroxine in treated Graves' disease. Effects on the level of antibodies to thyroid- stimulating hormone and on the risk of recurrence of hyperthyroidism. N Engl J Med. 324:947-53.

48. **Tamai H, Hayaki I, Kawai K, et al.** 1995 Lack of effect of thyroxine administration on elevated thyroid stimulating horone receptor antibody levels in treated Graves' disease patients. J Clin Endocrinol Metab. 80:1481-1484.

49. **Rizvi A, Crapo L.** 1996 Failure of thyroxine therapy for Graves' disease. Ann Intern Med. 124:694.

50. **McIver B, Rae P, Beckett G, Wilkinson E, Gold A, Toft A**. 1996 Lack of effect of thyroxine in patients with Graves' hyperthyroidism who are treated with an antithyroid drug. N Engl J Med. 334:220-224.

51. **Lucas A, Salinas I, Ruis F, et al.** 1997 Medical therapy of Graves' disease: does thyroxine prevent recurrence of hyperthyroidism? J Clin Endocrinol Metab. 82:2410-2413.

52. **Rittmaster R, Abbott EC, Douglas R, et al.** 1998 Effect of methimazole, with or without L-thyroxine, on remission rates in Graves' disease. J Clin Endocrinol Metab. 83:814-818.

53. **Suzuki S, Ichikawa K, Nagai M, et al.** 1997 Elevation of serum creatine kinase during treatment with antithyroid drugs in patients with hyperthyroidism due to Graves' disease. A novel side effect of antithyroid drugs. Arch Intern Med. 157:693-393.

54. **Jackson GL, Flickinger FW, Wells LW.** 1979 Massive overdosage of propylthiouracil. Ann Intern Med. 91:418-419.

55. **Reinwein D, Benker G, Lazarus JH, Alexander WD**, The European Multicenter Study Group on Antithyroid Drug Treatment. 1993 A prospective randomized trial of antithyroid drug dose in Graves' disease therapy. J Clin Endocrinol Metab. 76:1516-1521.

56. **Tajiri J, Noguchi S, Murakami T, Murakami N**. 1990 Antithyroid drug-induced agranulocytosis. The usefulness of routine white blood cell count monitoring. Arch Intern Med. 150:621-624.

57. **van der Klauw MN, Goudsmit R, Halie MR, et al.** 1999 A population-based case-cohort study of drug-associated agranulocytosis. Arch Intern Med. 159: 369-374.

58. **Cooper DS, Goldminz D, Levin AA et al.** 1983 Agranulocytosis associated with antithyroid drugs. Effects of patient age and drug dose. Ann Intern Med. 98:26-29.

59. **Fincher ME, Fariss BL, Plymate SR, Jones RE, Messier N.** 1984 Agranulocytosis and a small dose of methimazole. Ann Intern Med. 101:404-405.

60. **Mezquita P, Luna V, Mu±oz-Torres M, et al.** 1998 Methimazole-induced aplastic anemia in third exposure: successful treatment with recombinant human granulocyte colony-stimulating factor. Thyroid. 8:791-794.

61. **Tajiri J, Noguchi S, Okamura S, et al.** 1993 Granulocyte colony-stimulating factor treatment of antithyroid drug-induced granulocytopenia. Arch Intern Med. 153:509-514.

62. **Heinrich B, Gross M, Goebel FD.** 1989 Methimazole-induced agranulocytosis and granulocyte-colony stimulating factor. Ann Intern Med. 111:621-622.

63. **Liaw Y-F, Huang M-J, Fan K-D, Li K-L, Wu S-S, Chen T-J**. 1993 Hepatic injury during propylthiouracil therapy in patients with hyperthyroidism. A cohort study. Ann

Intern Med. 118:424-428.

64. **Arab D, Malatjalian D, Rittmaster R.** 1995 Severe cholestatic jaundice in uncomplicated hyperthyroidism treated with methimazole. J Clin Endocrinol Metab. 80:1083-1085.

65. **Nguyen LTH, Luong KVQ, Pham BV.** 1998 An antineutrophil cytoplasmic autoantibody associated with a propylthiouracil-induced adult respiratory distress-like syndrome: report of a case and review of the literature. Endocr Pract. 4:89-93.

66. **Reidy TJ, Upshaw JD, McChesney T.** 1982 Propylthiouracil-induced vasculitis: a fatal case. Southern Med J. 75:1297-1298.

67. **Griswold WR, Mendoza SA, Johnston W, Nichols S.** 1978 Vasculitis associated with propylthiouracil. Evidence for immune complex pathogenesis and response to therapy. Western J Med. 128:543-544.

68. **Gunton JE, Stiel J, Caterson RJ, McElduff A.** 1999 Anti-thyroid drugs and antineutrophil cytoplasmic antibody positive vasculitis. A case report and review of the literature. J Clin Endocrinol Metab. 84:13-16.

69. **Pillinger M, Staud R. 1998 Wegener's** granulomatosis in a patient receiving propylthiouracil for Graves' disease. Semin. Arthr. Rheum. 28:124-129.

70. **Bajaj S, Bell MJ, Shumak S, Briones-Urbina R.** 1998 Antithyroid arthritis syndrome. J Rheumatol. 1998 25:1235-1239.

11

RADIOIODINE THERAPY OF GRAVES' DISEASE

Milton D. Gross, John E. Freitas, James C. Sisson and B. Shapiro

INTRODUCTION

Over the past six decades radioiodine has played an important role in the diagnosis and therapy of Graves' disease. Early physiologic studies by Hamilton and Soley using [130]I and ^{131}I in 1940 were followed in 1941 by the first radioiodine therapy of Graves' hyperthyroidism by Hertz and Roberts (1,2). Since this first successful use, ^{131}I has now become the most common therapy for Graves' disease in adult patients in the United States (3). However, despite an extensive diagnostic and therapeutic experience in over 2 million patients of all ages and a demonstrable record of safety and efficacy many aspects of radioiodine therapy remain controversial and continue to generate lively debate concerning its use in the management of Graves' disease (4,5)(Table 1).

Table 1. Controversies in ^{131}I therapy of Grave's disease.

- What is the "best" therapy for Grave's disease (^{131}I, thyroidectomy, antithyroid drugs)?

- Who should be treated with [131]I?
    Women of child-bearing age (18 - 45 years)?
    Children?
    Adolescents?

- Should patients with Grave's disease be pre-treated with antithyroid drugs or ß-blockers prior to ^{131}I therapy? (in whom and for what duration?)

- What is the optimal method of dose estimation for ^{131}I therapy?

- What is the optimal dose vehicle for ^{131}I therapy (capsule vs. liquid)?

- Does ^{131}I therapy for Grave's disease exacerbate ophthalmopathy?

- Does ^{131}I therapy increase risk of malignancy (thyroid and extrathyroid), cause genetic defects in offspring or decrease fertility or increase mortality?

DIAGNOSIS

The classic presentation of Grave's disease includes: diffuse goiter, hyperthyroidism, ophthalmopathy and, in a minority of patients, pretibial myxedema and acropachy. However, with modern early diagnosis 50% of patients do not present with signs of infiltrative ophthalmopathy, pretibial myxedema or diffuse goiter. The hyperthyroidism of Grave's disease is confirmed by documentation of a suppressed serum thyroid stimulating hormone (TSH) (<0.05 mIU/L) and a elevated free thyroxine (free T4) and/or a free T3 to distinguish overt from subclinical disease (in which there is a normal free T4 and T3). Graves' disease is differentiated from other forms of thyrotoxicosis by clinical history and a Technetium (Tc99m) pertechnetate thyroid scan (5 min thyroid-salivary uptake estimate) or a ^{123}I or ^{131}I radioactive iodine uptake (RAIU) measurement of the percentage of administered radioiodine accumulated by the thyroid at 24 hours (Table 2). Patients with Graves' disease exhibit an elevated RAIU,

Table 2. Differential diagnosis of hyperthyroidism

- Grave's disease[*]

- Toxic multinodular goiter[*]

- Solitary thyroid nodule[*]

- Functional metastatic thyroid cancer[*+¶]

- Jod Basedow disease[†+]

- Factitious thyrotoxicosis[†+]

- Toxic struma ovarii[*+¶]

- Any form of hyperthyroidism following iodine exposure[†+]

- Subacute thyroiditis - painful granulomatosis[†+]

- Subacute thyroiditis – painless and postpartum[†+]

---

[*] potentially treatable with ^{131}I
[†] not suitable for ^{131}I therapy
[+] low neck 131I uptake (in case of iodine exposure uptake may rise after a suitable interval)
[¶] very rare

in contrast to subacute, postpartum or silent thyroiditis, Jod-Basedow's disease and thyrotoxicosis factitia all of which have decreased RAIU (< 5% in 24 hrs)(Figure 1). Patients with toxic nodular goiter may have normal or elevated RAIU with characteristic uni- or multinodular tracer accumulation on ^{99m}Tc pertechnetate, ^{123}I or

[131]I scans of the thyroid. Other laboratory tests can be used to exclude Grave's disease such as the serum thyroglobulin which is suppressed (<1.0 ng/ml) in thyrotoxicosis factitia (hyperthyroidism from surreptitious or inadvertent thyroid hormone ingestion) (6-9). The diagnosis of Grave's disease may be further confirmed by demonstration of the autoimmune pathogenesis by various assays of TSH-mimetic immunoglobulins.

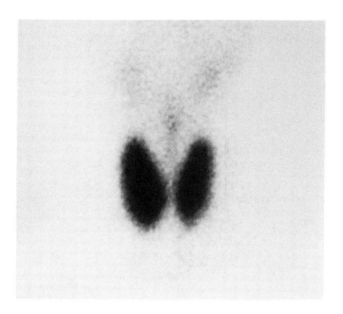

Figure 1. A Technetium-99m pertechnetate thyroid scan in a 42 year old woman with hyperthyroidism and a diffuse goiter estimated to weigh 40 grams. The scan depicts diffuse uptake (>60%) diagnostic of Grave's disease. Reproduced with permission; Freitas J.E. Quarterly J. Nucl. Med. 43:297-306, 1999.

MANAGEMENT

Although radioiodine has demonstrable efficacy and safety across the broad spectrum of patients to include a wide range of ages, both sexes and all degrees of severity of Grave's disease, patient preference must remain an important factor in the decision-making process that considers all available therapeutic options including antithyroid drugs (ATDs), surgery, and [131]I (7). Each has advantages and disadvantages and no one therapeutic option is unequivocally superior to the others for all patients with Graves' disease (Table 3).

Radioiodine is absolutely contraindicated in the treatment of Grave's disease in pregnant and breast-feeding patients. Women of child-bearing age are routinely asked to confirm that they are not pregnant or breast-feeding. When any uncertainty about the possibility of pregnancy arises, a sensitive pregnancy test (serum human chorionic gonadotropin) is mandatory. It is fortunate that when ^{131}I has been given inadvertently prior to 10-12 weeks of gestation (a time point before fetal thyroid iodine concentration occurs), no increase in fetal hypothyroidism or congenital malformations have been documented (8).

Table 3.   Alternative therapies for Grave's disease.

Therapy	Advantages	Disadvantages
Anti-thyroid drugs (> 1 year duration)	Permanent hypothyroidism is infrequent; if successful thyroid hormone replacement is avoided	After stopping treatment recurrence occurs in 50% or more of patients; toxicity in 3 to 4 %, serious side effects in 0.3 to 0.4%
Thyroidectomy	Effective with near total (98%) thyroidectomy; most rapid means of therapy for hyperthyroidism; relieves obstruction from large goiters	Hospitalization required; small risk to laryngeal nerves and parathyroid glands; post operative hypothyroidism is common with near total (98%) thyroidectomy
Radioiodine	Simplest therapy; optimally one dose is sufficient; outpatient therapy; no toxicity from radioiodine	Hypothyroidism is common; slow in action; improvement in 4 to 6 weeks; elimination of hyperthyroidism in 10 to 12 weeks

Modified and reproduced with permission from Sisson J.C. Treatment of Hyperthyroidism Section 2, in Principles of Nuclear Medicine 2nd Edition, Wagner NH, Szabo Z, Buchanan JW eds., W. B. Saunders, Philadelphia, 1995, pp 622.

After 12 weeks of gestation, however, radioiodine administration may be associated with fetal hypothyroidism (11). Furthermore, ^{131}I is actively secreted in breast milk for weeks after therapy and in nursing mothers resumption of breast-feeding after ^{131}I therapy is proscribed. Alternative therapies, either ATD or surgery are indicated for pregnant or breast-feeding patients with Grave's disease.

    Because of concerns about potential late, adverse radiation effects some therapists do not consider children and adolescents with Grave's disease for ^{131}I therapy and radioiodine treatment in this group of patients remains controversial (4). Long term follow-up evaluation of adolescents and children treated with ^{131}I has shown no increase in the incidence of leukemia, thyroid cancer, other malignancies or genetic abnormalities in their progeny (4,5). In 10 reported series (651 children), ATD therapy induced long term remission in 46.8% of patients, remission with subsequent relapse in 29%, and complications were reported in 17.8% (12). Failure to induce a remission was seen most often in children with large goiters, ophthalmopathy or markedly elevated serum thyroxine (> 20 ug/dl) or thyroglobulin (> 50 ng/ml) levels (12). Noncompliance and drug toxicity are common problems with ATD use in this group. In contrast, in 9 published series (555 children), thyroidectomy relieved hyperthyroidism in 90%, hypothyroidism was seen in 42%, and surgical complications occurred in 6.7% (12). Radioiodine (10 studies of 550 children) controlled hyperthyroidism in 98% (12% however required retreatment), with post-therapy hypothyroidism in 69% (12). Benign thyroid nodules were subsequently found in 4.4% of radioiodine treated patients which may be no more than the general population (12). Current American Thyroid Association and American Association of Clinical Endocrinologists treatment guidelines do not consider ^{131}I therapy to be contraindicated in children or adolescents (13,14). Despite these guidelines, most children continue to be treated initially with ATDs and are referred for subtotal or total thyroidectomy or ^{131}I therapy only after treatment failure (e.g. lack of remission or relapse)(4).

Although most patients with Graves' disease have evidence of ophthalmopathy (GO) when assessed by computed tomography (CT), clinically significant GO is present in only 10-25% of patients (15,16). The presence of GO is considered by some a relative contraindication to ^{131}I therapy because of concerns of further progression of ophthalmopathy after radioiodine (17). The relationship of GO progression to radioiodine therapy, its severity, significance and etiology is a subject of controversy (5). Worsening of GO following radioiodine must be considered with an understanding of the natural history of GO, a history of smoking and the presence of post-therapy hypothyroidism. In one series, 14% of patients had some degree of spontaneous worsening of their eye disease during one year of follow-up (18). Further, clinically significant GO is seen more frequently and is more severe in smokers than in non-smokers (19,20). Hypothyroidism following radioiodine therapy is also associated with progression of GO (21,22). Recent prospective studies have addressed the issue of whether ^{131}I causes exacerbation of Graves' ophthalmopathy (23,24). In a randomized study of the effect of radioiodine therapy upon the progression of GO (in which ^{131}I, ^{131}I and prednisone or methimazole were compared) ophthalmopathy progressed in 15% of ^{131}I treated patients, no progression was seen in the group treated with ^{131}I and prednisone, and progression was seen in 3 % of a methimazole-only treated group (24). Progression was more likely (24 % versus 8 %) in patients with pre-existing ophthalmopathy than in those with initially normal eye findings. Worsening of GO in ^{131}I treated patients was transient in two thirds and persistent in one third of patients. The degree of progression of GO is often only minor, but occasionally it may be severe. In the group with persistent GO, 87.5 % had findings of eye disease at presentation. It thus appears that radioiodine treatment may, in some patients, exacerbate GO within the first 1-5 months of therapy and is more likely to do so in those with pre-existing GO and a history of smoking. Corticosteroid therapy has been shown to prevent progression of GO when administered at the time of radioiodine therapy and a short time afterward. Further, control of hyperthyroidism is also important to prevent progression of GO and recurrent hyperthyroidism is less likely after ^{131}I than ATD therapy. Progressive ophthalmopathy is often associated with residual functioning thyroid tissues and this may be optimally treated with radioiodine ablation (25). At this time the data suggest that in smokers with active ophthalmopathy corticosteroids should be given in combination with radioiodine for therapy of Grave's disease.

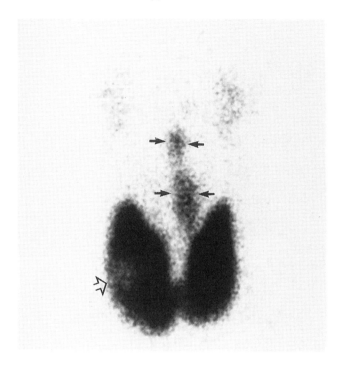

Figure 2. A Technetium-99m pertechnetate thyroid scan in a 47 year old man with hyperthyroidism and a goiter estimated to weigh 60 grams with a 2 cm nodule in the right lobe. The scan demonstrates diffuse increased uptake (>50%) and a pyramidal lobe (small arrows). A coincidental cold, colloid nodule (large arrow) is also depicted on the scan. Reproduced with permission; Freitas, JE. Quarterly J. Nucl. Med. 43:297-306, 1999.

Graves' disease can co-exist with a nodular goiter. Radionuclide thyroid scanning is useful to determine whether palpable nodularity in a patient with Grave's disease is cold (hypofunctioning) and to confirm the diagnosis (26)(Figure 2). When identified, cold nodules defined by thyroid scans should be evaluated by fine needle aspiration prior to radioiodine treatment to exclude the presence of concurrent thyroid cancer which appears to be more aggressive in Grave's disease than thyroid cancer in euthyroid patients (27). If the cytologic findings are suspicious or confirm malignancy, a surgical approach is the best choice for therapy of both conditions. In the presence of benign cytology, ^{131}I therapy is appropriate and will often result in a decrease or disappearance of thyroid nodule(s) after successful treatment of the Grave's disease.

In some patients, especially those with severe Grave's disease, the elderly with concomitant cardiovascular disease or other severe illnesses, may benefit from pre-treatment with ATDs to achieve initial control of thyrotoxicosis and to reduce the possibility of transient exacerbation of hyperthyroidism. Radioiodine therapy induces radiation thyroiditis and thus a release of preformed thyroid hormones within 1-2 weeks after therapy which may worsen the clinical status of some patients with Graves' disease. Furthermore, as the beneficial effects of ^{131}I on hyperthyroid symptoms are often delayed for at least 3-4 weeks, beta-blockade (propranolol; 40-160 mg/day or with a more cardio-selective blocker such as atenolol; 50-150 mg/day) can be used to reduce symptoms of uncontrolled hyperthyroidism and supplement the effects of the ATD therapy.

TREATMENT OF GRAVE'S DISEASE

Despite the proven efficacy and safety of radioiodine, thyroidologists continue to differ widely in their preference for therapy of Graves' disease based upon individual patient circumstances and local standards of care. Radioiodine is the preferred therapy of Grave's disease in approximately 70% of patients in the United States, but with considerable geographic variation and sex and age preference, while in Europe and Asia it is used much less frequently as initial therapy and is often restricted to patients older than 40 years (3,28). The costs of therapy vary from site to site, but ATD and ^{131}I therapies are roughly equivalent. Surgery (subtotal thyroidectomy) is approximately 4-fold more expensive than either ATD or [131]I (29).

Patient Preparation and Dose Selection

The majority of patients with Graves' disease can he treated with radioiodine without prior ATD therapy. However, opinions differ widely as to the value and necessity of ATD and for beta-blockade pre-treatment (30-32). Antithyroid drugs block thyroperoxidase-mediated iodination, reduce deiodinase-mediated intrathyroidal reuse of iodine, decrease intrathyroidal iodine stores and thus must be discontinued for at least 3 days prior to diagnostic studies to eliminate interference with 24 hour RAIU measurements. Similarly ATD therapy will prevent effective therapeutic radiation dose delivery without similar drug withdrawal. The decreased intrathyroidal iodine pool size induced by ATDs increases ^{131}I turnover, lowers effective ^{131}I half-life, reduces the effective radiation dose to the thyroid and significantly increases the failure rate of ^{131}I therapy (33,34). There also appear to be other, as yet unexplained, factors operative following ATD therapy which decrease the effectiveness of ^{131}I therapy even if the ATD exposure was remote.

Radioiodine (^{131}I) treats hyperthyroidism principally by beta particle irradiation of follicular cells, leading to acute organelle damage causing cellular necrosis (interphase cell death) and induction of sufficient irreversible deoxyribose nucleic acid (DNA) damage to the surviving thyroid cells to prevent cell division (replicative cell death). Long term follow-up studies indicate that regardless of the radiation absorbed dose or administered activity chosen for therapy, there is a high cumulative incidence of post-therapy hypothyroidism. It is unusual for a patient treated with radioiodine not to eventually require thyroid hormone replacement therapy, however, the quality of life in appropriately treated patients is no different from those free of thyroid disease

(10,35). Despite a clinical experience now amounting to many hundreds of thousands of patients treated with ^{131}I for Graves' disease, there is still no unanimity as to the selection of the appropriate dose of [131]I. Regardless of the method chosen to calculate the dose of administered radioiodine the radiation absorbed dose delivered to the thyroid gland is dependent on many factors including the RAIU, the effective half-life of ^{131}I in the gland and the volume of the gland. RAIU is a function of the size of the iodine pool and is influenced by dietary iodine intake. The iodine pool can be expanded (with a resultant reciprocal decrease in RAIU) by many factors including: administration of iodinated radiographic contrast media, kelp and other sea food ingestion and many drugs containing iodine (e.g. amiodarone). The effective half-life of ^{131}I can be estimated by serial measurements the neck performed over several days, but this procedure is usually not included in the routine pre-therapy evaluation of patients with Grave's disease.

Diagnostic ^{131}I thyroid uptake doses are often administered as a capsule while therapy doses may be given in liquid form. This is done because of a 3 to 4-fold greater cost of commercially supplied ^{131}I therapy capsules. However, it is important to recognize that a RAIU measurement performed after ingestion of a ^{131}I capsule may be lower than after a liquid dose (mean 44% versus 63%). Thus, patients treated with liquid ^{131}I doses calculated on the basis of RAIU-derived from ^{131}I administered in capsule form may receive a greater than intended radiation dose to the thyroid (36). Furthermore, the mean uptake of therapeutic doses tends to be less (absolute 8-15%) than diagnostic uptake measurements, most likely reflecting the radiation effects of the preceding diagnostic ^{131}I upon the accumulation of the therapy dose by the thyroid (i.e., thyroid stunning). In this situation the diagnostic dose fails to fulfill a major requirement for a tracer study, namely lack of a pharmacologic effect. Overall goiter size can be roughly estimated by palpation, but far more accurate determination by real-time ultrasound (RTUS), especially for large cervical and substernal goiters > 60 grams has been recommended (37,38). Volume also has been determines by CT, MRI, SPECT and PET. In the latter two methodologies the functional rather than anatomical volume is depicted.

Multiple therapeutic algorithms have been used to calculate therapy doses of [131]I. The most common dosing methods, their rationale and limitations are outlined in Table 4 (see also ref. 38). A direct relationship exists between the size of the administered dose of ^{131}I, the likelihood of cure of hyperthyroidism and the incidence of early permanent hypothyroidism. Regardless of the algorithm utilized, the majority of patients with Grave's disease become hypothyroid within 1-10 years of follow-up. Proponents of dosing protocols utilizing repetitive small doses of ^{131}I express the belief that postponing development of hypothyroidism for as long an interval as possible is a valuable goal even if control of hyperthyroidism requires months to achieve (39). The ablative approach is based upon the rapid elimination of hyperthyroidism for the majority of patients that justifies an increased incidence of radiation thyroiditis, a higher rate of hypothyroidism (often occurring within 12 weeks), and high radiation exposure for some patients as compared to other, more conventional approaches to radioiodine therapy (40,41). The other alternatives listed in Table 4 offer greater individualization of therapeutic doses. The sliding scale algorithm is designed to administer higher doses

Table 4. Comparison of ^{131}I dose schemes in thyrotoxicosis

Dose scheme	Therapy goals	Comments
Small fixed doses (2 -3 mCi) administered repeatedly as necessary	Minimize total radiation dose and incidence of hypothyroidism. Accepts need for repeated treatment	May require multiple doses and many months to control thyrotoxicosis
Largest possible outpatient dose (> 33 mCi in U.S.)	Prompt control of hyperthyroidism, minimize need for retreatment, high incidence of hypothyroidism	Early hypothyroidism in $\leq$ 12 weeks post thyroidectomy
Sliding scale*; 3 - 5 mCi for small glands; 7 -12 mCi for moderate size glands or moderate thyrotoxicosis; 20-30 mCi for large glands, severe thyrotoxicosis or thyrocardiac patients	Achieve prompt control of hyperthyroidism with a single dose of ^{131}I while limiting hypothyroidism	Some dose individualization with minimal effort
'First approximation dosimetry'* based on thyroid volume from palpation or ultrasound and single ^{131}I uptake (e.g., 100 - 200 mCi ^{131}I/gram retained in the thyroid at 24hours)	Prompt control of hyperthyroidism in majority of cases with a single dose while limiting the incidence of hypothyroidism	Dose individualization with minimal resource commitment
Higher precision dosimetry* (e.g., multiple ^{131}I uptake measurements, ^{124}I PET, ^{123}I SPECT; thyroid volume by ultrasound, CT or MRI	Prompt control of hyperthyroidism in majority of cases with single dose therapy while limiting incidence of hypothyroidism	Dose individualization with major commitment of resources

* Additional "fudge factors" may be assigned for age, cardiac disease, prior antithyroid drug therapy or pathology (e.g., toxic nodule or toxic multinodular goiter, presence of concomitant Hashimoto's thyroiditis). Modified and reproduced with permission J.

Nucl. Med. 1993; 34:1638-1641.

of ^{131}I radiation to larger goiters and a greater likelihood of cure, a benefit for patients with more severe Grave's disease and depending upon the uCi/gm dose selected, a larger proportion of patients can be controlled with a single dose of radioiodine (42). "First approximation" dosimetry is the most common therapeutic scheme employed. The selected desired dose per gram generally varies between 80-200 uCi retained at 24 hrs/gm with an additional 1-4 mCi of ^{131}I applied by some therapists for patients with a history of ATD pretreatment, pre-existing cardiac disease, multinodularity, severity of hyperthyroidism and advanced age.

Until recently the United States Nuclear Regulatory Commission (NRC) regulations required patients treated with > 30 mCi ^{131}I be hospitalized until the retained body burden fell below 30 mCi. In an effort to enhance the effect of administered ^{131}I, lithium carbonate, 900 mg in divided doses can be given for 3-4 days prior to radioiodine therapy and continued for 4-5 days thereafter to prolong radioiodine retention in the thyroid (43). The cure rate of hyperthyroidism with a single dose of radioiodine was 82%. Non-responders were retreated with higher doses of ^{131}I, 3-4 months later with an increase in cure rate to over 95% of patients (44). Greater precision in dosimetry requires more precise determinations of both thyroid volume by RTUS, CT or magnetic resonance imaging (MRI) and of effective ^{131}I half-life. Alternatively, thyroid volume and retained radioactivity can also be determined by ^{123}I single photon emission tomography (SPECT) or [124]I positron emission tomography (PET)(45). Determination of effective half-life is made from at least 3 measurements of RAIU typically at 24, 48, and 96 hours (33). When thyroid volume and effective ^{131}I half-life are known an appropriate dose of radioiodine can be administered to deliver a desired radiation absorbed dose (typically 7,000-30,000 rads). ATDs should not be resumed or initiated after therapy for at least several days to maximize the radiation effect of the administered [131]I (46).

POST ^{131}I THERAPY CONSIDERATIONS

In 1997 the Nuclear Regulatory Commission (NRC) release restrictions for outpatient radioiodine therapies in the United States were liberalized (47). The new guidelines provided for patient release after ^{131}I therapy when the radiation dose to members of the public are not likely to exceed 5 mSv (0.5 rem) in a year. In instances where the exposure to the public may exceed 1 mSv, written instructions concerning precautions must be provided to the patient explaining how to reduce radiation exposure to family members and the general public (Table 5). These regulatory changes now permit outpatient therapy for virtually all patients with Graves' disease, resulting in a reduction in health care costs. In contrast, radioiodine therapy is more stringently regulated in Europe where the maximal permissible dose to outpatients varies from 2 mCi (Germany), 5mCi (Switzerland, Austria, The Netherlands), 15 mCi (Poland, Finland, Greece, Hungary), 20 mCi (Belgium, France, United Kingdom), to 30 mCi (Italy) (48). However, in the year 2000 the emphasis of radiation protection will shift throughout the newly formed European Union from the dose administered to the patient to the restriction of radiation exposure to members of the public with a release threshold that will result in a maximal permissible dose no more than 1 mSv. The European Thyroid Association has provided recommendations for ^{131}I treated patients based upon this limit of 1 mSv, but direct dosimetry measurements on family members suggest that various degrees of isolation would he required to meet the 1 mSv standard (49). It is noteworthy that in those countries with restrictions that currently limit outpatient doses to < 5 mCi, the new regulations will allow more patients to be treated in an outpatient setting.

Table 5. Limiting ^{131}I radiation exposure to family and members of the general public.

Patient Instructions

For the first 3 days

- Avoid close contact with pregnant women and children.
- Restrict close proximity (e.g. 6 feet) to family members and other contacts
- Avoid mouth-to-mouth contact or sexual intercourse.
- Use separate eating utensils and wash them after each use. Do not share food or drink with anyone.
- Maintain good bathroom hygiene with proper disposal of all urine and stool. Avoid urine contamination. Flush the toilet 3 times after each use and rinse the sink after each use.
- Launder your clothing separately before reuse.

For the first 2 days

- Sleep alone in a separate room.
- Limit prolonged (> 2 hours) automobile trips with others.
- Do not travel by mass transportation (bus, train, airplane).

COMPLICATIONS AND POTENTIAL RISKS

The principal early side effects of ^{131}I therapy are acute radiation thyroiditis, exacerbation of thyrotoxicosis and progression of ophthalmopathy (4,5). Symptomatic radiation thyroiditis presents as anterior neck pain and swelling and is unusual with current doses of ^{131}I and is readily controlled with simple analgesics such as salicylates. In the majority of patients a radiation-induced release of stored thyroid hormone leading to a further elevation of free T4 levels is common, but usually clinically silent. More seriously ill patients can be protected by pretreatment with ATDs to deplete the intra-thyroidal hormone stores. ATDs can also be started early (5 to 7 days) after ^{131}I therapy to speed the control of hyperthyroidism. Progression of GO may occur, especially in those patients with signs of inflammatory or infiltrative disease at presentation. Corticosteroids (prednisone, 0.4 mg/kg/day) are recommended beginning within 3 days of ^{131}I therapy and continuing for 3-4 weeks with a rapid taper over 3 to 4 weeks (24). Progressive, severe GO in the face of corticosteroid therapy may warrant surgical intervention (i.e. orbital decompression) or orbital radiotherapy to control eye disease and preserve vision (50). Thyroid storm, transient hypocalcemia and hyper-parathyroidism have been reported after ^{131}I therapy, but are very uncommon (4,5).

Eventual hypothyroidism is an expected consequence of ^{131}I therapy for many patients with Graves' disease and can occur within a few weeks, months or years after treatment. Since permanent hypothyroidism eventually occurs in 5-20% of patients treated with ATDs, ^{131}I appears to exaggerate the natural history of Graves' disease (51). Higher doses of ^{131}I result in more frequent hypothyroidism earlier after therapy. Early post-therapy hypothyroidism is suggested by a rapid decrease in goiter size and patients should be alerted to typical symptoms (e.g. muscle cramps, cold intolerance, fatigue, constipation, and menorrhagia). The laboratory evaluation of the post ^{131}I therapy patient includes measurement of free T4 and serum TSH. The serum TSH may remain suppressed for 12-16 weeks post-^{131}I therapy despite falling or even subnormal free T4 levels and hypothyroid symptoms (52). Levothyroxine is administered at an initial replacement dose of 1.6 µg/kg of body weight for most adults unless a concomitant illnesses is present (e.g. cardiac), in which case a lower starting dose might be more prudent. Recently, combined regimens of T4 and T3 have been suggested as a means to more rapidly and completely return patients to a truly euthyroid state (53). Repeat measurements of free T4 and serum TSH measurements at 6 to 7 weeks following initiation of treatment can be used to assess the adequacy of thyroid hormone replacement. Patients with GO should be closely monitored and replacement therapy initiated as soon as free T4 levels begin to approach the lower range of normal as hypothyroidism is associated with progression of eye disease. After the first year after ^{131}I therapy, there is a steady 2-4% annual incidence of hypothyroidism in the remaining euthyroid patients (2,4,5).

A major controversy that persists is the concern of long-term risks associated with ^{131}I therapy in selected populations. The potential risks associated with ^{131}I therapy are carcinogenic effects including increased incidence of leukemia, increased long-term mortality, genetic effects and infertility. Available data demonstrates that none of these potential risks have been consistently demonstrated in the 60 years since ^{131}I has been used to treat Graves' disease. Neither has there been any definite evidence for increased risk of any cancer, leukemia, mortality from radioiodine therapy (54-57) or increased genetic risks or infertility (58,59).

SUMMARY

Radioiodine is a safe and effective therapy for the majority of patients with Graves' disease including children, adolescents and women of childbearing age. Prompt, consistent relief of hyperthyroidism with the development of hypothyroidism following a single dose are the expected consequences of successful ^{131}I therapy. Recent changes in U.S. NRC requirements have further liberalized the use of ^{131}I for Graves' disease, permitting more patients to be treated in an outpatient setting. The controversy concerning the role of ^{131}I in exacerbation of Grave's ophthalmopathy has been further clarified and effective preventive measures are available. Nevertheless, despite the large and growing body of evidence supporting the safety, efficacy and cost-effectiveness of ^{131}I therapy, controversy persists particularly in Europe and Asia in its use across the broad spectrum of patients with Grave's disease.

REFERENCES

10. **Hamilton JG, Soley MH.** 1939 Studies in iodine metabolism by the use of a new radioactive isotope of iodine. Am J Physiol. 126:P521-522
11. **Sawin CT, Becker DV.** 1997 Radioiodine and the treatment of hyperthyroidism: The early history. Thyroid 7:163-176
12. **Wartofsky L, Glinoer D, Solomon B, Nagataki S, LaGasse R, Nagayama Y, Izumi M.** 1991 Differences and similarities in the diagnosis and treatment of Graves' disease in Europe, Japan, and the United States. Thyroid 1:129-135
13. **Rivkees SA, Sklar C, Freemark M.** 1998 The management of Grave's disease in children, with special emphasis on radioiodine treatment. J. Clin. Endocrinol. Metab. 83: 3767-3776.
14. **Leech NJ, Dayan CM.** 1998 Controversies in the management of Grave's disease. Clin Endocrinol. 49: 273-280.
15. **Mariotti S, Martino E, Cupini C, et al.** 1982 Low serum thyroglobulin as a clue to the diagnosis of thyrotoxicosis factitia. N Engl J Med. 307:410-414
16. **Dabon-Almirante C, Surks MI.** 1998 Clinical and laboratory diagnosis of thyrotoxicosis. Endocrinol Metab Clin North Am. 27:25-35.
17. **Siegel RD, Lee SL.** 1998 Toxic nodular goiter: Toxic adenoma and toxic multinodular goiter. Endocrinol Metab Clin North Am. 27:151-168.
18. **Ross DS.** 1998 Syndromes of thyrotoxicosis with low radioactive iodine uptake. Endocrinol Metab Clin North Am. 27:169-185.
10. **Ljunggren J-G, Torring O, Wallin G, Taube A, Tallstedt L, Hamberger B, Lundell G.** 1998 Quality of life aspects and costs in treatment of Grave's hyperthyroidism with antithyroid drugs, surgery or radioiodine: results from a prospective, randomized study. Thyroid 8: 653-659.
11. **Stoffer SS, Hamburger JI.** 1976 Inadvertent I-131 therapy for hyperthyroidism in the first trimester of pregnancy. J Nucl Med. 17:146-149
12. **Zimmerman D, Lteif AN.** 1998 Thyrotoxicosis in children. Endocrinol Metab Clin North Am. 27:109-126.
13. **Garcia M, Baskin HJ, Feld S.** 1995 AACE clinical practice guidelines for the evaluation and treatment of hyperthyroidism. and hypothyroidism. Endocr Pract. 1:54-62
14. **Singer PA, Cooper DS, Levy EG, Landenson PW, Braverman LE, Daniels G, et al.** 1995 Treatment guidelines for patient with hyperthyroidism and hypothyroidism. JAMA. 273:808-812
15. **Forbes G, Gorman CA, Brennan MD, Gehring DG, Ilstrup DM, Earnest F 4th.** 1986 Ophthalmopathy of Graves' disease: computerized volume measurements of the orbital fat and muscle. Am J Neuroradiol. 7:651-656
16. **Burch HB, Wartofsky L.** 1993 Graves' ophthalmopathy: current concepts regarding pathogenesis and management. Endocr Rev. 14:747-793
17. **Degroot LJ, Gorman CA, Pinchera A, Bartelena L, Maroci C, Wiersinga WM, Prummel MF, Wartofsky L.** 1995 Therapeutic controversy. Radiation and Grave's ophthalmopathy J. Clin. Endocrinol. Metab. 80: 339-349.

18. **Perros P, Crombie AL, Kendall-Taylor P.** 1995 Natural history of thyroid associated ophthalmopathy. Clin Endocrinol. 42:45-50

19. Prummel MF, Wiersinga WM. 1993 Smoking and the risk of Graves' disease. JAMA 269:479-482

20. **Bartalena L, Bogazzi F, Tanda ML, Manetti L, Dell'Unto E, Martino E.** 1995 Cigarette smoking and the thyroid. Eur J Endocrinol. 133:507-512

21. **Tallstedt L, Lundell G, Blomgren H, Bring J.** 1994 Does early administration of thyroxine reduce the development of Graves' ophthalmopathy after radioiodine treatment? Eur J Endocrinol. 130:494-497

22. **Kung AW, Yau CC, Cheng A**. 1994 The incidence of ophthalmopathy after radioiodine therapy for Graves' disease; prognostic factors and the role of methimazole. J Clin Endocrinol Metab. 79:542-546

23. **Manso PG, Furlanetto RP, Wolosker AM, Paiva ER, de Abreu MT, Maciel RM.** 1998 Prospective and controlled study of ophthalmopathy after radioiodine therapy for Graves' hyperthyroidism. Thyroid 8;49-52

24. **Bartalena L, Marcocci C, Bogazzi F, Manetti L, Tanda ML, Dell 'Unto E, et al.** 1998 Relation between therapy for hyperthyroidism and the course of Graves' ophthalmopathy. N Engl J Med. 338:73-78

25. **DeGroot Q**. 1997 Radioiodine and the immune system. Thyroid 7:259-264

26. **Ripley S, Freitas JE.** 1984 Is thyroid scintigraphy necessary before I-131 therapy for hyperthyroidism? Concise Communication. J Nucl Med. 25:664-667

27. **Pellegriti G, Belfiore A, Giuffrida D, Lupo L, Vigneri R.** 1998 Outcome of differentiated thyroid cancer in Grave's patients. J. Clin. Endocrinol. Metab. 83:2805-2809

28. **Romaldini JH.** 1997 Case selection and restrictions recommended to patient with hyperthyroidism. in South America. Thyroid 7:225-228

29. **Levatan C, Wartofsky L.** 1995 A clinical guide to the management of Graves' disease with radioactive iodine. Endocr Pract. 1:205-212

30. **Franklyn JA.** 1994 The management of hyperthyroidism. N Engl J Med. 130:1731-1738

31. **Wartofsky L.** 1997 Radioiodine therapy for Graves' disease: Case selection and restrictions recommended to patients in North America. Thyroid 7:213-216

32. **Mechanick JI, Davies TF.** 1997 Medical management of hyperthyroidism: Theoretical and practical aspects. In Thyroid Disease, second edition, Falk SA, editor, Lippincott-Raven, Philadelphia, pp 253-296.

33. **Berg GEB, Annika MMK, Holmberg ECV, Fink M**. 1996 Iodine-131 treatment of hyperthyroidism: significance of effective half-life measurements. J Nucl Med. 37:228-232

34. **Tuttle RM, Patience T, Budd S**. 1995 Treatment with propylthiouracil before radioactive iodine therapy is associated with a higher treatment failure rate than therapy with radioactive iodine alone in Graves' disease. Thyroid 5:243-247.

35. **Peterson K, Bengtsson C, Lapidus L, Lindstedt G, Nystrom E**. 1990 Morbidity, mortality, and quality of life for patients treated with levothyroxine. Arch Inter Med. 150:2077-2081

36. **Rini JN, Vallabhajosua S, Zanzonico P, Hurley JR, Becker DV, Goldsmith SJ.** 1999 Thyroid uptake of liquid versus capsule ^{131}I tracers in hyperthyroid patients treated with liquid ^{131}I. Thyroid 9:347-352

37. **Wesche MFT, Teil-v.Buul MM, Smits NJ, Wiersinga WM.** 1998 Ultrasonographic versus scintigraphic measurement of thyroid volume in patients referred for ^{131}I therapy. Nucl Med Commun. 19:341-346.

37. **Shapiro B. 1993** Optimization of radioiodine therapy of thyrotoxicosis: what have we learned after 50 years? J Nucl Med. 34:1638-1641

38. **Flower M, Al-Saadi A, Harmer V, McCready R, Ott R.** 1994 Dose-response study on thyrotoxic patients undergoing positron emission tomography and radioiodine therapy. Eur

J Nucl Med. 21:531-536

39. **Safa AM, Skillern PG.** 1975 Treatment of hyperthyroidism with a large initial dose of sodium iodide 1-13 1. Arch Intern Med. 135:673-675

40. **Wise PH, Ahmad A, Burnet RB, Harding PE.** 1975 Intentional radioiodine ablation of Graves' disease. Lancet 2:1231-1232

41. **Sridama V, McCormick M, Kaplan EL, Fauchet R, DeGroot L.** 1984 Long-term follow-up study of compensated low dose I-131 therapy for Graves' disease. N Engl J Med. 311:426-432

43. **Bogazzi F, Bartelena L, Brogioni S, Scarcello G, Burelli A, Campomori A, Manetti L, Rosi G, Pinchera A, Martino E.** 1999 Comparison of radioiodine with radioiodine plus lithium in the treatment of Grave's hyperthyroidism. J. Clin. Endocrinol. Metab. 84: 499-503

44. **Kaplan MM, Meier DA, Dworkin HJ.** 1998 Treatment of hyperthyroidism with radioactive iodine. Endocr Metab Clin North Am. 27:205-223

45. **Crawford DC, Flower MA, Pratt BE, Hill C, Zweit J, McCready R, Harmer CL.** 1997 Thyroid volume measurement in thyrotoxic patients: comparison between ultrasonography and iodine-124 positron emission tomography. Eur J Nucl Med. 24: 1470-1478.

46. **Velkeniers B, Vanhaelst L, Cytryn R, Jockheer NM.** 1988 Treatment of hyperthyroidism with radioiodine: adjunctive therapy with antithyroid drugs reconsidered. Lancet 1:1127-1129

47. **US Nuclear Regulatory Commission.** 1997 1997 criteria for release of individuals administered radioactive materials. Federal Register 62:4120

48. **Beckers C.** 1997 Regulations and policies on radioiodine I-131 therapy in Europe. Thyroid 7;7:221-224

49. **Monsieurs M, Thierens H, Dierckx RA, Casier K De Baere E, De Ridder L, et al.** 1998 Real-life radiation burden to relatives of patients treated with Iodine-131. a study in eight centres in Flanders (Belgium). Eur J Nucl Med. 25:1368-1376.

50. **Gladstone GJ.** 1998 Ophthalmologic aspects of thyroid-related orbitopathy. Endocrinol Metab Clin North Am. 27:91-100

51. **Cooper DS.** 1998 Antithyroid drugs for the treatment of hyperthyroidism. Endocrinol Metab Clin North Am. 27:225-248

52. **Uy HL, Reasner CA, Samuels MH.** 1995 Pattern of recovery of the hypothalamic-pituitary-thyroid axis following radioactive iodine therapy in patients with Graves' disease. Am J Med. 99:173-179

53. **Bunevicius R, Kazanavicius G, Zalinkevicius R, Prange AJ.** 1999 Effects of thyroxine as compared with thyroxine and triiodothyronine in patients with hypothyroidism. N Engl J Med. 340: 424-429.

54. **Holm L-E, Dahlqvist 1, Israelsson A, Lundell G.** 1980 Malignant thyroid tumors after iodine-131 therapy. N Engl J Med. 303:188-191

55. **Holm L-E, Hall P, Wiklund K, Lundell G, Berg G, Bjelkengren G, et al.** 1991 Cancer risk after iodine-131 therapy for hyperthyroidism. J Natl Cancer Inst. 83:1072-1077

56. **Graham GD, Burman KD.** 1986 Radioiodine treatment of Graves' disease. An assessment of potential risks. Ann Intern Med. 105:900-905

57. **Hall P, Holm L-E.** 1997 Late consequences of radioiodine for diagnosis and therapy in Sweden. Thyroid 7:205-208

58. **Freitas JE, Swanson DP, Gross MD, Sisson JC.** 1979 Iodine I-131: Optimal therapy for hyperthyroidism in children and adolescents? J Nucl Med. 20:847-850

59. **Hamburger JI.** 1985 Management of hyperthyroidism in children and adolescents. J Clin Endocrinol Metab. 60:1019-1024

12

SURGICAL THERAPY OF GRAVES' DISEASE

Osamah Alsanea and Orlo H. Clark

INTRODUCTION

Despite major advances in molecular biology, the etiology of Graves' disease remains unknown and the treatment of Graves' disease is best described as empirical. Until a better understanding is achieved of the genetic or triggering events that result in autoimmune stimulation of the thyroid gland, physicians have to choose among imperfect treatment methods (1). In a survey of physicians at the American Thyroid Association, with a limited number of surgeons participating, only one percent chose surgery as a first treatment option for diffuse toxic goiter or Graves' disease (2). More than two thirds elected radioablation as the preferred method of treatment for their patients. Medical treatment with antithyroid drugs was reserved for the patient with a small goiter, and mild to moderate hyperthyroidism in the absence of high antibody titers; or in cases where radioablation could not be used. One might think that for patients with Graves' disease, surgery should be reserved for those patients who are no longer candidates for medical or radioablative treatment methods. A better understanding of the advantages and disadvantages of current surgical techniques employed in the treatment of Graves' disease would assist in the choice of the best selective treatment in Graves' disease.

HISTORICAL BACKGROUND

Caleb Hillier Parry (3,4) a physician in Bath, England was the first physician to report 8 patients with diffuse toxic goiter in 1786. His report was published after his death in 1825. In 1835, Robert James Graves' of the Meath Hospital in Dublin reported 6 pregnant patients who suffered from diffuse toxic goiter (5,6); hence the name given to the disease in the British Commonwealth and in the United States (7). During the same period, Carl A. Von Basedow of Merseburg, Germany described the disease in three females and his name was applied to the disease in Europe (8,9). Many physicians know the disease as Graves'-Basedow disease but that needs to be differentiated from Jod-Basedow which is hyperthyroidism as a result of excessive iodine intake usually in individuals with goiters.

Theodore Billroth, of Zurich and Vienna, was one of the first surgeons to treat a relatively large number of patients with thyroid disorders. His initial experience of 36 patients between 1860 and 1876 resulted in 16 deaths (36%) mostly as a result of sepsis.

The mortality rate decreased to 8% in 48 of his patients between 1877 and 1881 as a result of introducing antisepsis (10-12). Many consider Theodore Kocher to be the father of thyroid surgery (13,14). His operative mortality rate decreased from an initial 13% between 1872 and 1882 to an overall 0.5% between 1872 to 1917. More than 5000 thyroidectomies were performed in his unit in Berne Switzerland. Kocher was awarded the Nobel prize for his work on the physiology, pathology and surgery of the thyroid gland in 1909 (15).

Thyroid surgery represented the ultimate technical challenge to surgeons in the United States and Europe (16). The skill of surgeons like William Halsted of John Hopkins University, Charles H. and William J. Mayo of the Mayo clinic (17), George W. Crile of Cleveland, Frank H. Lahey of Boston and numerous others in dealing with a friable very vascular gland gained them their reputation as excellent surgeons (18). Their writings remain the principles of modern thyroid surgery (19).

PATHOPHYSIOLOGY

The etiology of Graves' disease remains to be elucidated. It is an autoimmune disorder of the thyroid gland (20). Antibodies against thyroperoxidase contribute to the lymphocyte infiltration of the gland (21). Thyroid stimulating antibodies (TSAb) induce cellular processes resulting in increased cyclic AMP levels, which in turn increase transcription and translation of thyroglobulin and thyroid peroxidase. Tri-iodothyronine and thyroxine are over produced and TSH receptor transcription is downregulated (22).

The association between TSAb titer and thyroid activity or recurrent hyperthyroidism has been debated for many years. A recent meta-analysis of 18 studies concluded that there is no evidence to support the role of these antibodies in predicting disease recurrence (23). This meta-analytic review was criticized for not considering the quality of the various assays used in the individual studies and absence of subgroup analysis such as in those with high antibody titers. Some physicians, however, believe that TSAb titers are sensitive markers for relapse with sensitivity approaching 90%. However, the positive predictive value of this test has not been shown to exceed the predictive value of other variables such as patient age, size of goiter and degree of ophthalmopathy. The cost of the test is probably not justified in the era of managed care since only a minority of patients benefit from it (24).

TSAb titers decrease dramatically after total thyroidectomy. Also recurrent or worsening ophthalmopathy is unlikely after total thyroidectomy as opposed to a 25% risk in patients who continue to have detectable antibodies following subtotal thyroidectomy (25,26).

Genetic susceptibility

Many hormonal disorders have been associated with HLA haplotypes, including Graves' disease. Supported by evidence from twin studies for polygenic inheritance in Graves' disease, recent work has focused on identifying the gene(s) responsible for this disease using linkage analysis (27). The thyrotropin receptor gene plays a minor role, if any, in susceptibility to Graves' disease (28). A polymorphism in the CTLA4 gene located on chromosome 2q33 is reported to be associated with susceptibility to Graves' disease (29-31). Recent work has revealed major loci at 14 q31 (termed GD-1) and at 20q11.2 that are linked to Graves' disease (32,33). The 14q31 locus is close to the recently identified multinodular goiter-1 locus. Preliminary work documented a locus on Xq21.33-22 linked to Graves' disease that may help explain the female predisposition to this disease. These data needs to be confirmed (34). It would also be interesting to know whether a particular gene is associated with aggressive thyroid cancer in Graves' disease patients.

PREOPERATIVE EVALUATION AND MANAGEMENT

Clinical presentation

Graves' disease primarily affects women (F:M 7-10:1). It is a disease of the childbearing age mostly around the 3rd or 4th decade of life. Patients' symptoms may wax and wane resulting from changes in the levels of circulating antibodies. Eventually, some patients with Graves' disease develop spontaneous hypothyroidism (35,36). Typical manifestations of Graves' disease include weight loss with a preserved appetite, heat intolerance, nervousness, anxiety, insomnia, proximal muscle weakness, fatigue, tremor, palpitation, increased frequency of bowel movements, and decreased menstrual flow. Many patients have a diffuse non tender goiter although some patients, especially elderly, have no goiter. Typical signs include hyperactivity, tachycardia, or atrial fibrillation, systolic hypertension, hyperreflexia, lid lag and lid retraction. The Marine-Lenhart syndrome is a variant of Graves' disease of surgical importance. Characterized by one or more nodules in a diffusely enlarged, overfunctioning gland, it occurs in up to 4.3% of patients with hyperthyroidism (37,38).

Laboratory and radiological evaluation

Documented elevated thyroid hormone levels and a depressed TSH level is the basis for the biochemical diagnosis of hyperthyroidism in clinically suspected individuals. Important tests that should not be overlooked in selected patients include:

1.   A pregnancy test in young woman before ^{131}I treatment is administered.
2.   Ultrasonography to evaluate palpable nodules (39,40).
3.   Fine needle aspiration for patients with solitary localized nodules in a Graves' gland or Marine-Lenhart disease to exclude malignancy (37,41).
4.   MRI imaging of the pituitary when TSH secreting pituitary tumor is suspected (42-44). A radioiodine body scan or computed tomography of the abdomen and pelvis to exclude a solid ovarian teratoma with toxic thyroid tissue (struma ovarii)(45), or an ultrasound examination to confirm an hCG/TSH secreting tumor of trophoblastic origin (46-48).

Medical preparation for surgery

Astwood first described thionamide medical therapy for hyperthyroidism in 1943 (49,50,51). Most clinicians recommend antithyroid medications to prepare patients for other treatments, as well for patients with T3 thyrotoxicosis, pregnant patients, those with a small goiter of short duration and with a low TSAb titer, or those who refuse other modalities of therapy. Antithyroid medications are likely to fail in young patients, those with large goiters, or those with high levels of thyroid hormones or high antibody titers (52,53). Early signs of remission include a reduction in goiter size, normalization of thyroid function tests and disappearance of TSH receptor antibodies (54,55).

The incidence of relapse correlates with the underlying disease process and duration of therapy, ranging from 87% after 3 months to 24% after 4 years of treatment (56). Despite its limited role in definitive therapy, medical treatment remains, in some studies, a valuable means of preparing patients for any form of thyroablative treatment. Understanding some of the differences between the different medications will help physicians in preparing their patients for definitive therapy (57). Thionamide medications can be associated with life threatening complications such as agranulocytosis or hepatic dysfunction (58). Fortunately, these complications are uncommon, but patients who develop fever or sore throat while taking propylthiouracil (PTU) or methimazole must immediately stop his or her medication pending a white blood count (59).

Thionamides

These drugs, which inhibit thyroperoxidase and prevent oxidation of iodine and iodotyrosine coupling, have a latency period of 2 to 6 weeks. Side effects occur in 3-7 % of patients, 0.1- 0.4% of these, such as agranulocytosis, being potentially life threatening. Endocrinologists prefer PTU to methimazole by a ratio of 3:1 because it has the added advantage of blocking peripheral conversion of T4 to T3. PTU is usually given as 100 to 300 mg in 3 to 4 doses, whereas methimazole is given as 10 to 30 mg in three doses initially. Once the patient becomes euthyroid, methimazole can be given once daily (55,60,61).

Iodide

Iodides transiently inhibit iodide organification and inhibit hormone release. They should be used for only 2 to 3 weeks prior to thyroidectomy because of loss of subsequent efficacy. Iodide is valuable for the emergency treatment of patients in thyroid storm (62) or for preparation for thyroidectomy. Iodides cause involution of the goiter, and probably decrease thyroid vascularity (63,64). They can be given either as Lugol's iodine solution, 3 drops in 2 doses (6mg iodine/ drop) or as SSKI (saturated solution of potassium iodide) given as 360 mg divided in 2 daily doses.

Beta-adrenergic blockers (Propranolol)

These drugs suppress the exaggerated sympathetic response and decrease peripheral conversion of T4 to T3 (65). Propranolol has been reported, like iodide, to decrease thyroid gland vascularity and therefore may make thyroid operations easier. The goal of treatment with beta blockers is to reduce the heart rate below 100 per minute. Propranolol is also useful in patients with uncontrolled hyperthyroidism; following 131I to relieve symptoms of hyperthyroidism; for patients in crises or with severe cardiac disease and for the preoperative preparation for elective or urgent surgery (66,67). It is given as 40 to 160 mg divided into 4 doses and titrated to abolish the sympathetic manifestations. Some patients may need doses as high as 320 mg per day. It should be started 1-2 days before surgery and continued for three days postoperatively because thyroxine has a 7 day half-life. When this regimen was used in 334 patients, none developed a perioperative crisis (68). Beta-blockers are contraindicated in patients with congestive heart disease and bronchospastic disorders, and should be avoided in pregnancy. Long lasting beta blockers may be preferable in patients prone to nausea and vomiting.

It is customary to use these medications in combination when preparing a patient for surgery depending on urgency of the condition, control of symptoms, compliance and contraindications of different medications. Commonly utilized combinations are (in order of popularity):

1. PTU- iodide- propranolol.
2. Iodide- propranolol.
3. Propranolol
4. PTU- iodide.
5. Iodide
6. PTU.

We do not recommend using iodide or propranolol alone (69) because when used together for 10 days thyroid function usually returns to normal (70).

SURGERY

Many surgical techniques have been recommended for patients with Graves' disease and can be grouped under three categories:

1. Subtotal bilateral thyroidectomy with or without ligation of the inferior thyroid arteries leaving 2-4 g of tissue on either side.
2. Hartley-Dunhill (71,72) procedure; namely, unilateral total lobectomy leaving 4-6 g on the contralateral side. We prefer this technique because we can leave a bigger remnant on one side. Management of recurrent disease is easier and safer because only one side needs to be explored.
3. Total thyroidectomy when the desired goal is to prevent any chance of persistent or recurrent disease.

The last approach is the preferred treatment in patients with evidence of coexisting malignancy; and probably in patients with severe exophthalmos or in those patients who have had severe complications from their antithyroid medications (73). Most surgeons recommend not ligating the inferior thyroid artery as it might decrease the blood flow to the parathyroid glands although there is no data to suggest it is detrimental. Total thyroidectomy probably represents minimal increased risk of complications versus subtotal thyroidectomy, but it avoids the possibility of relapse of hyperthyroidism (26, 74). Hence if the goal of surgery is to avoid recurrence, then this is the best alternative while if the aim was to achieve euthyroidism (74) then subtotal thyroidectomy becomes the procedure of choice. One must therefore balance a higher incidence of recurrence against a 100% risk of hypothyroidism (75).

During thyroid operations, it is advisable to autotransplant any parathyroid that is considered to have inadequate blood supply. This is usually done by placing 1 mm^3 pieces into the ipsilateral sternocleidomastoid muscle. The complication rate of thyroid operations depends upon the experience of the surgeon (76). Serious complications can include hypoparathyroidism (0-1%), recurrent laryngeal nerve injury (0-4%) and hematoma (0-1%). The overall complication rate including hematoma, keloid, and infection should be less than 2% (77).

As already mentioned recurrent or persistent hyperthyroidism and permanent hypothyroidism have an inverse correlation primarily related to remnant size. Other less important factors include degree of lymphocyte infiltration, fibrous stroma, and antibody titer.

Following subtotal thyroidectomy, most series report permanent hypothyroidism in as many as one third of their patients and recurrence ranging between 1.3- 18 % (78- 82). Postoperative hypothyroidism occurred in 31-36 % at 5 years if the remnant size was between 5 and 7 g. When a more extensive subtotal lobectomy was performed leaving less than 4 g on one side, hypothyroidism developed in 75% within 4-5 months of surgery and the recurrence rate was about 10% (83). Several surgeons, therefore, recommend total thyroidectomy as the method of choice since it avoids the risk of recurrence (78). We are reluctant to recommend total thyroidectomy for all patients with Graves' disease and use it selectively for patients with severe ophthalmopathy, serious allergies, coexisting thyroid cancers, and at patient request. In children, a smaller remnant must be left (2-3 g) as recurrence is more common.

Recent retrospective and prospective studies from Europe emphasize the importance of surgery as an excellent option in the management of difficult cases of Graves' disease, in fact, some clinicians recommended it as the initial treatment of choice for most patients who present with Graves' disease (26,84).

CLINICAL ISSUES RELATED TO SURGERY

Role of radioiodine in surgically treated patients

Hertz at Harvard University and Robert at the Massachusetts Institute of Technology first described ^{131}I ablative therapy in 1946 (85). Treatment with ^{131}I is safe and is reported to be less expensive than surgery in most but not all studies (86). It has become the mainstay of therapy for most patients with the exception of women who wish to become pregnant immediately following control of hyperthyroidism, women who are pregnant or breast feeding; those with coexisting thyroid nodules, and those who refuse ^{131}I for the fear of its potential mutagenicity (87-89). Patients with very large glands and with low radioiodine uptakes are probably best treated with thyroidectomy. [131]I is usually preferred in managing post operative recurrence given the likelihood that reoperation is associated with a higher complication rate and further recurrence of disease unless the entire thyroid gland is removed (90). One reason why we recommend the Hartley-Dunhill procedure is because if hyperthyroidism recurs, only one side of the neck needs to be explored to correct the hyperthyroidism. Hence those patients who are opposed to radioablation can be safely reoperated upon with only one recurrent laryngeal nerve and two parathyroid glands at risk. Several factors need to be emphasized before administering ^{131}I for therapy:-

1.   There is a 6 week to 6 month latency before treatment is effective.
2.   Need for pre-^{131}I treatment (usually a beta-blocker) till patient is euthyroid to avoid a postoperative arrhythmia and possible death.
3.   Some patients may require more than one treatment and others may refuse ^{131}I therapy.
4.   Benign thyroid tumors are more common after ^{131}I treatment (91-93).
5.   Ophthalmopathy progresses more commonly after ^{131}I than after thyroidectomy. Recent studies suggest, however, that when patients were given glucocorticoids and thyroid hormone to correct hypothyroidism, their ophthalmopathy did not progress versus controls (94,95).
6.   Women in childbearing age need to use birth control for 6 to 12 months after ^{131}I treatment. There is no evidence, however, to suggest a significant increase in birth defects or cancer risk in patients or their subsequent offspring (96).
7.   Several recent reports document an increase in mortality in patients treated with ^{131}I compared to untreated individuals living in the same area. It is unclear, however, whether such reports reflect the failure to control the disease or susceptibility to other disorders because most of the deaths were related to cardiac and cerebrovascular disorders as well as fractures (97-99).
8.   When thyroid cancers develop in patients who have been treated with ^{131}I for Graves' disease, the tumors are more aggressive (92).
9.   Hypothyroidism is an inevitable end result. Studies show that it will be impossible to modify ^{131}I therapy in a way to achieve both early control of hyperthyroidism and a low incidence of hypothyroidism. With surgical treatment, the operation can be tailored to suit the patient's condition and request (100,101).

Effect of surgery on ophthalmic Graves' disease

Total thyroidectomy appears to be very effective in controlling and sometimes reversing the eye manifestations of the disease in some patients (102). Ultimately, it cannot be over emphasized that the best treatment should focus on achieving the euthyroid state with or without hormone replacement since both hypothyroidism and recurrent hyperthyroidism aggravate ophthalmopathy (103).

Role of surgery in pregnant patients

The ideal treatment is to render the patient euthyroid with the lowest dose of thionamides because these drugs cross the placenta (104). Propranolol can be used transiently to control hyperthyroid symptoms (105). Subtotal thyroidectomy during the second trimester of pregnancy is indicated in patients who require high doses of thionamides or who have developed significant side effects from their antithyroid medications. Under treatment or suboptimal treatment of Graves' disease can cause premature labor (106). Hormonal treatment with thyroxine should be continued postoperatively to prevent maternal hypothyroidism (107). Radioiodine should never be used during pregnancy.

Surgery is indicated in juvenile Graves' disease

Neonatal hypothyroidism results from transplacental passage of TSH receptor autoantibodies from mother to infant. Antibody levels may remain elevated in infants for a few months. Infants with hyperthyroidism should be treated with antithyroid medications (108).

Graves' disease also occurs in children, usually in 11 to 16 year old females. Treatment is either with antithyroid medications or with subtotal thyroidectomy. Radioiodine should be avoided unless both former treatments have failed to control the disease. In children, as mentioned previously, a smaller thyroid remnant should be left because recurrence is more common. In a recent study of 232 adolescents, subtotal thyroidectomy was the best treatment with a 6.5% incidence of recurrence; 87% needed thyroxine to normalize serum TSH levels (109). The surgeons purposefully left very small remnants to prevent recurrence. The remnant size was determined by the amount of tissue needed to preserve the parathyroid glands rather than by estimation of residual tissue. Interestingly, 3 patients had occult thyroid malignancy, two of whom had metastasis to the lymph nodes (110,111).

Thyroid storm

As a result of better treatment and earlier disease recognition, thyroid storm has become a very rare entity. It should be suspected in patients who present with hyperthyroidism and central nervous system depression or agitation, cardiovascular dysfunction, fever and tachycardia > 130. It is a life threatening condition that requires immediate treatment in an intensive care unit. The caring physician should look for a precipitating factor such as an infection (112). Usual factors that precipitate thyroid storm are infections, trauma including operations and other factors causing stress (62,113). Treatment consists of:-

1.   Lugol's iodide orally or sodium ipodate (500 mg twice daily)(114) to block iodide uptake and, more importantly, release of hormone from the gland.
2.   Treatment of a precipitating cause, such as draining an abscess.
3.   Oxygen administration.
4.   PTU as a 600 mg initial dose followed by 200 mg every 6 hours.
5.   Hydrocortisone (decreases conversion of T4 to T3 and prevents adrenal exhaustion).
6.   Rapid cooling with ice packs.
7.   Thorazine, not aspirin, to prevent shivering (aspirin increases free thyroid hormone levels).

The above treatment along with supportive care has been shown to reduce mortality from nearly 100% to less than 10%.

Graves' disease and malignancy

TSH is one of the most important factors promoting normal thyroid tissue growth. Furthermore, TSH stimulates iodide transport, adenylate cyclase and growth of malignant thyroid cells. These reasons are the basis for post-operative TSH suppression with thyroxine in patients with thyroid cancer. In vitro, both TSH and TSAb increase cyclic AMP production in normal and neoplastic thyroid cells. It is, therefore, not surprising that TSAb is reported to promote the growth of coexistent thyroid cancer in patients with Graves' disease and to increase the aggressiveness of the tumor (115). Support for this concept is the observation of a positive correlation between the aggressiveness of thyroid cancer and the antibody titer in some, but not all, reports (116,117).

The relationship between Graves' disease and thyroid cancer is controversial. A review of seven reports between 1951 to 1986 showed an average cancer incidence of 0.06 % ranging up to 8.7 % (118). Such a difference is probably the result of selection bias, patient age, the extent of surgical treatment and thoroughness of pathological review. Some patients with thyroid cancer and Graves' disease have more aggressive tumors. Patients with Graves' disease and palpable nodules had a 22.2% incidence of carcinoma as opposed to 2.9% in patients with a recognized nodule. Thyroid cancers appear to be more virulent in the former group where the cancer is larger but not when they are occult (119). This difference might be explained on the basis that in some patients without palpable thyroid nodules, radioiodine treatment could ablate occult tumors. Belfiore et al. (116) documented a positive correlation between TSAb and the growth of thyroid cancers. They found that tumors in Graves' patients were most aggressive, followed by tumors in euthyroid patients who in turn had more aggressive tumors than tumors in patients with autonomous thyroid nodules. The last group obviously have suppressed TSH levels. Although hyperthyroid Graves' patients also had suppressed TSH levels, 92% of these patients also detectable TSAb. It seems logical that some form of immunotherapy should be used to decrease TSAb levels after thyroidectomy for an aggressive tumor. Because glucocorticoids have major side effects, some other forms of immunotherapy used in the field of transplantation may prove to be useful.

CONCLUSIONS

Thyroidectomy is an underutilized method of treatment for patients with Graves' disease. Surgery is technically somewhat more difficult than for non-toxic goiter because of increased tissue vascularity. Surgery should therefore be performed by surgeons experienced in thyroid surgery. The easiest Graves' glands to remove are the smaller glands but such patients, unless young, are often treated with radioiodine.

REFERENCES

1. **McIver B, Morris JC.** 1998 The pathogenesis of Graves' disease. Endocrinol Metab Clin North Am. 27:73-89.
2. **Solomon B, Glinoer D, Lagasse R, Wartofsky L.** 1990 Current trends in the management of Graves' disease. J Clin Endocrinol Metab. 70:1518-1524.
3. **Fye WB.** 1992 Caleb Hillier Parry. Clin Cardiol. 15:619-621.
4. **Jones B.** 1991 Caleb Hillier Parry. West Engl Med J. 106:101-102.
5. **Drury MI.** 1985 Robert Graves--150 years on. Ir J Med Sci. 154:470-475.
6. **Bloch H.** 1990 The Asclepiads of Dublin: a moment in Ireland's medical history. South Med J. 83:664-668.
7. **Taylor S.** 1986 Graves of Graves' disease, 1796-1853. J R Coll Physicians Lond. 20:298-300.
8. **Vereckei I.** 1980 [Karl Adolf von Basedow (1799-1854)]. Orv Hetil. 121:964-966.
9. **Hennemann G.** 1991 Historical aspects about the development of our knowledge of morbus Basedow. J Endocrinol Invest. 14:617-624.
10. **Rutledge RH.** 1995 Theodor Billroth: a century later. Surgery. 118:36-43.
11. **Giddings AE.** 1998 The history of thyroidectomy. J R Soc Med. 91 Suppl 33:3-6.
12. **Harrison TS.** 1970 Thyroid surgery in historical perspective. J Med Liban. 23:537-551.
13. **Gemsenjäger E.** 1993 [Goiter surgery from Kocher to today]. Schweiz Med Wochenschr. 123:207-213.
14. **Eastman CJ.** 1996 Graves' disease 150 years on [editorial]. Med J Aust. 165:467-468.
15. **Sulek K.** 1967 [Prize for T. Kocher in 1909 for his work on the physiology, pathology and surgery of the thyroid gland]. Wiad Lek. 20:1223.
16. **Welbourn RB.** 1996 Highlights from endocrine surgical history. World J Surg. 20:603-612.
17. **Nelson CW.** 1994 Thyroid surgical procedures and the Mayo brothers. Mayo Clin Proc. 69:1130.
18. **Halsted WS.** 1920 The operative story of goitre. John Hopkins Hospital Report. 19:171-257.
19. **Becker WF.** 1977 Presidential address: pioneers in thyroid surgery. Ann Surg. 185:493-504.
20. **Akamizu T, Mori T, Nakao K.** 1997 Pathogenesis of Graves' disease: molecular analysis of anti-thyrotropin receptor antibodies. Endocr J. 44:633-646.
21. **Gauna A, Segura G, Sartorio G, Soto R, Segal-Eiras A.** 1989 Immunological aspects of Graves' disease patients in different clinical stages. J Endocrinol Invest. 12:671-677.
22. **Cho BY, Oh SK, Shong YK, et al.** 1990 Changes in thyrotropin receptor antibody after subtotal thyroidectomy in Graves' disease: comparison with the degree of lymphocytic infiltration in the thyroid. Autoimmunity. 8:143-147.
23. **Feldt-Rasmussen U, Schleusener H, Carayon P.** 1994 Meta-analysis evaluation of the impact of thyrotropin receptor antibodies on long term remission after medical therapy of Graves' disease. J Clin Endocrinol Metab. 78:98-102.
24. **Davies TF, Roti E, Braverman LE, DeGroot LJ.** 1998 Thyroid controversy--stimulating antibodies. J Clin Endocrinol Metab. 83:3777-3785.
25. **Winsa B, Rastad J, Akerström G, Johansson H, Westermark K, Karlsson FA.** 1995 Retrospective evaluation of subtotal and total thyroidectomy in Graves' disease with and without endocrine ophthalmopathy. Eur J Endocrinol. 132:406-412.
26. **Miccoli P, Vitti P, Rago T, et al.** 1996 Surgical treatment of Graves' disease: subtotal or total thyroidectomy? Surgery. 120:1020-4; discussion 1024-1025.

27. **Brix TH, Kyvik KO, Hegedüs L.** 1998 What is the evidence of genetic factors in the etiology of Graves' disease? A brief review. Thyroid. 8:627-634.

28. **de Roux N, Shields DC, Misrahi M, Ratanachaiyavong S, McGregor AM, Milgrom E.** 1996 Analysis of the thyrotropin receptor as a candidate gene in familial Graves' disease. J Clin Endocrinol Metab. 81:3483-3486.

29. **Donner H, Rau H, Walfish PG, et al.** 1997 CTLA4 alanine-17 confers genetic susceptibility to Graves' disease and to type 1 diabetes mellitus. J Clin Endocrinol Metab. 82:143-146.

30. **Kotsa K, Watson PF, Weetman AP.** 1997 A CTLA-4 gene polymorphism is associated with both Graves disease and autoimmune hypothyroidism. Clin Endocrinol (Oxf). 46:551-554.

31. **Djilali-Saiah I, Larger E, Harfouch-Hammoud E, et al.** 1998 No major role for the CTLA-4 gene in the association of autoimmune thyroid disease with IDDM. Diabetes. 47:125-127.

32. **Tomer Y, Barbesino G, Greenberg DA, Concepcion E, Davies TF.** 1998 A new Graves disease-susceptibility locus maps to chromosome 20q11.2. International Consortium for the Genetics of Autoimmune Thyroid Disease. Am J Hum Genet. 63:1749-1756.

33. **Tomer Y, Barbesino G, Greenberg DA, Concepcion E, Davies TF.** 1998 Linkage analysis of candidate genes in autoimmune thyroid disease. III. Detailed analysis of chromosome 14 localizes Graves' disease-1 (GD-1) close to multinodular goiter-1 (MNG-1). International Consortium for the Genetics of Autoimmune Thyroid Disease. J Clin Endocrinol Metab. 83:4321-4327.

34. **Barbesino G, Tomer Y, Concepcion ES, Davies TF, Greenberg DA.** 1998 Linkage analysis of candidate genes in autoimmune thyroid disease. II. Selected gender-related genes and the X-chromosome. International Consortium for the Genetics of Autoimmune Thyroid Disease. J Clin Endocrinol Metab. 83:3290-3295.

35. **Tripp W, Rao V, Creary LB.** 1987 Various manifestations of hyperthyroidism in an ambulatory clinic: case studies. J Natl Med Assoc. 79:1167-1170.

36. **Wall J.** 1995 Extrathyroidal manifestations of Graves' disease [editorial; comment]. J Clin Endocrinol Metab. 80:3427-3429.

37. **Carnell NE, Valente WA.** 1998 Thyroid nodules in Graves' disease: classification, characterization, and response to treatment. Thyroid. 8:571-576.

38. **Nishikawa M, Yoshimura M, Yoshikawa N, et al.** 1997 Coexistence of an autonomously functioning thyroid nodule in a patient with Graves' disease: an unusual presentation of Marine-Lenhart syndrome. Endocr J. 44:571-574.

39. **Woeber KA.** 1995 Cost-effective evaluation of the patient with a thyroid nodule. Surg Clin North Am. 75:357-363.

40. **Burch HB, Shakir F, Fitzsimmons TR, Jaques DP, Shriver CD.** 1998 Diagnosis and management of the autonomously functioning thyroid nodule: the Walter Reed Army Medical Center experience, 1975-1996. Thyroid. 8:871-880.

41. **Pandolfi C, Colecchia M, Gianini A.** 1997 [Hyperfunctioning thyroid carcinoma. Description of a case]. Minerva Endocrinol. 22:79-82.

42. **Polak M, Bertherat J, Li JY, et al.** 1991 A human TSH-secreting adenoma: endocrine, biochemical and morphological studies. Evidence of somatostatin receptors by using quantitative autoradiography. Clinical and biological improve-ment by SMS 201-995 treatment. Acta Endocrinol (Copenh). 124:479-486.

43. **Scheithauer BW, Kovacs KT, Young WF, Jr., Randall RV.** 1992 The pituitary gland in hyperthyroidism. Mayo Clin Proc. 67:22-26.

44. **So WY, Yeung VT, Chow CC, Ko GT, Szeto CC, Cockram CS.** 1998 TSH secreting pituitary adenoma: a rare cause of thyrotoxicosis. Int J Clin Pract. 52:62-64.

45. **Bayot MR, Chopra IJ.** 1995 Coexistence of struma ovarii and Graves' disease. Thyroid. 5:469-471.

46. **Cavalieri RR, Gerard SK.** 1991 Unusual types of thyrotoxicosis. Adv Intern Med. 36:271-286.

47. **Gleason PE, Elliott DS, Zimmerman D, Smithson WA, Kramer SA.** 1994 Metastatic testicular choriocarcinoma and secondary hyperthyroidism: case report and review of the literature. J Urol. 151:1063-1064.

48. **O'Reilly S, Lyons DJ, Harrison M, Gaffney E, Cullen M, Clancy L.** 1993 Thyrotoxicosis induced by choriocarcinoma a report of two cases. Ir Med J. 86:124-127.

49. **Astwood EB.** 1984 Landmark article May 8, 1943: Treatment of hyperthyroidism with thiourea and thiouracil. By E.B. Astwood. JAMA. 251:1743-1746.

50. **McKenzie JM.** 1967 Symposium on hyperthyroidism. Etiology and clinical patterns. Appl Ther. 9:595-598.

51. **Astwood EB.** 1965 Thyroid disorders--a half century of innovation. Ann Intern Med. 63:553-558.

52. **Vitti P, Rago T, Chiovato L, et al.** 1997 Clinical features of patients with Graves' disease undergoing remission after antithyroid drug treatment. Thyroid. 7:369-375.

53. **Wang PW, Liu RT, Tung SC, et al.** 1998 Outcome of Graves' disease after antithyroid drug treatment in Taiwan. J Formos Med Assoc. 97:619-625.

54. **Glaser NS, Styne DM.** 1997 Predictors of early remission of hyperthyroidism in children [see comments]. J Clin Endocrinol Metab. 82:1719-1726.

55. **Gittoes NJ, Franklyn JA.** 1998 Hyperthyroidism. Current treatment guidelines. Drugs. 55:543-553.

56. **Wartofsky L.** 1973 Low remission after therapy for Graves disease. Possible relation of dietary iodine with antithyroid therapy results. JAMA. 226:1083-1088.

57. **Cooper DS.** 1998 Antithyroid drugs for the treatment of hyperthyroidism caused by Graves' disease. Endocrinol Metab Clin North Am. 27:225-247.

58. **Ichiki Y, Akahoshi M, Yamashita N, et al.** 1998 Propylthiouracil-induced severe hepatitis: a case report and review of the literature. J Gastroenterol. 33:747-750.

59. **Wartofsky L.** 1996 Treatment options for hyperthyroidism. Hosp Pract (Off Ed). 31:69-73, 76-78, 81-84.

60. **Benker G, Reinwein D, Kahaly G, et al.** 1998 Is there a methimazole dose effect on remission rate in Graves' disease? Results from a long-term prospective study. The European Multicentre Trial Group of the Treatment of Hyperthyroidism with Antithyroid Drugs. Clin Endocrinol (Oxf). 49:451-457.

61. **Kallner G, Vitols S, Ljunggren JG.** 1996 Comparison of standardized initial doses of two antithyroid drugs in the treatment of Graves' disease. J Intern Med. 239:525-529.

62. **Gavin LA.** 1991 Thyroid crises. Med Clin North Am. 75:179-193.

63. **Chang DC, Wheeler MH, Woodcock JP, et al.** 1987 The effect of preoperative Lugol's iodine on thyroid blood flow in patients with Graves' hyperthyroidism. Surgery. 102:1055-1061.

64. **Marigold JH, Morgan AK, Earle DJ, Young AE, Croft DN.** 1985 Lugol's iodine: its effect on thyroid blood flow in patients with thyrotoxicosis. Br J Surg. 72:45-47.

65. **Wiersinga WM.** 1991 Propranolol and thyroid hormone metabolism. Thyroid. 1:273-277.

66. **Melliere D, Etienne G, Becquemin JP.** 1988 Operation for hyperthyroidism. Methods and rationale. Am J Surg. 155:395-399.

67. **Lennquist S, Jörtsö E, Anderberg B, Smeds S.** 1985 Betablockers compared with antithyroid drugs as preoperative treatment in hyperthyroidism: drug tolerance, complications, and postoperative thyroid function. Surgery. 98:1141-1147.

68. **Lee TC, Coffey RJ, Currier BM, Ma XP, Canary JJ.** 1982 Propranolol and thyroidectomy in the treatment of thyrotoxicosis. Ann Surg. 195:766-773.

69. **Feely J, Crooks J, Forrest AL, Hamilton WF, Gunn A.** 1981 Propranolol in the surgical treatment of hyperthyroidism, including severely thyrotoxic patients. Br J Surg. 68:865-869.

70. **Feek CM, Sawers JS, Irvine WJ, Beckett GJ, Ratcliffe WA, Toft AD.** 1980 Combination of potassium iodide and propranolol in preparation of patients with Graves' disease for thyroid surgery. N Engl J Med. 302:883-885.

71. **Vellar ID.** 1974 Thomas Peel Dunhill, the forgotten man of thyroid surgery. Med Hist. 18:22-50.

72. **Taylor S.** 1997 Sir Thomas Peel Dunhill (1876-1957). World J Surg. 21:660-662.

73. **Abe Y, Sato H, Noguchi M, et al.** 1998 Effect of subtotal thyroidectomy on natural history of ophthalmopathy in Graves' disease. World J Surg. 22:714-717.

74. **Torre G, Borgonovo G, Arezzo A, et al.** 1998 Is euthyroidism the goal of surgical treatment of diffuse toxic goitre? Eur J Surg. 164:495-500.

75. **Sugino K, Mimura T, Ozaki O, et al.** 1995 Early recurrence of hyperthyroidism in patients with Graves' disease treated by subtotal thyroidectomy. World J Surg. 19:648-652.

76. **Sosa JA, Bowman HM, Tielsch JM, Powe NR, Gordon TA, Udelsman R.** 1998 The importance of surgeon experience for clinical and economic outcomes from thyroidectomy. Ann Surg. 228:320-330.

77. **Clark OH.** 1988 Total thyroidectomy: the preferred option for multinodular goiter [letter]. Ann Surg. 208:244-245.

78. **Kasuga Y, Sugenoya A, Kobayashi S, et al.** 1990 Clinical evaluation of the response to surgical treatment of Graves' disease. Surg Gynecol Obstet. 170:327-330.

79. **Davenport M, Talbot CH.** 1989 Thyroidectomy for Graves' disease: is hypothyroidism inevitable? Ann R Coll Surg Engl. 71:87-91.

80. **Cusick EL, Krukowski ZH, Matheson NA.** 1987 Outcome of surgery for Graves' disease re-examined. Br J Surg. 74:780-7833.

81. **Reid DJ.** 1987 Hyperthyroidism and hypothyroidism complicating the treatment of thyrotoxicosis. Br J Surg. 74:1060-1062.

82. **Sugino K, Mimura T, Toshima K, Ozaki O, Ito K.** 1993 [Outcome of surgical treatment for Graves's disease and a correlation between its clinical course and values of TSH receptor antibodies (TRAb)]. Nippon Geka Gakkai Zasshi. 94:611-614.

83. **Okamoto T, Fujimoto Y, Obara T, Ito Y, Aiba M.** 1992 Retrospective analysis of prognostic factors affecting the thyroid functional status after subtotal thyroidectomy for Graves' disease. World J Surg. 16:690-695; discussion 695-696.

84. **Linos DA, Karakitsos D, Papademetriou J.** 1997 Should the primary treatment of hyperthyroidism be surgical? Eur J Surg. 163:651-657.

85. **Sawin CT, Becker DV.** 1997 Radioiodine and the treatment of hyperthyroidism: the early history. Thyroid. 7:163-176.

86. **Ljunggren JG, Törring O, Wallin G, et al.** 1998 Quality of life aspects and costs in treatment of Graves' hyperthyroidism with antithyroid drugs, surgery, or radioiodine: results from a prospective, randomized study. Thyroid. 8:653-659.

87. **Wartofsky L.** 1997 Radioiodine therapy for Graves' disease: case selection and restrictions recommended to patients in North America. Thyroid. 7:213-216.

88. **Foley TP, Jr., Charron M.** 1997 Radioiodine treatment of juvenile Graves disease. Exp Clin Endocrinol Diabetes. 105 Suppl 4:61-65.

89. **Baxter MA, Stewart PM, Daykin J, Sheppard MC, Franklyn JA.** 1993 Radioiodine therapy for hyperthyroidism in young patients--perception of risk and use. Q J Med. 86:495-499.

90. **Sugino K, Mimura T, Ozaki O, et al.** 1995 Management of recurrent hyperthyroidism in patients with Graves' disease treated by subtotal thyroidectomy. J Endocrinol Invest. 18:415-419.

91. **Tezelman S, Grossman RF, Siperstein AE, Clark OH.** 1994 Radioiodine-associated thyroid cancers. World J Surg. 18:522-528.

92. **Katz N, Esik O, Füzy M, Gundy S.** 1998 [Cytogenetic study of thyroid patients treated with external irradiation or radioiodine]. Orv Hetil. 139:1521-6.

93. **Hall P, Holm LE.** 1997 Late consequences of radioiodine for diagnosis and therapy in Sweden. Thyroid. 7:205-208.

94. **Manso PG, Furlanetto RP, Wolosker AM, Paiva ER, de Abreu MT, Maciel RM.** 1998 Prospective and controlled study of ophthalmopathy after radioiodine therapy for Graves' hyperthyroidism. Thyroid. 8:49-52.

95. **Bartalena L, Marcocci C, Pinchera A.** 1997 Treating severe Graves' ophthalmopathy. Baillieres Clin Endocrinol Metab. 11:521-536.

96. **Evans PM, Webster J, Evans WD, Bevan JS, Scanlon MF.** 1998 Radioiodine treatment in unsuspected pregnancy. Clin Endocrinol (Oxf). 48:281-283.

97. **Franklyn JA, Maisonneuve P, Sheppard MC, Betteridge J, Boyle P.** 1998 Mortality after the treatment of hyperthyroidism with radioactive iodine. N Engl J Med. 338:712-718.

98. **Goldman MB, Maloof F, Monson RR, Aschengrau A, Cooper DS, Ridgway EC.** 1988 Radioactive iodine therapy and breast cancer. A follow-up study of hyperthyroid women. Am J Epidemiol. 127:969-980.

99. **Hall P, Lundell G, Holm L.** 1993 Mortality in patients treated for hyperthyroidism with iodine-131. Acta Endocrinol. 128:230-234.

100. **Nygaard B, Hegedüs L, Gervil M, et al.** 1995 Influence of compensated radioiodine therapy on thyroid volume and incidence of hypothyroidism in Graves' disease. J Intern Med. 238:491-497.

101. **Sridama V, McCormick M, Kaplan EL, Fauchet R, DeGroot LJ.** 1984 Long-term follow-up study of compensated low-dose 131I therapy for Graves' disease. N Engl J Med. 311:426-432.

102. **Winsa B, Rastad J, Larsson E, et al.** 1994 Total thyroidectomy in therapy-resistant Graves' disease. Surgery. 116:1068-1074; discussion 1074.

103. **Weetman AP, Wiersinga WM.** 1998 Current management of thyroid-associated ophthalmopathy in Europe. Results of an international survey [see comments]. Clin Endocrinol (Oxf). 49:21-28.

104. **Hamburger JI.** 1992 Diagnosis and management of Graves' disease in pregnancy. Thyroid. 2:219-224.

105. **Mestman JH.** 1998 Hyperthyroidism in pregnancy. Endocrinol Metab Clin North Am. 27:127-149.

106. **Stice RC, Grant CS, Gharib H, van Heerden JA.** 1984 The management of Graves' disease during pregnancy. Surg Gynecol Obstet. 158:157-160.

107. **Walfish PG, Chan JY.** 1985 Post-partum hyperthyroidism. Clin Endocrinol Metab. 14:417-447.

108. **Mandel S, Hanna C, LaFranchi S.** 1990 Thyroid function of infants born to mothers with Graves disease [letter; comment]. J Pediatr. 117:169-170.

109. **Söreide JA, van Heerden JA, Lo CY, Grant CS, Zimmerman D, Ilstrup DM.** 1996 Surgical treatment of Graves' disease in patients younger than 18 years. World J Surg. 20:794-799; discussion 799-800.

110. **Zimmerman D, Gan-Gaisano M.** 1990 Hyperthyroidism in children and adolescents. Pediatr Clin North Am. 37:1273-1295.

111. **Witte J, Goretzki PE, Röher HD.** 1997 Surgery for Graves disease in childhood and adolescence. Exp Clin Endocrinol Diab. 105 Suppl 4.58-60.

112. **Roth RN, McAuliffe MJ.** 1989 Hyperthyroidism and thyroid storm. Emerg Med Clin North Am. 7:873-883.

113. **Yoshida D.** 1996 Thyroid storm precipitated by trauma. J Emerg Med. 14:697-701.

114. **Robuschi G, Manfredi A, Salvi M, et al.** 1986 Effect of sodium ipodate and iodide on free T4 and free T3 concentrations in patients with Graves' disease. J Endocrinol Invest. 9:287-291.

115. **Pellegriti G, Belfiore A, Giuffrida D, Lupo L, Vigneri R.** 1998 Outcome of differentiated thyroid cancer in Graves' patients. J Clin Endocrinol Metab. 83:2805-2809.

116. **Filetti S, Belfiore A, Amir SM, et al.** 1988 The role of thyroid-stimulating antibodies of Graves' disease in differentiated thyroid cancer. N Engl J Med. 318:753-759.

117. **Röher HD, Goretzki PE, Frilling A.** 1988 Thyroid-stimulating antibodies of Graves' disease in thyroid cancer [letter]. N Engl J Med. 319:1669-1670.

118. **Mazzaferri EL.** 1990 Thyroid cancer and Graves' disease. J Clin Endocrinol Metab. 70:826-829.

119. **Kraimps JL, Bouin-Pineau MH, Maréchaud R, Barbier J.** 1997 [Thyroid nodules associated with Graves' disease: another argument for surgical treatment]. Chirurgie. 122:488-490.

13

MANAGEMENT OF GRAVES' DISEASE IN CHILDREN

Scott A. Rivkees

INTRODUCTION

Hyperthyroidism occurs much less commonly in children than hypothyroidism, yet is a far more pernicious illness (1,2). In children, Graves' disease is the most common cause of childhood thyrotoxicosis and is characterized by diffuse goiter, hyperthyroidism and occasionally ophthalmopathy (3-7). Untreated, Graves' disease is associated with excessive activity, tremor, tachycardia, flushing, palpitations, accelerated linear growth, weight loss, impaired skeletal mineralization, and poor school performance (3-6). Because Graves' disease only rarely spontaneously resolves within a short period (3-7), treatment of hyperthyroidism is essential.

Posthumous writings of Caleb Hiller Parry in 1825 first described the syndrome of thyroid enlargement, palpitations, and exophthalmos (8). Graves' later described the disease in 1835 and Basedow in 1840 (8). Medical treatment in the first half of the century consisted of bed rest, quinine, and iodine in the form of Lugol's solution (8). Partial thyroidectomy was used to provide permanent cures (8). With the advent of thiouracil and propylthiouracil (PTU) in the mid-1940s, medical therapy of Graves' improved markedly (1). Because of the relatively high incidence of toxic reactions that developed following the administration of thiouracil including agranulocytosis, leukopenia, and drug fever, PTU became the mainstay of medical therapy (1) and was later joined by methimazole (MMI) as an effective treatment option.

Chapman and co-workers introduced the use of radioactive iodine treatment of Graves' disease in the 1940s [see reference (9) for a wonderful perspective]. Radioiodine was not generally recommended for juvenile patients because of the theoretical possibility that radiation may induce malignancy (1). However, faced with unremitting hyperthyroidism in the face of toxic reactions to antithyroid medications, the first pediatric patients were treated with radioiodine in 1948 (J.D. Crawford, personal communication). When it became apparent that radioiodine was not associated with an increased risk of thyroid cancer, radioiodine therapy became widespread in adults and was extended to progressively younger children.

Despite continued advances in our understanding of the pathogenesis of Graves' disease and the risks and benefits of the different forms of therapy, the treatment of childhood Graves' disease remains a controversial issue. Potential complications are associated with each therapeutic option. Antithyroid drug therapy with thionamides is associated with potentially serious side effects and a high relapse rate (4,10-12). Thyroidectomy achieves high rates of remission, yet is a complex surgical procedure that can result in hypoparathyroidism or dysphonia (13). Radioiodine therapy achieves high rates of remission (12,14-18). Yet, the long term safety of 131-iodine in children and adolescents has been evaluated in less than 1,000 individuals (11,17,19-25).

The family and physician of a child or adolescent with Graves' disease are thus faced with a decision requiring thoughtful consideration of the treatment options detailed below and the impact these treatments have on the lifestyle of child and parent.

THYROIDECTOMY

Before the introduction of antithyroid drugs in the mid-1940s, nearly all cases of hyperthyroidism in children were treated surgically (2). Whereas subtotal (partial) thyroidectomy was advocated in previous years for children and adults (26,27), total (near-total) thyroidectomy is now recommended to reduce the risk of recurrent hyperthyroidism (28-30).

In preparation for surgery, the child should be rendered euthyroid. This is typically done with either PTU or MMI. One week before surgery, adding iodine to the treatment may be desirable because it causes the gland to become firmer and less vascular, thereby facilitating surgery.

Following subtotal thyroidectomy, relief of hyperthyroidism is achieved in about 80% of children and adults, and hypothyroidism develops in about 60% of individuals (26,27). Hyperthyroidism recurs in about 10-15% of patients after subtotal thyroidectomy (26,29). In comparison, hyperthyroidism recurs in less than 3% of children and adults who undergo total thyroidectomy, and hypothyroidism is nearly universal (27-31).

Complication rates are comparable following subtotal or total thyroidectomy (29). The most comprehensive survey of the complications of thyroid surgery was based on results of 24,108 thyroid operations on adults and children performed in 1970 (13). These cases were estimated to represent one third of the thyroidectomies performed that year in the United States (13). In-hospital mortality rates were 0.5% for adults and 0.08% (1 death in about 1,000 operations) for children (13). The most frequent non-lethal complications included pain and transient hypocalcemia (13). Less common problems (1-4%) include hemorrhage, permanent hypoparathyroidism, and vocal cord paralysis (13). Other studies describing complications of thyroid surgery in children involved far fewer subjects (26,28,32), but showed similar rates of complications (26,28,32).

More recent large follow-up studies describing the incidence of complications and deaths after thyroid surgery are not available. Yet, with advances in anesthesia, surgery, and postoperative care, it is possible that complication rates have decreased. However, with increasing use of radioiodine, less thyroid surgery is now performed and fewer surgeons can develop and maintain their skills than in the past (33). Thus, if a child is operated on, it should be by a surgeon with expertise in performing thyroidectomies in children.

ANTITHYROID DRUG THERAPY

Despite disappointing long-term rates of remission, treatment with antithyroid drugs has remained the first line of therapy for children with Graves' disease in many centers. Mainstays of antithyroid therapy include the thionamide derivatives PTU and MMI. These compounds reduce thyroid hormone synthesis by inhibiting the oxidation and organic binding of thyroid iodide (34,35). These medications do not cure Graves' disease, rather they control the hyperthyroid state until the disease runs it course.

MMI is tenfold more potent than PTU and has a longer half-life (34,35). Recommended doses for initial therapy are 5-10 mg/kg per day for PTU and 0.5 to 1.0 mg/kg per day for MMI (36). However, even lower doses of PTU or MMI may be effective for induction or maintenance therapy.

To control the hyperthyroid state, PTU and MMI are typically given every eight hours. However, once-a-day dosing may bring remission as rapidly as divided doses (37,38) and is especially well suited for maintenance therapy (39,40). Because MMI pills (5 or 10 mg) are smaller than PTU tablets (50 mg), and fewer MMI pills are generally needed, MMI may be more convenient.

In contrast to oral iodine therapy (see below), thiouracil drugs do not prevent thyroid gland hyperplasia. Thus, thyroid enlargement may occur during therapy. The thyroid gland may become softer and the outlines of the gland more difficult to distinguish (1). Because radioiodine is less effective in large than in small glands (41), thyroid size should be continuously monitored for progressive thyroid enlargement that may make the patient an unsuitable candidate for radioiodine treatment. If the gland enlarges, this may also be due to hypothyroidism. Thus, patients should be monitored for TSH elevations.

Although MMI and PTU promptly inhibit hormone formation, they do not inhibit hormone release. Thus, levels of circulating thyroid hormones may remain elevated for several weeks as stored hormone is released. Until circulating levels of thyroid hormones normalize, the signs and symptoms of hyperthyroidism may be controlled with beta blockers such as atenolol (25 or 50 mg, QD or BID) or propranolol (2.5-10 mg BID or TID). If the child has reactive airway disease, beta blocker therapy may trigger acute exacerbations of asthma. Thus, beta blockers should be avoided in asthmatic children. If beta blocker therapy is needed in a severely symptomatic child with a history of asthma, inpatient observation and use of $beta_1$-adrenergic receptor-selective agents (e.g., metoprolol) should be considered. Beta blockers should also be used with caution in children with diabetes and cardiac disease.

Thyrotoxicosis can be controlled more quickly than with thionamides using solutions of saturated potassium iodine (SSKI or Lugol's solution; 1-3 drops TID) which block the release of stored hormones. Side effects of iodine are uncommon and include acneiform eruptions, fever, coryza, and salivation (1). Severe, and fatal reactions to iodine have also been observed (1). When combined thionamide and iodine therapy is used, PTU or MMI should be given a few hours before iodine to prevent iodine-induced increases in thyroid hormone synthesis (1).

After initiation with PTU or MMI, maximal clinical responses are seen after 4 to 6 weeks, at which time biochemical hypothyroidism develops and the thionamide dose can be reduced 30-50%. To achieve a euthyroid state, the dose of MMI or PTU can either be reduced further, or supplemented with levo-thyroxine (36). The latter approach is generally preferred because titrating doses of antithyroid drugs is difficult and requires frequent testing (36). When adjunctive levo-thyroxine therapy is used, treatment is started when T4 or free-T4 values fall below normal (36).

Complications of PTU and MMI

Despite the common use of PTU or MMI in treating childhood Graves' disease, these medications can have toxicity and 1% of children will develop serious complications (6,10,11,42). To date, 36 serious adverse events and two deaths from liver failure due to antithyroid drug therapy of childhood Graves' disease have been reported to the FDA MedWatch Program which is very prone to under-reporting (S. Malozowski, personal communication). Childhood deaths associated with antithyroid drug therapy have also been described in published reports (11).

Published studies including 500 children (4,11,12,26,43,44), show that complications of drug therapy include increases in liver enzymes (28%) and leukopenia (25%). However, changes in liver enzymes and mild leukopenia or granulocytopenia commonly also occur in untreated and uncomplicated Graves' disease (35,45). Other complications include rashes (9%), granulocytopenia (4.5%) and arthritis (2.4%),

The far more serious complications of drug therapy are agranulocytosis (0.4%), and hepatitis (0.45%). Fortunately, these complications occur in less than 1% of treated patients. Agranulocytosis is usually reversible when the drug is stopped and is rarely fatal (46-48). Severe hepatitis, however, may not be reversible and may progress to end stage liver disease requiring transplantation (45) (FDA MedWatch data). Other rare and serious adverse effects of thionamide drugs include periarteritis nodosa, other forms of vasculitis, nephrotic syndrome, hypothrombinemia, and aplastic anemia (49).

Most side effects of antithyroid drugs develop within eight weeks of starting therapy. However, adverse effects may develop later. Parents should be instructed to contact their endocrinologist or local physician promptly if fever, sore throat, oral ulceration, rash, joint pain, nausea, abdominal pain, or other unusual symptoms develop. When side effects of MMI or PTU develop, medication is often discontinued and radioiodine or surgery is considered. Some clinicians will change to another thionamide when a mild toxic reaction occurs. However, published data about the risks and benefits of changing medications in children are limited, and medication changes should be made with caution. If a serious complication develops, such as hepatitis or agranulocytosis, it is best not to resume antithyroid drug therapy.

Long-term efficacy of antithyroid drugs

In children, published remission rates after several years of drug therapy are usually less than 30 to 40% (4,11,12,26,43,44,50). It has also been shown that after two years of treatment, remission rates in children are 25%, and four years of drug therapy are needed to achieve 50% remission rates (10). It is projected that 10 years of drug therapy are needed to achieve remission in 75% of children (10).

When responses to medical therapy between prepubertal and pubertal children are compared, 1-year remission rates are much less in prepubertal (17%) than in pubertal children (30%) (50). Thus, the chance of a favorable long-term outcome following drug therapy in young children is not high.

The efficacy of antithyroid drugs is inversely related to serum levels of thyrotropin receptor antibodies (TRAbs), including thyroid-stimulating antibodies (TSAb) (51-55). After several years of antithyroid therapy, remission rates in adults range from 15% in individuals with high levels of TRAb at the time of diagnosis, to 50% in individuals with low pretreatment TRAb levels (51).

It has also been suggested that long-term remission rates can be predicted by observing responses to short-term (ca. 6 months) antithyroid drug therapy (56-61). Short-term therapy appears to work as well as long-term therapy in patients with mild hyperthyroidism and small goiters, but neither short- nor long-term antithyroid drug therapy is likely to lead to a lasting remission in patients with severe thyrotoxicosis and a large goiter (M. Greer, personal communication)(56,57). Although most of the evidence supports the efficacy of short term therapy, some investigators have noted higher relapse rates after short-term than long-term treatment (60,62).

Risks of cancer after drug therapy

Antithyroid drugs are preferred to radioiodine therapy by many clinicians based on the assumption that cancer risk is less after drug therapy than after radioiodine. However, available data suggest that this assumption is not correct.

The largest long term follow-up study of thyroid cancer risks after treatment of Graves' disease, the Collaborative Thyrotoxicosis Study Group (CTSG), revealed that the incidence of thyroid carcinomas over 10-20 years of follow-up (not lifetime incidences) was fivefold higher in adults with Graves' disease treated with thionamide drugs (follow-up period normalized incidence rate = 1 case per 332 individuals) than in patients treated with 131-iodine (1 /1,783), and eightfold higher than in patients treated surgically (1/2,820) (63). The incidence of thyroid adenomas were also 10 and 20 times higher among the adults treated with antithyroid drugs (1/76) than in patients treated with 131-iodine (1/802) or surgery (1/1,692), respectively (63). Rather than reflecting a causative role for medical therapy in the pathogenesis of thyroid neoplasia, these observations may reflect the persistence of more thyroid tissue in patients treated with drugs than in individuals treated with radioiodine or surgery.

Although CTSG data showed an increased rate of thyroid cancer in the drug-treated patients (63), it is important to note that thyroid cancer mortality rates were not increased in the CTSG patients treated with drugs (64). Thyroid cancer has also not been reported in the large number of children treated with antithyroid drugs.

RADIOACTIVE IODINE

The use of 131-iodine to treat Graves' disease makes this therapy one of the most widespread therapeutic uses of a systemically administered radionuclide. The therapeutic effects of radioiodine are dependent on the trapping of iodine by the thyroid. Because the uptake of 131-iodine is indistinguishable from ordinary iodine, 131-iodine is trapped in thyroid cells which are destroyed by internal radiation.

Thyroid destruction is strongly influenced by rates of iodine uptake and the amount of thyroid tissue. Doses of radioiodine administered to the patient are thus based upon gland size and iodine uptake using standard formulas [dose (mCi) = (uCi 131I/gm of thyroid x estimated thyroid weight)/ 24-hour radioiodine uptake] (65-67). For example, if a dose of 200 uCi/gm of thyroid tissue is desired for a patient with a 40 gm thyroid gland with 50% radioiodine uptake at 24-hours, the administered dose will be 16 mCi.

Thyroid size can be assessed clinically relative to the size of a normal thyroid gland size (0.5-1 gm per year of age; 15-20 gm for adults), or more precisely by ultrasound (68,69). However, even when accurate gland size, uptake, and effective 131-iodine half-times are measured and a high degree of accuracy of delivered doses is obtained, the outcome is still imprecise due to individual variation in the sensitivity of the thyroid to radioiodine (70). Thus, clinical estimate of thyroid size is usually sufficient.

It has been suggested that doses (administered activities) delivering 30,000 to 40,000 cGy (rad) to the thyroid are required to ablate the thyroid gland (71,72). However, doses delivering 10,000 to 20,000 cGy to the thyroid are more commonly used and may result in complete or partial destruction of the thyroid (72). Administered thyroid doses of 150 uCi/gm (5.5 MBq/gm) yield radiation doses of 12,000 cGy to the thyroid (73). Exposures to the stomach, marrow, liver, and gonads will be about 14, 6.8, 4.8, and 2.5 cGy per organ, respectively. The total body exposure will be about 4.0 cGy (73).

Because of the risk to the fetus of radioiodine therapy, 131-iodine should not be given to pregnant women. A negative pregnancy test should be documented before the dose is given. If a patient is taking antithyroid medication, as often happens, treatment can be stopped 5-7 days before the administration of radioiodine.

Within 4 to 10 days after 131-iodine administration, circulating levels of thyroid hormones may rise as thyroid hormone is released from degenerating follicular cells (74). Symptoms of hyperthyroidism during this time can be controlled using beta-blockers (75,76). SSKI or Lugol's solution will attenuate biochemical hyperthyroid-ism during this period and will not adversely affect the outcome of radioiodine therapy (76). Six to 8 weeks after treatment, the thyroid gland shrinks and biochemical hypothyroidism, which can be transient, often develops (77). In up to 20% of patients, hyperthyroidism will persist beyond two months of therapy; a second dose of radioiodine is recommended for these patients (14). However, this second dose of radioiodine is not usually given until 6 months after initial therapy.

The details of 131-iodine therapy for childhood Graves' disease have been reported in several studies (11,17,19-25). Patients as young as 1 year of age have been treated with 131-iodine (24). The reported 131-iodine doses in children and adolescents have ranged from 100 to 250 uCi/gm of thyroid tissue (11,17,19-25).

Long-term cure rates

Long term cure rates are higher in patients treated with larger than with smaller amounts of radioiodine (7). There also is considerable variability in rates of hyper- and hypothyroidism among different centers using the same administered doses (74).

In adult patients treated with low doses of 131-iodine (50-75 uCi/gm), hyperthyroidism persists in 30-50% one year after therapy (78-81). The incidence of hyperthyroidism declines progressively afterwards (82).   The incidence of hypothyroidism in patients treated with lower doses ranges from 7 to 20% at one year, and increases with time (80,82). In comparison, after treatment with higher 131-iodine doses (150-250 uCi/gm), only 5-10% of patients are hyperthyroid at one year, and 40-80% become hypothyroid (63,73,83).

In children treated with 50-100 uCi/gm of thyroid tissue, 25 to 40% are hyperthyroid several years after therapy (84). In comparison, in children treated with a single dose of 150-200 uCi/gm thyroid, hyperthyroidism persists in 5-20%, and 60-90% become hypothyroid (14,23,24,85).

The success of radioiodine therapy is influenced by the size of the thyroid gland and possibly by circulating levels of TRAb (86). Responses to 131-iodine therapy are lower in patients with very large glands (>80 g) and high TRAb levels than in patients with smaller glands (41,86-88). Thus, total surgical thyroidectomy may be associated with higher cure rates than radioiodine therapy for persistently large glands. There is also some evidence that responses to radioiodine are less favorable after treatment with PTU (88-90), but not after MMI (91).

Complication rates

Acute complications of 131-iodine therapy have been reported, but the incidence of these is low and not well defined (74).   In children, very few acute adverse responses to 131-iodine therapy of Graves' disease have been described (11,17,19-25).

In adults, transient nausea has been reported after radioiodine administration, and mild pain over the thyroid gland, reflecting radiation thyroiditis, may develop 1 to 3 days after a therapeutic dose (74). These side-effects are self-limited and respond to treatment with non-steroidal anti-inflammatory agents (74). Severe neck swelling and tracheal compression have been reported rarely in patients with very large goiters after 131-iodine administration and can be controlled with large doses of corticosteroids (74). Neck swelling after radioiodine treatment typically occurs with doses greater than 50,000 cGy; such doses are above those needed for ablative therapy (92). Vocal cord paresis occurs very rarely (93).

Thyroid storm has been reported to develop between 1 and 14 days after 131-iodine treatment in a very small number of patients (94-96). This complication is rare and no cases were reported among 7,000 patients treated with 131-iodine at one center (14). Patients with severe thyrotoxicosis and very large goiters may be at higher risk for thyroid storm. In this setting, antithyroid drugs can be administered for several weeks before radioiodine therapy to ensure that the thyroid has been depleted of stored hormones before radioiodine therapy (96).

Recent discussions have focused on the association of 131-iodine therapy of Graves' disease with the development or progression of ophthalmopathy in adult patients (97,98). In contrast to adults, children rarely develop severe ophthalmopathy and proptosis is generally mild (3,42,99). Of 87 children treated with 131-iodine for

Graves' disease at one center, eye signs improved in 90% of children, did not change in 7.5%, and worsened in 3% after treatment (24). In 45 children with ophthalmopathy at the onset of treatment, eye disease improved in 73% and worsened in 2% after one year or more of drug therapy (4). Following subtotal thyroidectomy in 80 children, eye disease worsened in 9% (29). In contrast, eye disease was stable in 60 (75%) children after total surgical thyroidectomy (29). Thus, eye disease worsens in only a small percentage of children following medical, radioiodine, or surgical therapy of Graves' disease.

Data presented in one recent report suggested that the development and progression of ophthalmopathy are prevented by treatment with prednisone for 3 months after radioiodine therapy (100). However, adjunctive prednisone therapy is not routinely   recommended for most children since long-term progression of ophthalmopathy occurs infrequently and unpredictably after radioiodine (100). Prolonged prednisone administration is also associated with weight gain, immune suppression, and growth failure in children. On the other hand, prednisone may be useful after radioiodine therapy for the rare pediatric patient with severe eye disease.

Thyroid Cancer Risks

The increased risk of thyroid cancer after thyroid irradiation in childhood has been recognized for nearly 50 years (101). Thus, a major concern of 131-iodine therapy relates to the risks of thyroid and non-thyroid cancers (7).

Studies of the effects of external radiation, diagnostic 131-iodine use, and environmental radioiodine and gamma ray exposure have provided important insights regarding the risks of radiation exposure and thyroid carcinomas (102-108). These studies show that the risk of thyroid cancer is increased with exposure to low or moderate levels of external radiation (20-2000 cGy). In contrast, thyroid cancer risks are much lower following high-level irradiation that results in cell death (108,109).

External radiation data
The risk of thyroid malignancy following thyroid irradiation is higher in younger children than in older children or adults (103,106,110,111).
Studies of external thyroid irradiation show that when exposure occurs after 20 years of age, the risk of thyroid malignancy is not significantly increased (106,110). Yet, when exposure occurs before 20 years of age, thyroid cancer rates increase at progressively younger ages (103,106,110). Atomic bomb survivor data show that thyroid cancer relative risks/Gy are 9.4, 3.0, 0.34, and -0.23 for ages 0-9, 10-19, 20-39, and >40 years, respectively, at the time of exposure (E. Ron, personal communication). For individuals exposed to head and neck irradiation, thyroid cancer relative risks/Gy were 9.0, 5.4, and 1.8, when exposure occurred between 0-5, 5-10, 10-15 years of age, respectively [Ref (110); E. Ron; personal communication].

Following the nuclear disaster at Chernobyl, the greatest number of cases of thyroid cancer occurred in infants less than one year of age at the time of the accident (112). When patients were between 0 and 5 years of age at the time of exposure, thyroid carcinoma predominated relative to thyroid adenomas (112). After 6 years of age, thyroid adenomas occurred more frequently than carcinomas (112). The number of cases of thyroid cancer decreased progressively through 12 years of age (112). However, it is not clear whether 131-iodine exposure alone had a major contribution to the possible radiation effect (108,111).

Even after external radiation exposure between 1 and 15 years of age, thyroid malignancies occur infrequently (1 to 4 cases per 10,000 person-years) (110). The most common form of neoplasia developing after radiation exposure is papillary carcinoma, which has an excellent prognosis in children and is almost never fatal (113).

Radioiodine data

Studies involving children less than 16 years of age show that thyroid cancer risks are not increased if relatively high, ablative doses of radioiodine are used. Yet, if low doses of radioiodine are given, the risk of thyroid neoplasia is increased.

CTSG data showed that thyroid adenomas developed in 30% of 30 children treated in one center with low doses of 131-iodine (50 uCi/gm) estimated to result in thyroid exposure of 2,500 cGy (63,84). Yet, in the other centers where children were treated with higher doses of 131-iodine (100-200 uCi/gm), the incidence of thyroid neoplasms was not increased (63).   Among adult patients in the CTSG cohort treated with radioiodine for Graves' disease, a small increase thyroid cancer mortality was observed, which was thought to reflect the nature of the underlying thyroid disease (64).

There are four reported cases of thyroid malignancy in children previously treated with 131-iodine (5-years-of-age at treatment with 50 uCi/gm; 9-years-of-age at treatment with 5.4 mCi; 11-years-of-age at treatment with 1.25 mCi; 16-years-of-age at treatment with 3.2 mCi) (21,84,114-116). Three of these individuals were treated with relatively low doses of 131-iodine, and one patient was treated with a moderate dose of 131-iodine.

In contrast to children treated with low doses of radioiodine, there is currently no evidence suggesting that children treated with high doses of radioiodine have increased risks of thyroid cancer.   Outcomes after 131-iodine treatment of children and adolescents with hyperthyroidism have been reported for approximately 1,000 individuals treated with higher doses of radioiodine (11,17,19-25). The duration of follow-up in these studies ranged from less than 5 years to 15 years, with some subjects followed for more than 20 years. These studies have not revealed an increased risk of thyroid malignancy; there have been no reports of thyroid cancer in patients treated with high doses of radioiodine for childhood Graves' disease.

It is therefore imperative that higher doses of 131-iodine (>150 uCi/gm of thyroid tissue) be used in children. Ablation of the thyroid gland will decrease the risks of radioiodine-induced tumors and is clearly preferable to lower dose therapy.

Although radioiodine is being used in progressively younger ages, we do not know if there is an age below which high-dose 131-iodine therapy should be avoided. Risks of thyroid cancer after external irradiation are highest in children less than 5 years of age, and progressively decline with advancing age (106,110). Thus, if there is residual thyroid tissue in young children after radioiodine treatment, there is a risk of thyroid cancer. It may therefore be prudent to avoid radioiodine therapy in children less than 5 years. However, children as young as one year have been treated with radioiodine with excellent outcomes (24).

Non-thyroid cancer risks

131-Iodine therapy is associated with a whole body exposure rate of about 0.45 cGy per mCi (117). Thus, it is estimated that the average child treated with 131-iodine will receive about 4 cGy of whole body irradiation (7,117). Radiation exposure will be slightly higher in the non-thyroidal tissues that accumulate iodine, including the salivary glands, stomach and bladder (117). However, detecting increases in cancer risk associated with such low doses will be very difficult even if very large populations of children are studied, and any increases in the incidence of non-thyroid cancers are likely to be very small (118).

In adults treated with 131-iodine for Graves' disease, increased rates of cancer mortality are not seen (64). Several long-term follow-up studies involving more than 60,000 patients also have not revealed substantive increases in rates of leukemia or other cancers (63,119-122).

Health of Offspring

Radiation exposure of the gonads during 131-iodine therapy approximates 2.5 cGy, which is comparable to the gonadal exposure from a barium enema or an intravenous pyelogram (123). The literature contains data on 500 offspring born to approximately 370 subjects treated with iodine-131 for hyperthyroidism during childhood and adolescence (11,17,19,20,22-24). The incidence of congenital anomalies reported among the offspring of patients treated with radioiodine does not differ from the incidence in the general population. In addition, there was no increased prevalence of congenital anomalies in the offspring of 77 patients treated in childhood with 80-700 mCi of 131-iodine (124). Furthermore, there was no evidence of an increased rate of birth defects in survivors of the Hiroshima and Nagasaki atomic bomb blasts who were exposed to higher levels of external irradiation of the gonads than are associated with radioiodine therapy (125).

Our approach

When treating children, we use radioiodine doses of 200-250 uCi/gm and aim to minimize the amount of residual thyroid tissue. When radioiodine is being used to treat a hyperthyroid child who is not on antithyroid medication, symptoms of hyperthyroidism are controlled before and after radioiodine therapy with atenolol (25-50 mg BID; unless there is asthma). For the patient with profound hyperthyroidism and a large gland at presentation desiring radioiodine therapy, we often use antithyroid drugs for one month or more to achieve biochemical eu- or hypothyroidism before 131-iodine treatment; one week before 131-iodine treatment, antithyroid drugs are stopped.

Patients who cannot be treated with beta-blockers and become symptomatic after radioiodine are treated with SSKI (2 drops in orange juice for 7 days, started 7 days after radioiodine).

Thyroid hormone levels are checked every 2-4 weeks after treatment. Levothyroxine replacement therapy is generally started when the circulating T4 concentration drops to less than 5 ug%. If there is persistent hyperthyroidism after radioiodine treatment, patients may be treated with either SSKI or antithyroid medication for several weeks and thyroid function assessed 2-4 weeks after the medication is stopped.

In our experience, about 10% of children and adolescents will require a second course of radioiodine for persistent hyperthyroidism. We have observed more initial treatment failures in pubertal than in prepubertal children and in children previously treated with antithyroid drugs than in those who have not received antithyroid medications.

COMPARATIVE RISKS AND BENEFITS OF TREATMENT OPTIONS

When considering simplicity of treatment, complication rates, cancer risk, and long-term remission rates, each treatment option for Graves' disease differs.

Surgery is the oldest effective treatment of Graves' disease, has very favorable cure rates (90%), and reverses the hyperthyroid state rapidly. Total thyroidectomy is a complex surgical procedure with definite surgical risks, including death in about 1 per 1,000 operations in children (13). Of concern is the fact that the number of skilled thyroid surgeons has declined over the past several decades (33).

When radioiodine therapy is not desired, surgery is useful for the patient who develops drug-related complications or does not achieve lasting remission with drug treatment. Surgery may also be preferable when the thyroid gland is very large (>80 gm), which makes the child a poor candidate for radioiodine therapy (41).

Medical therapy of childhood Graves' disease is associated with disappointing long term remission rates after several years of treatment (4,10-12,44). Although thionamide therapy is associated with mild side effects in some patients, serious side effects are seen in less than 1% of treated children.

Drug therapy is often a first line therapy in many centers (42) and is especially useful when TRAb levels are low and the thyroid gland is small (51,52). Thionamide treatment is also useful for controlling hyperthyroidism while more definitive forms of therapy are being considered, or until the child is considered old enough for radioiodine treatment.

Radioiodine is associated with high cure rates and is the simplest and least expensive treatment option for Graves' disease (126). Whereas childhood deaths have been associated with surgery or drug therapy, there are no reported childhood deaths associated with radioiodine treatment of hyperthyroidism.

The fear of cancer leads many clinicians to avoid radioiodine therapy of childhood Graves' disease. Yet, studies of children with Graves' disease treated with ablative doses of 131-iodine have not revealed an increased risk of thyroid neoplasia (11,17,19-25).

TREATMENT APPROACHES FOR CHILDREN

In many centers, a uniform approach to the treatment of Graves' disease is applied to children irrespective of the child's age. However, based on what is now known about the risks and benefits of different treatments and the pathogenesis of Graves' disease, we can now be more selective in our approach to therapy. To reduce treatment risks and expedite cures, the therapy of the child or adolescent with Graves' disease can be guided by the patients age and the nature of the intrinsic autoimmune disease.

For children less than five years of age, antithyroid medications should be considered as a first line therapy. Although radioiodine has also been successfully used in this age group without an apparent increase in cancer rates (24), it is best to defer radioiodine therapy because of the possible increased risks of thyroid cancer after radiation exposure in very young children.

Because young children are less likely to have remission than older children on drug treatment (50), prolonged drug therapy may be needed. If there are no toxic effects, continuing antithyroid drugs is reasonable until the child is considered old enough for radioiodine therapy. Alternatively, thyroidectomy or ablative radioiodine therapy can be considered if reactions to medications develop or there is the desire to avoid prolonged drug use. Fortunately, less than 5% of children with Graves' disease present at five years of age or younger (2).

Fifteen percent of children with Graves' disease will present between 6 and 10 years of age (2). Considering drug therapy as a first line measure for this age group is reasonable. Yet, as 10 years of age are approached, either radioiodine or drug therapy can be considered as initial therapy.

Children ten years of age and older account for 80% of the pediatric cases of Graves' disease. For this age group, radioiodine or antithyroid drugs can be considered as first line treatment options. In determining if drug therapy is likely to be successful, TRAb levels may be predictive of remission rates. The presence of low TRAb levels suggests the possibility of remission on medical therapy. Yet, if TRAb levels are high, the odds of spontaneous remission are low (51,53-55). However, TRAb levels may not always be indicative of remission likelihood (53). We have also observed relapsing thyrotoxicosis after medication is stopped in children with low initial TRAb levels.

The critical issue about drug therapy is whether a lasting cure can be achieved after using medications to palliate the hyperthyroid state. Thus, rather than basing treatment on TRAb levels, it seems reasonable for to treat for 6-12 months and stop the drug when a clinical remission, normal gland size, and a normal TSH have been achieved. If a relapse occurs, medical treatment can be resumed or an alternative form of therapy chosen. If drug treatment is resumed, available evidence suggests that several years of therapy will be needed (2 years for 25% and 4 years for 50% chance of cure) until spontaneous remission occurs (10).

When radioiodine is used, it is essential that higher doses of 131-iodine be used in children. The goal of radioiodine therapy in children should be to ablate the thyroid gland.

Finally, irrespective of the treatment option selected, careful follow up is needed for all patients treated for Graves' disease. Long-term follow-up should include regular examination of the thyroid gland and measurement of circulating levels of thyroid hormones once or twice a year. All newly appearing thyroid nodules should be biopsied or excised.

AREAS FOR FUTURE INVESTIGATION

Treating children with Graves' disease is controversial because we do not have answers to many of the fundamental issues discussed above. Additional investigation is needed to more fully compare long term cancer risks among children treated with antithyroid drugs and radioiodine. Based on current estimates of thyroid cancer risks and power calculations, several thousand children in each treatment group, more than ten years post-therapy, will be needed for such a study (Charles Land; personal communication). In the short-term, establishing a registry for reporting thyroid neoplasms in patients treated for childhood Graves' disease may provide useful information.

We also do not know how much thyroid tissue remains after the different therapies of childhood Graves' disease. If patients with Graves' disease have a higher rate of thyroid cancer as suggested (127), treatments that minimize the amount of residual thyroid tissue may be favored. Studies are therefore needed to assess the amount of thyroid tissue that persists years after remission is achieved using either radioiodine or drugs.

Although serious side effects to medical therapy occur in less than 1% of children, drug-related fatalities can occur. With the advent of new areas of pharmacology research, such as pharmacogenomics, it will be important to develop novel approaches for identifying children at risk for serious adverse reactions to thionamide medications. We also need to develop additional strategies to predict the likelihood of drug therapy success in children and adolescents with Graves' disease.

REFERENCES

1. **Talbot NB, Sobel EH, McArthur JW, Crawford JD** 1952 The Thyroid. p. 1-51. In Functional Endocrinology: From Birth Through Adolescence. Harvard University Press, Cambridge.
2. **Wilkins L** 1965 Hyperthyroidism. p. 141-150. In The Diagnosis and Treatment of Endocrine Disorders in Children and Adolescence. Charles Thomas, Springfield.
3. **Saxena KM, Crawford JD, Talbot NB** 1964 Childhood thyrotoxicosis: a longer term perspective. Br Med J. 2:1153-1158.
4. **Barnes HV Blizzard RM** 1977 Antithyroid drug therapy for toxic diffuse goiter (Graves disease): thirty years experience in children and adolescents. J Pediatr. 91:313-320.
5. **Fisher DA** 1994 Graves' disease in children. Curr Ther Endocrinol Metab. 5:71-4:71-74.
6. **Zimmerman D, Lteif AN** 1998 Thyrotoxicosis in children. Endocrinol Metab Clin North Am. 27:109-125.
7. **Rivkees SA, Sklar C, Freemark M** 1998 Clinical review 99: The management of Graves' disease in children, with special emphasis on radioiodine treatment. J Clin Endocrinol Metab. 83:3767-3776.
8. **Osler W** 1935 Graves' Disease. p. 900-907. In The Practice of Medicine. D. Appleton, New York.
9. **Chapman EM** 1983 History of the discovery and early use of radioactive iodine. JAMA. 250:2042-2044.
10. **Lippe BM, Landaw EM, Kaplan SA** 1987 Hyperthyroidism in children treated with long term medical therapy: twenty-five percent remission every two years. J Clin Endocrinol Metab. 64:1241-1245.
11. **Hamburger JI** 1985 Management of hyperthyroidism in children and adolescents. J Clin Endocrinol Metab. 60:1019-1024.
12. **Crawford JD** 1981 Hyperthyroidism in children. A reevaluation of treatment. Am J Dis Child. 135:109-110.
13. **Foster RS, Jr.** 1978 Morbidity and mortality after thyroidectomy. Surg Gynecol Obstet. 146:423-429.
14. **Levy WJ, Schumacher OP, Gupta M** 1988 Treatment of childhood Graves' disease. A

review with emphasis on radioiodine treatment. Cleve Clin J Med. 55:373-382.

15. **Crile G, Jr. Skillern PG** 1968 Advantages of radioiodine over thyroidectomy in the treatment of Graves' disease. Cleve Clin Q. 35:73-77.

16. **Dobyns BM** 1973 Radioiodine versus thyroidectomy for hyperthyroidism. Del Med J. 45:300-303.

17. **Freitas JE, Swanson DP, Gross MD, Sisson JC** 1979 Iodine-131: optimal therapy for hyperthyroidism in children and adolescents? J Nucl Med. 20:847-850.

18. **Hall P, Berg G, Bjelkengren G, Boice JD, Jr., Ericsson UB, Hallquist A, Lidberg M, Lundell G, Tennvall J, Wiklund K** 1992 Cancer mortality after iodine-131 therapy for hyperthyroidism. Int J Cancer. 50:886-890.

19. **Starr P, Jaffe HL, Oettinger L, Jr.** 1969 Later results of 131-I treatment of hyperthyroidism in 73 children and adolescents: 1967 followup. J Nucl Med. 10:586-590.

20. **Starr P, Jaffe HL, Oettinger LJ** 1964 Late results of 131I treatment of hyperthyroidism in 73 children and adolescents. J Nucl Med. 5:81-89.

21. **Kogut MD, Kaplan SA, Collipp PJ, Tiamsic T, Boyle D** 1965 Treatment of hyperthyroidism in chidlren: analysis of fourty-five patients. N Engl J Med. 272:217-222.

22. **Crile G, Jr. Schumacher OP** 1965 Radioactive iodine treatment of Graves' disease. Results in 32 children under 16 years of age. Am J Dis Child. 110:501-504.

23. **Hayek A, Chapman EM, Crawford JD** 1970 Long-term results of treatment of thyrotoxicosis in children and adolescents with radioactive iodine. N Engl J Med. 283:949-953.

24. **Safa AM, Schumacher OP, Rodriguez-Antunez A** 1975 Long-term follow-up results in children and adolescents treated with radioactive iodine (131I) for hyperthyroidism. N Engl J Med. 292:167-171.

25. **Moll GW, Jr. Patel BR** 1997 Pediatric Graves' disease: therapeutic options and experience with radioiodine at the University of Mississippi Medical Center. South Med J. 90:1017-1022.

26. **Buckingham BA, Costin G, Roe TF, Weitzman JJ, Kogut MD** 1981 Hyperthyroidism in children. A reevaluation of treatment. Am J Dis Child. 135:112-117.

27. **Ching T, Warden MJ, Fefferman RA** 1977 Thyroid surgery in children and teenagers. Arch Otolaryngol. 103:544-546.

28. **Altman RP** 1973 Total thyroidectomy for the treatment of Graves' disease in children. J Pediatr Surg. 8:295-300.

29. **Miccoli P, Vitti P, Rago T, Iacconi P, Bartalena L, Bogazzi F, Fiore E, Valeriano R, Chiovato L, Rocchi R, Pinchera A** 1996 Surgical treatment of Graves' disease: subtotal or total thyroidectomy? Surgery. 120:1020-1024.

30. **Perzik SL** 1976 Total thyroidectomy in Graves' disease in children. J Pediatr Surg. 11:191-194.

31. **Rudberg C, Johansson H, Akerstrom G, Tuvemo T, Karlsson FA** 1996 Graves' disease in children and adolescents. Late results of surgical treatment. Eur J Endocrinol. 134:710-715.

32. **Thompson NW, Dunn EL, Freitas JE, Sisson JC, Coran AG, Nishiyama RH** 1977 Surgical treatment of thyrotoxicosis in children and adolescents. J Pediatr Surg. 12:1009-1018.

33. **Argov S Duek D** 1982 The vanishing surgical treatment of Graves' disease: review of current literature and experience with 50 patients. Curr Surg. 39:158-162.

34. **Cooper DS** 1986 Which anti-thyroid drug? Am J Med. 80:1165-1168.

35. **Cooper DS** 1984 Antithyroid drugs. N Engl J Med. 311:1353-1362.

36. **Dallas JS Foley TP** 1996 Hyperthyroidism. p. 401-414. In F. Lifshitz. (ed.), Pediatric Endocrinology. Marcel Dekker,Inc. New York.

37. **Mashio Y, Beniko M, Ikota A, Mizumoto H, Kunita H** 1988 Treatment of

hyperthyroidism with a small single daily dose of methimazole. Acta Endocrinol (Copenh). 119:139-144.

38. **Mashio Y, Beniko M, Matsuda A, Koizumi S, Matsuya K, Mizumoto H, Ikota A, Kunita H** 1997 Treatment of hyperthyroidism with a small single daily dose of methimazole: a prospective long-term follow-up study. Endocr J. 44:553-558.

39. **Greer MA, Meihoff W, Studer H** 1965 Treatment of hyperthyroidism with a singe daily dose of propylthiouracil. N Engl J Med. 272:888-891.

40. **Shiroozu A, Okamura K, Ikenoue H, Sato K, Nakashima T, Yoshinari M, Fujishima M, Yoshizumi T** 1986 Treatment of hyperthyroidism with a small single daily dose of methimazole. J Clin Endocrinol Metab. 63:125-128.

41. **Peters H, Fischer C, Bogner U, Reiners C, Schleusener H** 1997 Treatment of Graves' hyperthyroidism with radioiodine: results of a prospective randomized study. Thyroid. 7:247-251.

42. **LeFranchi S, Mandel SH** 1995 Graves' disease in the neonatal period and childhood. p. 1237-1246. In L. E. Braverman and R. D. Utiger. (ed.), The Thyroid: A Fundamental and Clinical Text. J.B. Lippincott, Philadelphia.

43. **Hung W, Wilkins L, Blizzard RM** 1962 Medical therapy of thyrotoxicosis in children. Pediatrics. 30:17-26.

44. **Vaidya VA, Bongiovanni AM, Parks JS, Tenore A, Kirkland RT** 1974 Twenty-two years' experience in the medical management of juvenile thyrotoxicosis. Pediatrics. 54:565-570.

45. **Hanson JS** 1984 Propylthiouracil and hepatitis. Two cases and a review of the literature. Arch Intern Med. 144:994-996.

46. **Amrhein JA, Kenny FM, Ross D** 1970 Granulocytopenia, lupus-like syndrome, and other complications of propylthiouracil therapy. J Pediatr. 76:54-63.

47. **Tajiri J, Noguchi S, Murakami N** 1997 Usefulness of granulocyte count measurement four hours after injection of granulocyte colony-stimulating factor for detecting recovery from antithyroid drug-induced granulocytopenia. Thyroid. 7:575-578.

48. **Magner JA Snyder DK** 1994 Methimazole-induced agranulocytosis treated with recombinant human granulocyte colony-stimulating factor (G-CSF). Thyroid. 4:295-296.

49. **Bartalena L, Bogazzi F, Martino E** 1996 Adverse effects of thyroid hormone preparations and antithyroid drugs. Drug Saf. 15:53-63.

50. **Shulman DI, Muhar I, Jorgensen EV, Diamond FB, Bercu BB, Root AW** 1997 Autoimmune hyperthyroidism in prepubertal children and adolescents: comparison of clinical and biochemical features at diagnosis and responses to medical therapy. Thyroid. 7:755-760.

51. **Vitti P, Rago T, Chiovato L, Pallini S, Santini F, Fiore E, Rocchi R, Martino E, Pinchera A** 1997 Clinical features of patients with Graves' disease undergoing remission after antithyroid drug treatment. Thyroid. 7:369-375.

52. **Kim WB, Chung HK, Lee HK, Kohn LD, Tahara K, Cho BY** 1997 Changes in epitopes for thyroid-stimulating antibodies in Graves' disease sera during treatment of hyperthyroidism: therapeutic implications. J Clin Endocrinol Metab. 82:1953-1959.

53. **Davies TF, Roti E, Braverman LE, DeGroot LJ** 1998 Thyroid controversy--stimulating antibodies. J Clin Endocrinol Metab. 83:3777-3785.

54. **Wilson R, McKillop JH, Henderson N, Pearson DW, Thomson JA** 1986 The ability of the serum thyrotrophin receptor antibody (TRAb) index and HLA status to predict long-term remission of thyrotoxicosis following medical therapy for Graves' disease. Clin Endocrinol (Oxf). 25:151-156.

55. **Rapoport B, Greenspan FS, Filetti S, Pepitone M** 1984 Clinical experience with a human thyroid cell bioassay for thyroid-stimulating immunoglobulin. J Clin Endocrinol Metab. 58:332-338.

56. **Bouma DJ, Kammer H, Greer MA** 1982 Follow-up comparison of short-term versus 1-year antithyroid drug therapy for the thyrotoxicosis of Graves' disease. J Clin Endocrinol Metab. 55:1138-1142.

57. **Greer MA, Kammer H, Bouma DJ** 1977 Short-term antithyroid drug therapy for the thyrotoxicosis of Graves's disease. N Engl J Med. 297:173-176.

58. **DeGroot LJ** 1977 Short-term antithyroid drug therapy. N Engl J Med. 297:212-213.

59. **Bing RF Rosenthal FD** 1982 Early remission in thyrotoxicosis produced by short courses of treatment. Acta Endocrinol (Copenh). 100:221-223.

60. **Allannic H, Fauchet R, Orgiazzi J, Madec AM, Genetet B, Lorcy Y, Le Guerrier AM, Delambre C, Derennes V** 1990 Antithyroid drugs and Graves' disease: a prospective randomized evaluation of the efficacy of treatment duration. J Clin Endocrinol Metab. 70:675-679.

61. **Garcia-Mayor RV, Paramo C, Luna Cano R, Perez Mendez LF, Galofre JC, Andrade A** 1992 Antithyroid drug and Graves' hyperthyroidism. Significance of treatment duration and TRAb determination on lasting remission. J Endocrinol Invest. 15:815-820.

62. **Ford HC, Feek CM, Delahunt JW** 1991 Once daily, low dose, short term antithyroid drug treatment of Graves' disease is followed by an unacceptably high relapse rate. N Z Med J. 104:97-98.

63. **Dobyns BM, Sheline GE, Workman JB, Tompkins EA, McConahey WM, Becker DV** 1974 Malignant and benign neoplasms of the thyroid in patients treated for hyperthyroidism: a report of the cooperative thyrotoxicosis therapy follow-up study. J Clin Endocrinol Metab. 38:976-998.

64. **Ron E, Doody MM, Becker DV, Brill AB, Curtis RE, Goldman MB, Harris BS, 3rd, Hoffman DA, McConahey WM, Maxon HR, Preston-Martin S, Warshauer ME, Wong FL, Boice JD, Jr.** 1998 Cancer mortality following treatment for adult hyperthyroidism. Cooperative Thyrotoxicosis Therapy Follow-up Study Group [see comments]. JAMA. 280:347-355.

65. **Cunnien AJ, Hay ID, Gorman CA, Offord KP, Scanlon PW** 1982 Radioiodine-induced hypothyroidism in Graves' disease: factors associated. J Nucl Med. 23:978-983.

66. **de Bruin TW, Croon CD, de Klerk JM, van Isselt JW** 1994 Standardized radioiodine therapy in Graves' disease: the persistent effect of thyroid weight and radioiodine uptake on outcome. J Intern Med. 236:507-513.

67. **Dobyns BM** 1975 Radiation effects of radiodine on the thyroid. Effects vary with dosage and sensitivity of the gland to radiation. R I Med J. 58:94-7, 122-5.

68. **Vitti P, Martino E, Aghini-Lombardi F, Rago T, Antonangeli L, Maccherini D, Nanni P, Loviselli A, Balestrieri A, Araneo G** 1994 Thyroid volume measurement by ultrasound in children as a tool for the assessment of mild iodine deficiency. J Clin Endocrinol Metab. 79:600-603.

69. **Ueda D** 1990 Normal volume of the thyroid gland in children. J Clin Ultrasound. 18:455-462.

70. **Peters H, Fischer C, Bogner U, Reiners C, Schleusener H** 1995 Radioiodine therapy of Graves' hyperthyroidism: standard vs. calculated 131iodine activity. Results from a prospective, randomized, multicentre study. Eur J Clin Invest. 25:186-193.

71. **Maxon HR, Thomas SR, Hertzberg VS, Kereiakes JG, Chen IW, Sperling MI, Saenger EL** 1983 Relation between effective radiation dose and outcome of radioiodine therapy for thyroid cancer. N Engl J Med. 309:937-941.

72. **Goolden AWG Davey JB** 1963 The ablation of normal thyroid tissue with iodine-131. Br J Radiol. 36:340-345.

73. **Graham GD Burman KD** 1986 Radioiodine treatment of Graves' disease. An assessment of its potential risks. Ann Intern Med. 105:900-905.

74. **Becker DV Hurley JR** 1971 Complications of radioiodine treatment of hyperthyroidism.

Semin Nucl Med. 1:442-460.

75. **Refetoff S, Demeester-Mirkine N, Ermans AM, DeGroot LJ** 1977 Rapid control of thyrotoxicosis with combined 131I, anthithyroid drugs and KI therapy. J Nucl Med Allied Sci. 21:23-29.

76. **Ross DS, Daniels GH, De Stefano P, Maloof F, Ridgway EC** 1983 Use of adjunctive potassium iodide after radioactive iodine (131I) treatment of Graves' hyperthyroidism. J Clin Endocrinol Metab. 57:250-253.

77. **Aizawa Y, Yoshida K, Kaise N, Fukazawa H, Kiso Y, Sayama N, Hori H, Abe K** 1997 The development of transient hypothyroidism after iodine-131 treatment in hyperthyroid patients with Graves' disease: prevalence, mechanism and prognosis. Clin Endocrinol (Oxf). 46:1-5.

78. **Goolden AW Stewart JS** 1986 Long-term results from graded low dose radioactive iodine therapy for thyrotoxicosis. Clin Endocrinol (Oxf). 24:217-222.

79. **McCullagh EP, Jelden GL, Rodriguez-Antunez A** 1976 Incidence of hypothyroidism following small doses of 131I in the treatment of Graves' disease. Ohio State Med J. 72:538-540.

80. **Rapoport B, Caplan R, DeGroot LJ** 1973 Low-dose sodium iodide I 131 therapy in Graves disease. JAMA. 224:1610-1613.

81. **Sridama V, McCormick M, Kaplan EL, Fauchet R, DeGroot LJ** 1984 Long-term follow-up study of compensated low-dose 131I therapy for Graves' disease. N Engl J Med. 311:426-432.

82. **Sridama V DeGroot LJ** 1989 Treatment of Graves' disease and the course of ophthalmopathy. Am J Med. 87:70-73.

83. **Safa AM Skillern PG** 1975 Treatment of hyperthyroidism with a large initial dose of sodium iodide I 131. Arch Intern Med. 135:673-675.

84. **Sheline GE, Lindsay S, McCormack KR, Galante M** 1962 Thyroid nodules occuring late after treatment of thyrotoxicosis with radioiodine. J Clin Endocrinol Metab. 22:8-17.

85. **Snyder S** 1978 Vocal cord paralysis after radioiodine therapy. J Nucl Med. 19:975-976.

86. **Chiovato L, Fiore E, Vitti P, Rocchi R, Rago T, Dokic D, Latrofa F, Mammoli C, Lippi F, Ceccarelli C, Pinchera A** 1998 Outcome of thyroid function in Graves' patients treated with radioiodine: Role of thyroid -stimulating and thyrotropin-blocking antibodies and of radioiodine-induced thyroid damage. J Clin Endocrinol Metab. 83:40-46.

87. **Murakami Y, Takamatsu J, Sakane S, Kuma K, Ohsawa N** 1996 Changes in thyroid volume in response to radioactive iodine for Graves' hyperthyroidism correlated with activity of thyroid-stimulating antibody and treatment outcome. J Clin Endocrinol Metab. 81:3257-3260.

88. **Hancock LD, Tuttle RM, LeMar H, Bauman J, Patience T** 1997 The effect of propylthiouracil on subsequent radioactive iodine therapy in Graves' disease. Clin Endocrinol (Oxf). 47:425-430.

89. **Tuttle RM, Patience T, Budd S** 1995 Treatment with propylthiouracil before radioactive iodine therapy is associated with a higher treatment failure rate than therapy with radioactive iodine alone in Graves' disease. Thyroid. 5:243-247.

90. **Yoshida K, Aizawa Y, Kaise N, Fukazawa H, Kiso Y, Sayama N, Mori K, Hori H, Abe K** 1996 Relationship between thyroid-stimulating antibodies and thyrotropin-binding inhibitory immunoglobulins years after administration of radioiodine for Graves' disease: retrospective clinical survey. J Endocrinol Invest. 19:682-686.

91. **Imseis RE, Vanmiddlesworth L, Massie JD, Bush AJ, Vanmiddlesworth NR** 1998 Pretreatment with propylthiouracil but not methimazole reduces the therapeutic efficacy of iodine-131 in hyperthyroidism. J Clin Endocrinol Metab. 83:685-687.

92. **Goolden AW, Kam KC, Fitzpatrick ML, Munro AJ** 1986 Oedema of the neck after ablation of the thyroid with radioactive iodine. Br J Radiol. 59:583-586.

93. **Craswell PW** 1972 Vocal cord paresis following radioactive iodine therapy. Br J Clin Pract. 26:571-572.

94. **Benua RS, Becker DV, Hurley JR** 1994 Thyroid storm. Curr Ther Endocrinol Metab. 5:75-7:75-77.

95. **Creutzig H, Kallfelz I, Haindl J, Thiede G, Hundeshagen H** 1976 Letter: Thyroid storm and iodine-131 treatment. Lancet. 2:145

96. **McDermott MT, Kidd GS, Dodson LE, Jr., Hofeldt FD** 1983 Radioiodine-induced thyroid storm. Case report and literature review. Am J Med. 75:353-359.

97. **DeGroot LJ, Gorman CA, Pinchera A, Bartalena L, Marcocci C, Wiersinga WM, Prummel MF, Wartofsky L, Marocci C,C.** 1995 Therapeutic controversies. Retro-orbital radiation and radioactive iodide ablation of the thyroid may be good for Graves' ophthalmopathy. J Clin Endocrinol Metab. 80:339-340.

98. **Tallstedt L Lundell G** 1997 Radioiodine treatment, ablation, and ophthalmopathy: a balanced perspective. Thyroid. 7:241-245.

99. **Bartley GB, Fatourechi V, Kadrmas EF, Jacobsen SJ, Ilstrup DM, Garrity JA, Gorman CA** 1996 Chronology of Graves' ophthalmopathy in an incidence cohort. Am J Ophthalmol. 121:426-434.

100. **Bartalena L, Marcocci C, Bagozzi F, Manetti L, Tanda ML, Dell'Unto E, Bruno-Bossio G, Nardi M, Bartolomei MP, Lepri A, Rossi G, Martino E, Pincehra A** 1998 Relation between therapy for hyperthyroidism and the course of Graves' ophthalmopathy. N Engl J Med. 338:73-78.

101. **Duffy BJ, Jr. Fitzgerald PJ** 1950 Cancer of the thyroid in children: a report of twenty-eight cases. J Clin Endocrinol Metab. 10:1296-1308.

102. **Becker DV, Robbins J, Beebe GW, Bouville AC, Wachholz BW** 1996 Childhood thyroid cancer following the Chernobyl accident: a status report. Endocrinol Metab Clin North Am. 25:197-211.

103. **Dolphin GW** 1968 The risk of thyroid cancers following irradiation. Health Phys. 15:219-228.

104. **Goldman MB, Monson RR, Maloof F** 1990 Cancer mortality in women with thyroid disease. Cancer Res. 50:2283-2289.

105. **Ron E Saftlas AF** 1996 Head and neck radiation carcinogenesis: epidemiologic evidence. Otolaryngol Head Neck Surg. 115:403-408.

106. **Shore RE** 1992 Issues and epidemiological evidence regarding radiation-induced thyroid cancer. Radiat Res. 131:98-111.

107. **Thompson DE, Mabuchi K, Ron E, Soda M, Tokunaga M, Ochikubo S, Sugimoto S, Ikeda T, Terasaki M** 1994 Cancer incidence in atomic bomb survivors. Part II: Solid tumors, 1958-1987. Radiat Res. 137:S17-67.

108. **Boice JD, Jr.** 1998 Radiation and thyroid cancer-what more can be learned? Acta Oncol. 34:321-324.

109. **Tucker MA, Jones PH, Boice JD, Jr., Robison LL, Stone BJ, Stovall M, Jenkin RD, Lubin JH, Baum ES, Siegel SE** 1991 Therapeutic radiation at a young age is linked to secondary thyroid cancer. The Late Effects Study Group. Cancer Res. 51:2885-2888.

110. **Ron E, Lubin JH, Shore RE, Mabuchi K, Modan B, Pottern LM, Schneider AB, Tucker MA, Boice JD, Jr.** 1995 Thyroid cancer after exposure to external radiation: a pooled analysis of seven studies. Radiat Res. 141:259-277.

111. **Kumpusalo L, Kumpusalo E, Soimakallio S, Salomaa S, Paile W, Kolmakow S, Zhukowsky G, Ilchenko I, Nissinen A** 1996 Thyroid ultrasound findings 7 years after the Chernobyl accident. A comparative epidemiological study in the Bryansk region of Russia. Acta Radiol. 37:904-909.

112. **Nikiforov Y, Gnepp DR, Fagin JA** 1996 Thyroid lesions in children and adolescents after the Chernobyl disaster: implications for the study of radiation tumorigenesis. J Clin

Endocrinol Metab. 81:9-14.

113. **Zimmerman D, Hay ID, Gough IR, Goellner JR, Ryan JJ, Grant CS, McConahey WM** 1988 Papillary thyroid carcinoma in children and adults: long-term follow-up of 1039 patients conservatively treated at one institution during three decades. Surgery. 104:1157-1166.

114. **Farbota LM, Calandra DB, Lawrence AM, Paloyan E** 1985 Thyroid carcinoma in Graves' disease. Surgery. 98:1148-1153.

115. **Karlan MS, Pollock WF, Snyder WH** 1964 Carcinoma of the thyroid following treatment of hyperthyroidism with radioactive iodine. Calif Med J.. 101:196-201.

116. **Gorman CA Robertson JS** 1978 Radiation dose in the selection of 131I or surgical treatment for toxic thyroid adenoma. Ann Intern Med. 89:85-90.

117. **Utiger RD** 1992 Pathogenesis of Graves' ophthalmopathy. N Engl J Med. 326:1772-1773.

118. **Land CE** 1980 Estimating cancer risks from low doses of ionizing radiation. Science. 209:1197-1203.

119. **Hall P, Holm LE, Lundell G, Bjelkengren G, Larsson LG, Lindberg S, Tennvall J, Wicklund H, Boice JD, Jr.** 1991 Cancer risks in thyroid cancer patients. Br J Cancer. 64:159-163.

120. **Holm LE, Hall P, Wiklund K, Lundell G, Berg G, Bjelkengren G, Cederquist E, Ericsson UB, Hallquist A, Larsson LG** 1991 Cancer risk after iodine-131 therapy for hyperthyroidism. J Natl Cancer Inst. 83:1072-1077.

121. **Pochin EE** 1968 Leukemia following radioiodine treatment of thyrotoxicosis. Br Med J. 11:1545-1550.

122. **Werner SC, Gittleshon AM, Brill AB** 1961 Leukemia following radioiodine therapy of hyperthyroidism. JAMA. 177:646-648.

123. **Robertson JS Gorman CA** 1976 Gonadal radiation dose and its genetic significance in radioiodine therapy of hyperthyroidism. J Nucl Med. 17:826-835.

124. **Sarkar SD, Beierwaltes WH, Gill SP, Cowley BJ** 1976 Subsequent fertility and birth histories of children and adolescents treated with 131I for thyroid cancer. J Nucl Med. 17:460-464.

125. **Schull WJ, Otake M, Neel JV** 1981 Genetic effects of the atomic bombs: a reappraisal. Science. 213:1220-1227.

126. **Spencer RP, Kayani N, Karimeddini MK** 1985 Radioiodine therapy of hyperthyroidism: socioeconomic considerations. J Nucl Med. 26:663-665.

127. **Mazzaferri EL** 1990 Thyroid cancer and Graves' disease. J Clin Endocrinol Metab. 70:826-829.

14

PREGNANCY AND GRAVES' DISEASE

John H Lazarus

INTRODUCTION

The prevalence of Graves' disease is approximately 3.0/1000 with an incidence of about 0.5/1000/year. The prevalence and incidence in women during child bearing years is not known but thyrotoxicosis is said to occur in 2/1000 pregnancies and Graves' disease would be expected to account for at least 80% of these cases. While these figures are low, Graves' hyperthyroidism can have a dramatic effect on the mother as well as the fetus. The thyroid hormone changes and immunological effects of normal pregnancy will be reviewed as a background to the discussion of Graves' disease in pregnancy and the postpartum period. The subject has been reviewed (1-4)

PREGNANCY AND THE THYROID

Hormonal Changes

It has been known for some time that pregnancy has an appreciable effect on thyroid economy (5). There are significant changes in iodine metabolism characterised by increased excretion of iodine in the urine accounting for the increase in thyroid volume even in areas of moderate dietary iodine intake (6). Thyroid hormone transport proteins, particularly TBG, increase due to enhanced hepatic synthesis and a reduced degradation rate due to oligosaccharide modification. Serum concentrations of thyroid hormones have been reported to be decreased, increased or unchanged during gestation. The increase in thyroid volume already referred to is substantially greater in iodine deficient areas (7).

The placenta secretes hCG, a glycoprotein hormone sharing a common alpha subunit with TSH but having a unique beta subunit, which confers specificity. Evidence derived both from *in vitro* studies on thyroid tissue and on eucaryotic cells stably expressing the human TSH receptor (TSHR), suggests that hCG, or a molecular variant, is able to act as a TSH agonist although this is controversial (8). Whether hCG has any effect on thyroid antibody expression during pregnancy is unknown.

Immune Changes

Pregnancy has a profound effect on the immune system in order to maintain the fetal/maternal allograft, which is not rejected despite displaying paternal histocompatability antigens. This effect is partly mediated by the placenta since the trophoblast (the layer of cells at the interface) does not express classical MHC class I and II. HLA-G, a non-classical MHC molecule which is expressed on the trophoblast, may be a ligand for the natural killer (NK) cell receptor and so protect the fetus from NK cell damage whilst allowing these cells to secrete their cytokines which have pleiotropic effects (9).

Apart from these localised mechanisms of protection, more systemic controls are also in operation. The Th1 (cell mediated) and Th2 (humoral) immune responses are characterised by their cytokine profile (Th1 - gamma interferon, tumor necrosis factor and IL-2; Th2 - principally IL-4 and IL-10). Whether a Th1 or Th2 response prevails seems to be determined by the cytokines elaborated at the induction of the response and there seems to be mutual antagonism between the two. In pregnancy there appears to be a bias towards a Th2, humoral response, since Th1 cytokines are potentially harmful to the fetus. This seems to be achieved by the fetal/placental unit producing Th2 cytokines which inhibit the production of Th1 cytokines (10). The consequence may be a successful pregnancy but it may increase the susceptibility of the mother to certain infections, particularly those which are combatted by a cell mediated response, such as tuberculosis. However, the Th1 and Th2 status in pregnancy may not be clear cut: for example, TSHR antibodies decline during gestation (11) which is not in keeping with a Th2 response. Recently it has been shown that there is a switch in the type of antibody production during pregnancy in patients with Graves' disease from the stimulating to the blocking variety (12).

Apart from the bias towards Th2, there is thymic involution and a reduction in the production of new B lymphocytes and their export to the periphery (13). This implies that B cells responsible for producing antibodies were already in existence before pregnancy and that a disruption in the maintenance of tolerance can occur. In autoimmune thyroiditis as in Graves' disease there is usually a fall in the titre of thyroid antibodies during gestation, indicating the importance of Th1 cell mediated help in the production of pathogenic anti-thyroid peroxidase (TPO) antibodies. Modifications in the balance of ' helper' and 'suppressor' T lymphocytes have been observed (14-16) with an increase in the numbers of the former, CD4+CD45RA+, and a decrease in the latter, CD4+CD29+, coupled with a reduction in T lymphocyte proliferative response to mitogens (17). In addition there are alterations in cellular immunity characterised by a fall in the $CD4^{+}/CD8^{+}$ ratio in late pregnancy and an increase in NK activity in postpartum autoimmune thyroid disease (18) which may result in immune depression (19). The balance which exists between Th1- and Th2-type responses is also vital in determining the susceptibility of an individual to develop autoimmune disease.

Whether individual humans have a tenancy to mount a Th1 or Th2 response to a given (auto) antigen remains to be determined. Considerable efforts have been made to determine the MHC haplotype which confers the greatest risk of developing autoimmune thyroid disease (AITD) in general and pregnancy associated AITD in particular. Results vary considerably with the ethnic background of the population studied but broadly speaking HLADR3/DR5 heterozygosity is associated with Graves' disease (20) in a caucasian population.

Just as the immune system is geared to maintaining the fetus throughout pregnancy, there is an abrupt change at parturition and the separation of the placenta may be achieved by immune mechanisms (21) with a rapid switch back to a Th1-type response. Immediately postpartum, IgG1 levels are suppressed and this period is usually associated with a flare up in Th1 disorders such as Hashimoto's thyroiditis, insulin dependent diabetes mellitus and non-Graves' postpartum thyroiditis.

Outcome of poorly treated or untreated Graves' hyperthyroidism in pregnancy

Prompt diagnosis and treatment are essential to avoid both maternal and fetal complications. Maternal complications include, miscarriage, placenta abruptio and preterm delivery. Congestive heart failure and thyroid storm may also occur and the risk of pre-eclampsia is significantly higher in women with poorly controlled hyperthyroidism (22,3,4). From the fetal aspect, hyperthyroidism, neonatal hyperthyroidism, prematurity and intra-uterine growth retardation may be observed. Hamburger (23) cited 11 reports that collectively documented a 5.6% incidence of fetal death or stillbirth in 249 pregnancies and a further 5% fetal and neonatal abnormalities. These figures are greater than those expected in normal pregnancy. However many of these reports are relatively old. With better recognition of the treatment requirements of the pregnant Graves' patient these complications should become less frequent. There is therefore no doubt that hyperthyroidism should be treated although it is true to state that Graves' disease may ameliorate during gestation in similar fashion to some other autoimmune diseases.

This gestational amelioration is often associated with a reduction in titer of TSHR autoantibodies and, as has been stated, a change from stimulatory to blocking antibody activity is observed in Graves' disease during pregnancy in some cases (12). It should also be noted that a variety of thyroid related antibodies may occur in patients with Graves' disease. Zakarija et al (24) for example reported the presence of two species of stimulating antibody in a patient who gave birth to three children with transient neonatal hyperthyroidism. In addition to the classical TSAb, another stimulating antibody was observed whose *in vitro* stimulating activity was not inhibited by a TSH binding inhibitory antibody also present in this particular patient in appreciable amounts. This report emphasises the concept that patients with Graves' hyperthyroidism often possess more than one antibody directed against the TSHR. To emphasize this point, a recent report has documented in a patient with Graves' disease in late pregnancy the appearance of a blocking antibody to the TSHR, suggested to be the cause of the development of primary hypothyroidism (25).

Clinical Aspects

While the commonest cause of hyperthyroidism in pregnancy is Graves' disease other causes such as toxic multinodular goiter, toxic adenoma and subacute thyroiditis may occur. Rarer causes include struma ovarii and hydatidiform mole. The clinical presentation of hyperthyroidism may not be obvious as symptoms of tachycardia, sweating, dyspnea and nervousness may be seen in normal pregnancy. Cardiac systolic flow murmurs occur in normal pregnancy as well as hyperthyroidism. The diagnosis of Graves' disease is made clinically by a family history of autoimmune thyroid disease and/or by a diffuse goiter together with extrathyroidal signs of ophthalmopathy or dermopathy.

The diagnosis of hyperthyroidism in pregnancy is made by measurement of serum thyroid hormone levels and of TSH using a sensitive assay (26). Free T4 and T3 as, opposed to total T4 andT3, assays are preferred as the former compensate for an estrogen stimulated increase in TBG concentration. However free hormone concentrations decline during gestation and a normal range should be established in pregnancy. Also, TSH may be suppressed in early pregnancy due to the secretion of hCG which is a weak thyroid stimulatory. Thus the serum TSH alone is usually not adequate to assess thyroid status in early gestation but has a high specificity in later pregnancy (27). Radioiodine uptake studies are contra-indicated during pregnancy but thyroid ultrasound will indicate the diffuse nature of the thyroid gland. The diagnosis of Graves' disease may be confirmed if the clinical picture is unclear by measurement of TSHR antibodies (optimally measured as the TSHR stimulating antibody - TSAb). Because of the immune changes already referred to, TSAb titers decline during gestation along with those of anti-TPO antibodies. Thus at 36 weeks TSAb may be undetectable. If still positive at this time the risk of neonatal hyperthyroidism consequent to transplacental passage of maternal antibody is increased. Measurement of TSAb is particularly important in a woman previously treated for Graves' hyperthyroidism and who is euthyroid during gestation (28). In this situation a false sense of security in relation to the development of neonatal hyperthyroidism may be engendered if TSAb is not measured at 36 weeks. Cases of neonatal hyperthyroidism have been recorded whose mothers were receiving thyroxine therapy for post-surgical hypothyroidism while pregnant.

Management

Prior to conception

There is a good case for a preconception clinic for patients with Graves' hyperthyroidism who wish to become pregnant. Firstly, education about the effects of the disease on maternal health and fetal well-being can be given to allay fears which are commonly present in these women. The patient's thyroid status should be checked frequently to minimise risk of miscarriage should she be hyperthyroid at the time of conception. If treatment had been commenced with methimazole or carbimazole a change to propylthiouracil (PTU) is recommended to reduce the admittedly rare occurrence of aplasia cutis reported following the administration of the former drugs (29) although a cause and effect relationship is disputed (3). During gestation the patient management will be as detailed below.

Previously treated patients with Graves' disease

These patients may have received antithyroid drugs, surgery or radioiodine therapy and be euthyroid on or off thyroxine therapy. The important concern here is the realisation that neonatal hyperthyroidism may still occur. Recent guidelines state that if the patient is in remission after receiving only antithyroid drugs, there is no need to measure TSHR antibodies as the maternal thyroid function gives a reliable estimate of fetal thyroid status and the risk of neonatal hyperthyroidism is very low (28). TSHR antibodies should be measured in euthyroid pregnant women previously treated by either radioiodine or surgery early in pregnancy. If the antibody level is high at this time the fetus should be evaluated carefully during gestation and the antibodies measured again in the last trimester (see Table 1).

Table 1: Guidelines for measurements of TSH-receptor antibodies in a pregnant woman with Graves' disease

Patient Status	Measurement
Euthyroid - previous AITD	Not necessary
Euthyroid, with or without T4 therapy; previous [131] I treatment or surgery	Check in early pregnancy: - if low or absent, no further testing - if high, check fetus and check antibodies in last trimester
Receiving AITD during pregnancy	Measure in last trimester

AITD - Antithyroid drugs
Adapted from Laurberg et al 1998 (28)

Graves' hyperthyroidism inadvertently treated with radioiodine in early gestation.
The practical procedures surrounding the administration of radioiodine therapy for Graves' disease vary widely (30). In many clinics, routine pregnancy testing is not performed before ^{131}I administration. Despite denial of pregnancy, several reports of inappropriate radioiodine administration have highlighted the concern about the fetal radiation risk (31). The maternal thyroid uptake, the gestational age and the ability of the fetal thyroid to concentrate iodine are all vital in determining the radioiodine exposure in utero (32). The fetal thyroid concentrates iodide after 10 to 12 weeks gestation and is relatively more avid for iodine than the maternal thyroid. The fetal tissues are also more radio-sensitive. Administration of up to 15 mCi (555 MBq)[131]I for hyperthyroidism up to 10 weeks gestation does not compromise fetal thyroid function and the low fetal whole body irradiation is not considered sufficient to justify termination of pregnancy although this is often performed. However, from limited clinical data, ^{131}I given after that gestational age results in biochemical hypothyroidism and even cretinism in the neonate (33). In these circumstances termination of pregnancy may be advised but dosimetry studies should be performed. If the pregnancy continues to term intra-uterine hypothyroidism may be diagnosed by umbilical cord sampling.

The neonate should be evaluated at birth specifically for hypothyroidism and for malformations which are more common with higher doses of radiation.

Patients found to have hyperthyroid Graves' disease in early pregnancy.

Medical therapy is preferred by most clinicians as radioiodine is contra-indicated and surgery requires pretreatment with antithyroid drugs to render the patient euthyroid. Treatment is essential to minimise the adverse outcomes associated with Graves' disease (see above). PTU should be given in a dose of 100 to 150mg three times daily until the patient becomes euthyroid at which time the dose should be reduced to the lowest amount to maintain the euthyroid state. However, in terms of rapidity of action and fetal hypothyroidism inducing potential, there is probably little reason to choose PTU over methimazole (MMI)(34,35). The so-called 'block and replace' regime in which thyroxine is given with antithyroid drug should not be used because the dose of antithyroid drug would inevitably be too high and cause fetal goiter and hypothyroidism. The aim of treatment should be to maintain the serum T4 concentration at the upper end of the normal range. Hashizume et al. (36) have reported that T4 administration to pregnant women with Graves' hyperthyroidism during pregnancy and after delivery, together with MMI, effectively reduced the incidence of postpartum recurrence of hyperthyroidism (see below), but these results have not been confirmed. PTU has a shorter half-life in plasma than MMI but is not present in as high a concentration in breast milk. Hence women receiving PTU can breast feed without significant risk to the neonate (37,38). PTU should be continued in low dose throughout gestation and up to, and through, labor. Common complications of thionamide therapy include skin rash, arthralgia and nausea in about 2% of patients. Methimazole (or carbimazole) may be used as an alternative in this situation with only a 33% chance of cross-reaction. Agranulocytosis is rare and is an indication for immediate withdrawal of the drug and possible treatment with granulocyte colony stimulating factor although the results are not always satisfactory (39). There is no benefit in routinely monitoring the white blood count as the fall in this count may be very rapid. Available evidence suggests that there is no significant effect of antithyroid drugs in utero on the long-term health of the neonate or child, assuming the dose during gestation has not cause iatrogenic fetal hypothyroidism. Thus, Messer et al. (40) compared 17 children of 13 hyperthyroid mothers with 25 children of 15 euthyroid mothers 7 to 11 years postpartum and found no differences between these groups in their clinical status, mental development or psychomotor development. These data confirm results of similar studies (41,42) in which the intellectual capacity of subjects whose mothers had received antithyroid drugs during pregnancy was examined. These drugs did not adversely affect intellectual capacity of the offspring. Beta-adrenergic blocking agents such as propranolol may be used for a few weeks to ameliorate the peripheral sympathomimetic actions of excess thyroid hormone but prolonged use can result in retarded fetal growth, impaired response to anoxic stress together with postnatal bradycardia and hypoglycaemia (43). These drugs can be used in the uncommon instance of intolerance to both of the available thionamide drugs.

Surgery

Subtotal thyroidectomy is indicated if control of the hyperthyroidism is poor on account of poor compliance or inability to take drugs. Patients with a very large goiter may also require surgery because of pressure symptoms in the neck. Surgery is preferred in the second trimester because of a higher risk of associated abortion earlier in gestation. In general, surgery should be avoided if it is considered that medical therapy has a reasonable chance of success.

Severe hyperthyroidism

This term refers to patients who have been non-compliant with previously prescribed drug therapy as well as patients presenting for the first time late in gestation with severe hyperthyroidism. Rarely an episode of infection or the development of pre-eclampsia may precipitate thyroid storm. This is a medical emergency requiring the use of thionamides, iodides, beta blockers, fluid replacement and possibly steroid therapy and plasmapheresis to achieve euthyroidism (44).

Postpartum Graves' Disease

Patients with Graves' disease may develop Graves' hyperthyroidism followed by transient hypothyroidism due to co-existing destructive autoimmune thyroiditis during the early postpartum period despite increasing TSAb activity (45). This consideration may be important when considering postpartum relapse of the disease. The pathogenesis of postpartum hyperthyroidism is related to the so-called 'immune rebound phenomenon' in which the immune system, depressed during gestation, becomes activated postpartum with an accompanying elevation of thyroid antibodies. This phenomenon has been well shown by the dramatic postpartum rise in anti-TPO antibodies in women found to be anti-TPO antibody positive in early pregnancy (46). Gonzalez-Jimenez et al (11) have shown that TSHR antibodies tend to decrease during late gestation in Graves' disease patients but a significant rebound is observed in the late postpartum period. Individual patients at high risk of postpartum onset of Graves' disease can be found in early pregnancy by the detection of TSAb (47). Tada et al (48) reported that at least 37 of 92 patients with Graves' disease who were of child bearing age showed clear evidence of postpartum onset of the disease. Thus, in this selected group of 20-39 year old women, at least 40% developed their disease during the postpartum period.

It is important to differentiate postpartum Graves' disease with accompanying hyperthyroidism from the other causes of postpartum hyperthyroidism detailed above. Clinical examination, the presence of TSHR antibodies, and the thyroid radioiodine uptake and scintiscanning will usually resolve any diagnostic difficulty. However, a comprehensive study in Japan (49) in which 96 episodes of postpartum hyperthyroidism were studied suggested that silent thyroiditis (i.e. postpartum thyroiditis) commonly develops concomitantly with the activation of Graves' disease and may delay or mask the development of Graves' hyperthyroidism. The serum thyroglobulin concentration, which is raised in postpartum destructive thyroiditis with hyperthyroidism (50,51), has also been shown to be useful for the differentiation of this condition from Graves' hyperthyroidism following delivery.

Therapy of postpartum Graves' hyperthyroidism should be carried out by the usual methods (52) remembering that radioiodine is contra-indicated during breast feeding. Clearly, prevention of postpartum patients Graves' hyperthyroidism may be achieved by adequate treatment of the condition before the onset of gestation (53).

REFERENCES

1. **Lazarus JH.** 1993 Treatment of hyper- and hypothyroidism in pregnancy. J Endocrinol Invest. 16: 391-396.
2. **Roti E, Minelli R, Salvi M.** 1996 Clinical Review 80 Management of hyperthyroidism and hypothyroidism in the pregnant woman. J Clin Endocrinol Metab. 81: 1679-1685.
3. **Mestman JH.** 1998 Hyperthyroidism in pregnancy. Endocrinol Metab Clin North Am. 27: 127-149.
4. **Maziukiewicz UR, Burrow GN.** 1999 Hyperthyroidism in pregnancy, diagnosis and treatment. Thyroid (in press).
5. **Burrow GN, Fisher DA, Larsen PR.** 1994 Maternal and fetal thyroid function. N Engl J Med. 331: 1072-1078.
6. **Smyth PPA, Hetherton AMT, Smith DF, Radcliffe M.** 1997 Maternal iodine status and thyroid volume during pregnancy: Correlation with neonatal iodine intake. J Clin Endocrinol Metab. 82: 2840-2843.
7. **Glinoer D, Lemone M.** 1992 Goiter and pregnancy: a new insight into an old problem. Thyroid 2: 65-70.
8. **Hoermann R, Poertl S, Liss I et al.** 1995 Variation in the thyrotropic activity of human chorionic-gonadotropin in Chinese-hamster ovary cells arises from differential expression of the human thyrotropin receptor and microheterogeneity of the hormone. J Clin Endocrinol Metab 80: 1605-1610.
9. **Carosella ED, Dausset J, Kirszenbaum M.** 1996 HLA-G revisited. Immunol Today 17: 407-409.
10. **Wegmann TG, Lin H, Guilbert L, Mosmann TR.** 1993 Bidirectional cytokine interactions in the maternal-fetal relationship: is successful pregnancy a T_h2 phenomenon? Immunology Today 14: 353-356.
11. **Gonzalez-Jimenez A, Fernandez-Soto ML, Escobar-Jimenez F, Glinoer D, Navarrete L.** 1993 Thyroid function parameters and TSH-receptor antibodies in healthy subjects and Graves' disease patients: a sequential study before, during and after pregnancy. Thyroidology. 5: 13-20.
12. **Kung AWC, Jones BM** 1998 A change from stimulatory to blocking antibody activity in Graves' disease during pregnancy J Clin Endocrinol Metab 83:514-518.
13. **Kincade PW, Medina KL, Smithson G, Scott DC** 1994 Pregnancy: a clue to normal regulation of B lymphopoiesis. Immunology Today 15: 539-544.
14. **Sridama V, Pacini F, Yang SL et al** 1982 Decreased levels of helper T-cells: a possible cause of immunodeficiency in pregnancy. N Engl J Med. 307: 352-356.
15. **Barnett MA, Learmonth RP, Pihl E, Wood EC** 1983 T helper lymphocyte depression in early pregnancy. J Reproductive Immunol. 5: 55-57.
16. **Iwatani Y, Amino N, Tachi J et al** 1988 Changes of lymphocyte subsets in normal pregnant and postpartum women: postpartum increase of NK/K (Leu 7) cells. Am J Reproductive Immunol. 18: 52-55.
17. **Matthiesen L, Berg G, Ernerudh J, Hakansson L** 1996 Lymphocyte subsets and mitogen stimulation of blood-lymphocytes in normal pregnancy. Am J Reproductive

Immunol. 35: 70-79.

18. **Hidaka Y, Amino N, Iwatani Y** *et al* 1992 Increase in peripheral natural killer cell activity in patients with autoimmune thyroid disease. Autoimmunity 11: 239-246.

19. **Rich KC, Siegel JN, Jennings C** *et al* 1995 CD4^{+} Lymphocytes in perinatal human- immunodeficiency-virus (HIV) infection - evidence for pregnancy-induced immune depression in uninfected and HIV-infected women. J Infectious Dis. 172:1221-1227.

20. **Boehm BO, Kuhnl P, Manfras BJ** *et al* 1992 HLA-DRB3 gene alleles in caucasian patients with Graves' disease. Clin Investigator 70: 956-960.

21. **DeJongh AU, Jorens R, Student P, Heylen R** 1996 The contribution of the immune-system to parturition. Mediators of Inflammation 5: 173-182.

22. **Miller LK, Wing DA, Leung AS, Koonings PP, Montoro MN** *et al* 1994 Low birth weight and pre-eclampsia in pregnancies complicated by hyper-thyroidism. Obstet Gynecol. 80: 946-949.

23. **Hamburger JI** 1992 Diagnosis and management of Graves' disease in pregnancy. Thyroid 2: 219-224.

24. **Zakarija M, De Forteza R, McKenzie JM, Ghandur-Mnaymneh L** 1994 Characteristics and clinical correlates of a novel thyroid-stimulating autoantibody. Autoimmunity 19: 31-37.

25. **Ueta Y, Fukui H, Murakami H, Yamanoughi Y, Yamamoto R** 1999 Development of primary hypothyroidism with the appearance of blocking-type antibody to thyrotropin receptor in Graves' disease in late pregnancy. Thyroid 9:179-182.

26. **Brent GA** 1997 Maternal thyroid function: interpretation of thyroid function tests in pregnancy. Clin Obstet Gynecol. 40: 3-15.

27. **Bobrowski RA Streicher P Dzieczkowski JS Dombrowski MP Gonik B** 1998 Applicability of the third-generation, thyroid-stimulating hormone assay in pregnancy J Matern Fetal Med. 7: 65-67.

28. **Laurberg P, Nygaard B, Glinoer D, Grussendorf M, Orgiazzi J** 1998 Guidelines for TSH-receptor antibody measurements in pregnancy: results of an evidence-based symposium organized by the European Thyroid Association. Eur J Endocrinol. 139:584-590.

29. **Mandel SJ, Brent GA Larsen PR** 1994 Review of antithyroid drug use during pregnancy and report of case of aplasia cutis. Thyroid 4:129-133.

30. **Hedley AJ, Lazarus JH, McGhee SM, Jones RB, Sharp PF, Naven LM, Beardwell CG, Hall R** 1992 Treatment of hyperthyroidism by radioactive iodine. Summary of a UK National Survey prepared for the Royal College of Physicians Committee on Endocrinology and Diabetes. J Royal Coll Phys Lond. 26:348-351.

31. **Evans PMS, Webster J, Evans WD, Bevan JS, Scanlon MF** 1998 Radioiodine treatment in unsuspected pregnancy Clin Endocrinol. 48: 281-283.

32. **Zansonico PB** 1997 Radiation dose to patients and relatives incident to ^{131}I therapy. Thyroid. 7: 199-204.

33. **Gorman CA.** 1999 Radioiodine and Pregnancy. Thyroid 1999 (in press).

34. **Wing DA, Miller LK, Koonings PP, Montoro MN, Mestman JH.** 1994 A comparison of propylthiouracil versus methimazole in the treatment of hyperthyroidism in pregnancy. Am J Obstet Gynecol. 170: 90-95.

35. **Momotani N, Noh JY, Ishikawa N, Ito K.** 1997 Effects of anti-thyroid drugs on fetal thyroid function during the treatment of pregnant hyperthyroid women. J Clin Endocrinol Metab. 82: 3633-3636.

36. **Hashizume K, Ichikawa K, Nishii Y.** *et al* 1992 Effect of administration of thyroxine on the risk of postpartum recurrence of hyperthyroid Graves' disease. J Clin Endocrinol Metab. **75**: 6-10.

37. **Kampmann JP, Johansen K, Hansen JM.** *et al.* 1980 Propylthiouracil in human milk : revision of dogma. Lancet 1 : 736-737.

38. **Momotani N, Yamashita R, Yoshimoto M** *et al* 1989 Recovery from fetal hypothyroidism: Evidence for the safety of breast feeding while taking propylthiouracil. Clin Endocrinol. **31:** 591-595.

39. **Fukata S, Kanji K, Sugawara M** 1999 Granulocyte Colony-Stimulating Factor (G-CSF) does not improve recovery from antithyroid drug-induced agranulo-cytosis: A prospective study. Thyroid 9: 29-31.

40. **Messer PM, Hauffa BP, Olbricht T, Benker G, Kotulla P, Reinwein D** 1990 Antithyroid drug treatment of Graves' disease in pregnancy: long-term effects on somatic growth, intellectual development and thyroid function of the offspring. Acta Endocrinol. 123: 311-316.

41. **McCarroll GN, Hutchinson M, McAuley R** *et al* 1976 Long term assessment of children exposed in utero to carbimazole. Arch Dis Child. 51: 532-536.

42. **Eisenstern Z, Weiss M, Katz Y, Bank H.** 1992 Intellectual capacity of subjects exposed to methimazole or propylthiouracil in utero. Euro J Pediatr. 151:558-559.

43. **Pruyn SC Phelan JP Buchanan GC** 1979 Long term propranolol therapy in pregnancy: Maternal and fetal outcome Am J Obstet Gynecol. 135: 485-489.

44. **Wartofsky L** 1996 Thyrotoxic storm. In: Werner and Ingbar's The Thyroid 7th edition , Braverman LE Utiger RD (eds) Lippincott Co, Philadelphia, p701-707.

45. **Shigemasa C, Mitani Y, Taniguchi S** *et al* 1990 Development of postpartum spontaneously resolving transient Graves' hyperthyroidism followed immediately by transient hypothyroidism. J Int Med. 228: 23-28.

46. **Lazarus JH, Hall R, Othman S** *et al* 1996 The clinical spectrum of postpartum thyroid disease. Quart J Med. 89: 429-435.

47. **Hidaka Y, Tamaki H, Iwatani Y** *et al* 1994 Prediction of postpartum Graves' thyrotoxicosis by measurement of thyroid stimulating antibody in early pregnancy. Clin Endocrinol. 41: 15-20.

48. **Tada H, Hidaka Y, Tsuruta E** *et al* 1994 Prevalence of postpartum onset of disease within patients with Graves' disease of child-bearing age. Endocrine J. 41: 325-327.

49. **Momotani N, Noh J, Ishikawa N, Ito K** 1994 Relationship between silent thyroiditis and recurrent Graves' disease in the postpartum period. J Clin Endocrinol Metabol. 79: 285-289.

50. **Parkes AB, Black EG, Adams H** *et al* 1994 Serum thyroglobulin- an early indicator of auto immune postpartum thyroiditis. Clin Endocrinol. 441: 9-14.

51. **Hidaka Y, Nishi I, Tamaki H** *et al* 1994 Differentiation of postpartum thyrotoxicosis by serum thyroglobulin: usefulness of a new multisite immunoradiometric assay. Thyroid 4: 275-278.

52. **Cooper DS** 1996 Treatment of thyrotoxicosis. In: Werner & Ingbar's, The Thyroid. Braverman LE, RD Utiger (eds). 7th Edition, JB Lippincot Co.,Philadelphia, p713-734.

53. **Singer PA** 1992 Will postpartum recurrence of Graves' hyperthyroidism become a thing of the past? J Clin Endocrinol Metab. 75: 5A-5B.

15

NEONATAL GRAVES' DISEASE

Margita Zakarija and J. Maxwell McKenzie

INTRODUCTION

The syndrome that is now commonly called neonatal Graves' disease, i.e., hyperthyroidism of limited duration and occasionally associated with goiter and ophthalmopathy, was first reported in 1910 (1), followed by a case presentation in 1912 (2). Until 1974 an additional 75 cases were described (3) and since then the number has approximately doubled. As can be seen, the condition is not common. Considering that Graves' disease occurs in about 0.2% of pregnant women (4) and overt thyrotoxicosis in approximately 2% of their offspring (4,5), the overall prevalence is of the order of 1 per 25,000 neonates (4) or even, as estimated by Fisher (6), 1 per 200,000. Still, the timely diagnosis of the syndrome is very important, since it can have dire consequences if left untreated (3,7).

That hyperthyroidism of Graves' disease might be due to a thyroid-stimulating substance distinct from TSH was recognized in 1956 (8). Shortly afterwards the substance was named long-acting thyroid stimulator (LATS) and it was shown to be an IgG. By 1964 it was postulated that LATS was the cause of neonatal hyperthyroidism (9-11). In 1967 an IgG, that protected LATS from neutralization by human thyroid tissue, was described in sera of patients with Graves' disease who were LATS-negative (12) and the term LATS-protector (LATS-P) was coined. Subsequently, LATS-P was also implicated as the cause of neonatal hyperthyroidism (13). Although positive assay results were reported from both mother and neonate when neonatal Graves' disease occurred, there were several features that were difficult for some (3) to reconcile with the simple concept of transplacental passage of a thyroid stimulator. For example, LATS was detected in only a minority of subjects with Graves' disease, the duration of hyperthyroidism in the affected neonates was from several days to 2-6 months, while the half-life of maternal IgG was thought to be only 6 days, and there were instances of hyperthyroidism diagnosed in neonates who needed treatment for several years thereafter (3). Development of more sensitive assays and cloning of the TSH receptor (reviewed in 14) helped to clarify these issues. With the use of human thyroid slices and measurement of cyclic AMP as the end-point of the assay, we have shown that while LATS-negative Graves' disease IgG were stimulatory in this system, LATS-positive IgG gave much higher responses (15). Similarly, the stimulator, by now renamed thyroid-stimulating antibody (TSAb), had to be of a certain titer in the maternal circulation to induce hyperthyroidism in the neonate (16), but this experience was not uniform (17). In more sophisticated assays, multiple stimulating and blocking antibodies, all directed at the TSH receptor, have been detected in patients with autoimmune thyroid disease

(18-22). These antibodies are collectively classified as TSH receptor antibodies or TRAb, and all have a potential of influencing fetal thyroid function (23).

In contrast to the antibody-induced neonatal syndromes, protracted neonatal hyperthyroidism, persisting for years and usually found in children from mothers without a history of autoimmune thyroid disease (3), was probably due to activating mutations of the TSH receptor (24). Germline mutations causing non-autoimmune autosomal dominant (25) and sporadic hyperthyroidism (26,27) were described, as well as a somatic mutation as a cause of a solitary toxic adenoma, resulting in congenital hyperthyroidism (28). The prevalence of non-autoimmune hyper-thyroidism is unknown, but the condition obviously is quite rare.

The pathogenesis of ophthalmopathy is still being debated, but when present in a neonate is usually a consequence of maternal Graves' disease. Therefore, the description of a child harboring an activating germline mutation of the TSH receptor and presenting with severe hyperthyroidism, goiter and ocular signs, including proptosis (27), is quite intriguing. The extraocular muscles were not enlarged, but there was hypertrophy of the retroorbital tissue (27). This might be relevant to the recent recognition of a functional TSH receptor expressed on differentiated orbital adipocytes (29).

FETAL THYROID FUNCTION AND TRANSPLACENTAL PASSAGE OF MATERNAL IgG

The effect of maternal Graves' disease on fetal thyroid status is dependent on many factors, including how mature is the fetal thyroid, the permeability of the placenta for substances affecting thyroid function, the titer of TSAb and, in some instances, of other TRAb in the maternal circulation, and if the mother is being treated with an anti-thyroid drug or not.

The fetal thyroid gland is discernible in a 16 to 17 day embryo, by 10 weeks colloid and thyroglobulin are present (6) and by 12 weeks very small amounts of total T_4 and free T_4 are found in the fetal circulation (6,30). Full thyroid function is established by 22-24 weeks of gestation, although the maturation of the pituitary-thyroid axis continues nearly till term (6,30). For example, the increase in free T_4 concentration, that reaches adult levels by 36 weeks of gestation, parallels the increase in TSH levels, that continue to rise through term (30).

Substances that easily cross the placenta are iodide and anti-thyroid drugs, methimazole and PTU (6). The placenta is impermeable to TSH and T_3, while a small, but physiologically important, amount of maternal T_4 reaches the fetal circulation (6). Of all immunoglobulin isotypes only IgG crosses the placenta and the passage starts at approximately 3 months of gestation (31). At 16 weeks, fetal serum IgG is only 5-8% of the adult concentration, 10-20% until 17-22 weeks, 50-60% at 8 months, and then, due to an abrupt change in placental permeability, reaches the maternal concentration at term. Throughout gestation, there is a minimal contribution of IgG by the fetus. Significant synthesis of IgG starts after birth and adult levels are achieved by late adolescence (31). The decay of maternal IgG in the child's circulation is exponential, but the concentration of IgG, that is highly variable in the population, also influences its half-life (reviewed in 32). Therefore, it is not surprising that reported half-lives vary from as short as 12 days to as long as 90 days, with the majority quoting 30-50 days. Sarvas et al. (32) found that 7% of the original maternal IgG1 was still present at 6 months and the calculated half-life was 48.4 days. From these data and taking into account the onset of fetal thyroid function (Fig. 1), it can be postulated that the highly-potent maternal TRAb may influence the fetal thyroid function as early as 16-20 weeks of gestation and the effect in the child may persist for 6 or more months.

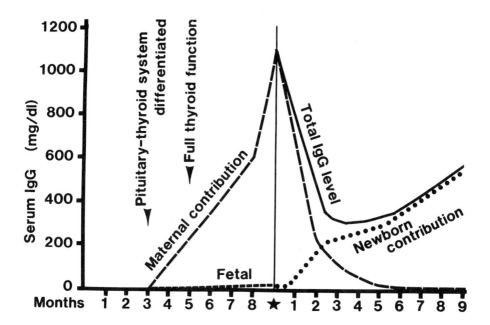

Figure 1. Development of pituitary-thyroid system and IgG levels with age. Adapted from Stites (31) (who modified from Allansmith et al. 1968 J Pediatr. 72:289; with permission from the publishers of J Pediatr., C.V. Mosby Co.).

An important factor that can modulate the course of maternal Graves' disease is suppressed immune function during pregnancy (33-37). Typically, autoimmune diseases ameliorate as pregnancy progresses, with frequently a rebound in the postpartum period (36,37). Titers of anti-thyroid antibodies, TSAb (16) and anti-microsomal and thyro-globulin antibodies (38), decline during pregnancy and rise postpartum (16,38). In Graves' disease, amelioration is reflected in a lower dose of anti-thyroid drug required to control hyperthyroidism.

FETAL AND NEONATAL CONSEQUENCES OF MATERNAL GRAVES' DISEASE AND THEIR PREVENTION

As discussed earlier, the influence of maternal TSAb on fetal thyroid function can be expected from approximately the middle of the second trimester. Since pregnant women with overt Graves' disease are being treated with anti-thyroid drugs, their effect on the fetal thyroid prevents intrauterine thyrotoxicosis, i.e., mother and fetus are treated simultaneously. In contrast, most instances of fetal hyperthyroidism were documented (39-50) in mothers who had Graves' disease in the past, underwent ablative therapy with either [131]I (39-45) or surgery (46-50) and during pregnancy were euthyroid with or without replacement therapy. Most distressing is the fact that in the majority of cases the right diagnosis was established only after at least one fetus/neonate was affected, culminating in 11 stillbirths per 5 mothers (40,42,48-50). Fetal and neonatal hyperthyroidism has also been described in 3 mothers with Hashimoto's thyroiditis (16,51,52), who had no history of Graves' hyperthyroidism, although 2 presented with ophthalmopathy (16,51). Two children of these 3 mothers died shortly after birth and 1 was stillborn. This brings the total number of reported fetal/neonatal deaths, attributable to fetal hyperthyroidism, to 15 per 9 mothers (16,39,40,42,48-52).

Clinical features of fetal hyperthyroidism encompass one or more of the following, which largely depend on the time of onset, i.e., the duration of the condition: tachycardia; hyperactivity; growth retardation; advanced bone age; goiter (not always present); hepatosplenomegaly; jaundice; heart failure; non-immune hydrops and, in extreme cases, death. In neonates born with hyperthyroidism, there is also increased mortality and morbidity, and, if left untreated, premature craniosynostosis can have a deleterious effect on brain development.

When fetal hyperthyroidism is anticipated or suspected, in utero evaluation of thyroid function consists of: monitoring heart rate; measurement of thyroid hormones and TSH in samples obtained by ultrasound-guided percutaneous fetal umbilical cord blood sampling (cordocentesis, funipuncture); use of ultrasound to assess maturity and presence of a goiter. An heart rate over 160 per minute is indicative of hyperthyroidism and the earliest reported tachycardia was in a 16 weeks old fetus (52). A more direct method of monitoring fetal thyroid status is measurement of thyroid hormone and TSH in the cord blood. In one report (45), an elevated free T4 level and suppressed TSH were found in a 20 weeks old fetus in whom tachycardia developed 4 weeks later.

Attempts to treat fetal hyperthyroidism in mothers who are not on an anti-thyroid drug were quite successful (39-42,44-48,50-52). This treatment consisted of prescribing for the mother PTU (in 2 instances carbimazole was used) in doses that varied from 100 mg to 300 mg daily, 600 mg being an exception. (At this point, thyroid replacement therapy has to be initiated in mothers who are euthyroid and are not taking thyroid hormone.) Higher doses were tapered when the fetal heart rate returned to normal or when repeat cord blood sampling showed a decrease in the fetal thyroid hormone level. Through term, PTU doses ranged from 50-150 mg daily. Most neonates were euthyroid at birth but developed hyperthyroidism a few days to a week later. This possibility has to be kept in mind if the mother and child are discharged 2 days postpartum and an early follow-up appointment should be given. At least the mother should be warned to look for signs of hyperthyroidism in her child.

Treatment of neonatal hyperthyroidism (reviewed in ref. 23) is similar to that of an adult and in the case of severe hyperthyroidism iodide, as SSKI solution, may be added to the regimen for 1 to 3 weeks (23). The length of therapy (usually 1 to 3 months) is also related to the severity of the hyperthyroidism, which in turn reflects the potency of TSAb. Therefore, if a TSAb assay is readily available, the therapy should be continued as long as TSAb persists in the child's circulation (52).

In considering the treatment of a hyperthyroid pregnant woman, it has been agreed that the dose of PTU (preferred over methimazole in pregnancy [4,53]) should be the minimum required to control hyperthyroidism and to keep maternal thyroid hormone indices just above normal (4,53). This strategy usually results in a euthyroid fetus/neonate. Indeed, it has been shown that there is a direct inverse correlation between the PTU concentration in maternal serum in the third trimester and the free T4 index in the cord blood (54). As mentioned earlier, the requirement for PTU decreases as the pregnancy progresses and, therefore, our practice is to monitor maternal thyroid status every 4-6 weeks, with adjustment of the PTU dose as required. Inadvertent over-treatment of the mother can cause fetal goiter and hypothyroidism (55,56), which can be treated with intra-amniotic administration of thyroxine, 250 µg once a week, until the findings in the fetus normalize (55,56). Concerns have been expressed about the possible adverse effect of the exposure to PTU in utero, i.e., of even a subtle hypothyroxinemia, on the development of the central nervous system and sequelae later in life (57). Testing children exposed to PTU or methimazole in utero, all of whom were euthyroid at birth, and comparing them with unexposed siblings, showed no difference in intellectual capacity between the two groups (58), suggesting that, when used judiciously, the treatment is quite safe.

As far as the neonates of hyperthyroid treated women are concerned, the same guidelines apply as for non-hyperthyroid treated mothers, since neonatal hyper-thyroidism can occur once the protective effect of PTU wears off, i.e., a few days postpartum.

ASSAYS FOR TSAb, UNUSUAL NEONATAL PRESENTATIONS AND MOTHERS TO BE SCREENED

All of the existing assays for TSAb have been developed as research procedures (14) and only a limited number is commercially available, while the others are still in the domain of research laboratories (14, 20-22). The assays are based on the ability of TSAb to either stimulate thyroid cells in culture to increase their production of cyclic AMP or to inhibit binding of ^{125}I-labeled TSH to a preparation of thyroid cell membranes (59). Commercially, a rat thyroid cell line, FRTL5 cells, is used for the stimulation type assay and solubilized porcine thyroid membranes for the TSH-binding inhibition (TBI assay), employing a single concentration of the crude IgG preparation for the former and the patient's serum for the latter. While the studies, in a research setting, of TSAb in pregnant women with Graves' disease using both assays (60) or only TBI assays (61), have shown that the results correlated with (60), or could predict (61), neonatal hyperthyroidism, the overall picture is not that simple. Besides documented multiple stimulating antibodies in patients with Graves' disease (20) and purely blocking antibodies (14), primarily in patients with Hashimoto's thyroiditis, it has been established that these antibodies can coexist in either type of autoimmune thyroid disease (14,18,19,21,62,63). This coexistence is reflected in a biphasic response to a patient's IgG in a stimulating type of assay (14,18,19,52,63) and a higher inhibition of the TSH binding than would be expected from a pure TSAb. An example of such a response in the TSAb assay, in this instance using Chinese hamster ovary cells transfected with the human recombinant TSH receptor (16), is shown in Fig. 2.

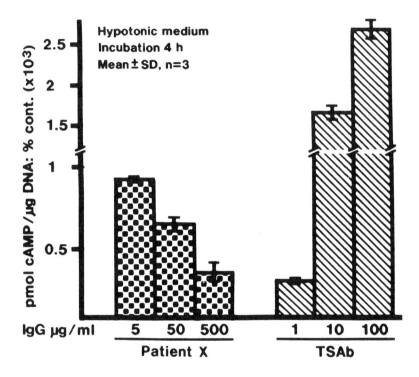

Figure 2. Cyclic AMP assay with JP-26 Chinese hamster ovary cells expressing the recombinant TSH receptor. After incubation of cells with indicated concentrations of IgG, cAMP was measured in the medium and expressed as pmol cAMP/μg DNA/well, % of control. Control refers to cells incubated with the medium alone.

As can be seen, IgG from patient X was less stimulatory at a higher IgG concentration, unlike the IgG from a patient containing only TSAb, and it was much more potent in inhibiting TSH binding than TSAb-IgG (18,63). Unusual clinical features of patient X were that she had long-standing hypothyroidism, but her 3 live-born (1 stillborn) children had fetal (52) and delayed onset neonatal hyperthyroidism (63), due to the interaction of multiple TSH receptor antibodies (18,62,63). The original report on this patient claimed that her serum was LATS- and LATS-P-negative (64). In our hands, once the serum was diluted the LATS-P value was one of the highest ever obtained (63). We have encountered more instances of such unusual presentations, but none was as dramatic as in the patient X's children.

Another instance of delayed onset of neonatal hyperthyroidism and the TSAb assay of maternal and neonatal IgG is illustrated in Fig.3, this time using human thyroid cells in hypotonic medium as the assay system.

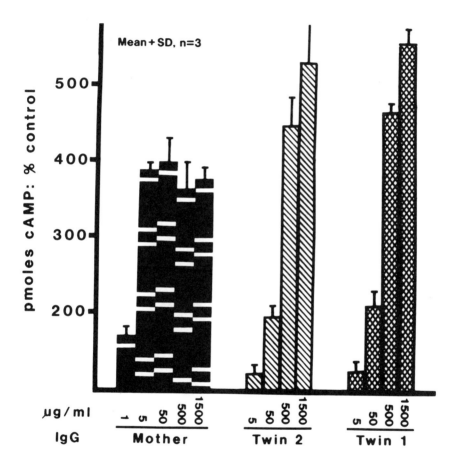

Figure 3. Cyclic AMP assay with human thyroid cells. After incubation of cells with the indicated concentrations of IgG, cAMP was measured in the medium and expressed as pmol cAMP, % control. Control refers to cells incubated with the medium alone.

The mother developed Graves' hyperthyroidism at 20 weeks of gestation and was placed on PTU, 100 mg, and propranolol, 40 mg, three times per day, until delivery (65). T4 levels in the twins were normal on the third day postpartum, but they developed severe hyperthyroidism at 23 days of age, when maternal and twins' blood was drawn for TSAb assay (65). As seen in Fig. 3, response to maternal IgG was maximal at 5µg/ml, while the IgG from the twins elicited concentration-dependent cAMP accumulation. A similar response with maternal IgG was obtained in FRTL5 cells. The striking feature of this IgG is its very high potency at 5 µg/ml. The delayed onset of hyperthyroidism in the twins cannot be explained by their exposure to PTU in utero, since its effect wears off a few days postpartum. The lesson from this case and that of mother X is, that if their IgG were assayed at a usual single higher concentration of IgG, the stimulation would have been low or non-existent, and a potential effect on neonates or, in the latter case, on the fetal and neonatal thyroid function, would have been discounted. We have found that at least 33% of patients with Graves' disease have both stimulating and blocking antibodies, with biphasic responses in TSAb assays (59). The full understanding of TRAb interactions and how they affect clinical presentations will have to await their further characterization and elucidation of the exact binding sites on the TSH receptor.

Considering the low prevalence of fetal/neonatal hyperthyroidism it is unrealistic to suggest screening for TSAb all pregnant women with Graves' disease. However, the consequences of missed diagnosis can be life-threatening for the fetus/neonate. We, therefore, recommend screening for TSAb in a select population. This population includes:

1. Previous child with neonatal hyperthyroidism, even if maternal diagnosis is Hashimoto's thyroiditis
2. Graves' disease
   a) On anti-thyroid therapy, requiring relatively high dosage in the third trimester
   b) Postablation (^{131}I or surgery), euthyroid
   c) Postablation, hypothyroid on T4

It is important to recognize that highly potent TSAb usually remains at a same titer over the years and does not decline appreciably even during pregnancy (52). This is underscored by sequential occurrences of neonates with hyperthyroidism in the same mother (39-42,46-52). Another important aspect of the management is the need for close interaction between endocrinologist and obstetrician.

The preferred assay for screening is the measurement of TSAb, because it is more specific and sensitive than the TBI assay. If the result from a commercial laboratory does not agree with the clinical assessment of, e.g., the fetal thyroid function, consideration should be given to enlisting expertise of a research laboratory.

REFERENCES

1. **Schmauch, quoted by Ochner AJ, Thompson RL.** 1910 The surgery and pathology of the thyroid and parathyroid glands. St. Louis: Mosby ; p 192.
2. **White C**. 1912 A foetus with congenital hereditary Graves' disease. J Obstet Gynaec Brit Emp. 21:231.
3. **Hollingsworth DR, Mabry CC.** 1976 Congenital Graves' disease. Four familial cases with long-term follow-up and perspective. Am J Dis Child. 130:148-155.
4. **Burrow GN.** 1985 The management of thyrotoxicosis in pregnancy. N Engl J Med. 313:562-565.

5. **Mitsuda N, Tamaki H, Amino N, Hosono T, Miyai K, Tanizawa O**. 1992 Risk factors for developmental disorders in infants born to women with Graves disease. Obstet Gynecol. 80:359-364.

6. **Fisher DA**. 1997 Fetal thyroid function: diagnosis and management of fetal thyroid disorders. Clin Obstet Gynecol. 40:16-31.

7. **Daneman D, Howard NJ**. 1980 Neonatal thyrotoxicosis: intellectual impairment and craniosynostosis in later years. J Pediatr. 97:257-259.

8. **Adams DD, Purves HD**. 1956 Abnormal responses in the assay of thyrotrophin. Proc Univ Otago Med Sch. 34:11-12.

9. **McKenzie JM**. 1964 Neonatal Graves' disease. J Clin Endocrinol Metab. 24:660-668.

10. **Adams DD, Lord JM, Stevely HAA**. 1964 Congenital thyrotoxicosis. Lancet. 2:497-498.

11. **Sunshine P, Kusumoto H, Kriss JP**. 1965 Survival time of circulating long-acting thyroid stimulator in neonatal thyrotoxicosis: implications for diagnosis and therapy of the disorder. Pediatrics. 36:869-876.

12. **Adams DD, Kennedy TH**. 1967 Occurrence in thyrotoxicosis of a gamma globulin which protects LATS from neutralization by an extract of thyroid gland. J Clin Endocrinol Metab. 27:173-177.

13. **Dirmikis SM, Munro DS**. 1975 Placental transmission of thyroid-stimulating immunoglobins. Br Med J. 2:665-666.

14. **McKenzie JM, Zakarija M**. 1996 Antibodies in autoimmune thyroid disease. In: Braverman LE, Utiger RD, eds. The Thyroid. 7th ed. New York: Lippincott-Raven; 416-432.

15. **McKenzie JM, Zakarija M**. 1978 Pathogenesis of neonatal Graves' disease. J Endocrinol Invest. 2:183-189.

16. **Zakarija M, McKenzie JM**. 1983 Pregnancy-associated changes in the thyroid-stimulating antibody of Graves' disease and the relationship to neonatal hyperthyroidism. J Clin Endocrinol Metab. 57:1036-1040.

17. **Rapoport B, Greenspan FS, Filetti S, Pepitone M**. 1984 Clinical experience with a human thyroid cell bioassay for thyroid-stimulating immunoglobulins. J Clin Endocrinol Metab. 58:332-338.

18. **Zakarija M, Garcia A, McKenzie JM**. 1985 Studies on multiple thyroid cell membrane-directed antibodies in Graves' disease. J Clin Invest. 76:1885-1891.

19. **Zakarija M, McKenzie JM, Eidson MS**. 1990 Transient neonatal hypothyroidism: characterization of maternal antibodies to the thyrotropin receptor. J Clin Endocrinol Metab. 70:1239-1246.

20. **Nagayama Y, Rapoport B**. 1992 Thyroid stimulatory antibodies in different patients with autoimmune thyroid disease do not all recognize the same components of the human thyrotropin receptor: selective role of amino acids Ser^{25} - Glu^{30}. J Clin Endocrinol Metab. 75: 1425-1430.

21. **Kosugi S, Ban T, Akamizu T, Valente W, Kohn LD**. 1993 Use of thyrotropin receptor (TSHR) mutants to detect stimulating TSHR antibodies in hypothyroid patients with idiopathic myxedema, who have blocking TSHR antibodies. J Clin Endocrinol Metab. 77:19-24.

22. **Watanabe Y, Tahara K, Hirai A, Tada H, Kohn LD, Amino N**. 1997 Subtypes of anti-TSH receptor antibodies classified by bio- and conversion assays using CHO cells expressing wild type human TSH receptor or TSH receptor-LH/CG receptor chimera. Thyroid. 7:13-19.

23. **McKenzie JM, Zakarija M**. 1992 Fetal and neonatal hyperthyroidism and hypothyroidism due to maternal TSH receptor antibodies. Thyroid. 2:155-159.

24. **Van Sande J, Parma J, Tonacchera M, Dumont J, Vassart G**. 1995 Somatic and germline mutations of the TSH receptor gene in thyroid disease. J Clin Endocrinol Metab. 80:2577-2585.

25. **Duprez L, Parma J, Van Sande J, et al.** 1994 Germline mutations in the thyrotropin receptor gene cause non-autoimmune autosomal dominant hyperthyroidism. Nature Genet. 7:396-401.

26. **Kopp P, Van Sande J, Parma J, et al.** 1995 Brief report: Congenital hyperthyroidism caused by a mutation in the thyrotropin receptor gene. N Engl J Med. 332:150-154.

27. **De Roux N, Polak M, Couet J, et al.** 1996 A neomutation of the thyroid-stimulating hormone receptor in a severe neonatal hyperthyroidism. J Clin Endocrinol Metab. 81:2023-2026.

28. **Kopp P, Muirhead S, Jourdain N, Gu W-X, Jameson JL, Rodd C.** 1997 Congenital hyperthyroidism caused by a solitary toxic adenoma harboring a novel somatic mutation (serine 281 →isoleucine) in the extracellular domain of the thyrotropin receptor. J Clin Invest. 100:1634-1639.

29. **Valyasevi RW, Ericson DZ, Harteneck DA, et al.** 1999 Differentiation of human orbital preadipocyte fibroblasts induces expression of functional thyrotropin receptor. J Clin Endocrinol Metab. 84:2557-2562.

30. **Thorpe-Beeston JG, Nicolaides KH, McGregor AM.** 1992 Fetal thyroid function. Thyroid. 2:207-217.

31. **Stites DP.** 1980 Clinical laboratory methods for detection of antigens & antibodies. In: Fudenberg HH, Stites DP, Caldwell JL, Wells JV, eds. Basic & clinical immunology. 3rd ed. Los Altos, California: Lange Medical Publishers; 343-381.

32. **Sarvas H, Seppala I, Kurikka S, Siegberg R, Makela O.** 1993 Half-life of the maternal IgG1 allotype in infants. J Clin Immunol. 13:145-151.

33. **Hunt JS.** 1992 Immunobiology of pregnancy. Curr Opin Immunol. 4:591-596.

34. **Sargent IL.** 1993 Maternal and fetal immune responses during pregnancy. Exp Clin Immunogenet. 10:85-102.

35. **Medina KL, Smithson G, Kincade PW.** 1993 Suppression of B lymphopoeisis during normal pregnancy. J Exp Med. 178:1507-1515.

36. **Iwatani Y, Amino N, Tachi J, et al.** 1988 Changes in lymphocyte subsets in normal pregnant women and postpartum women: postpartum increase of NK/K (Leu 7) cells. Am J Reproduct Immunol. 18:52-56.

37. **Stagnaro-Green A, Roman SH, Cobin RH, El-Harazy E, Wallenstein S, Davies TF.** 1992 A prospective study of lymphocyte-initiated immunosuppression in normal pregnancy: evidence of a T-cell etiology for postpartum thyroid dysfunction. J Clin Endocrinol Metab. 74:645-653.

38. **Amino N, Kuro R, Tanizawa O, et al.** 1978 Changes of serum anti-thyroid antibodies during and after pregnancy in autoimmune thyroid disease. Clin Exp Immunol. 31:30-37.

39. **Volpe R, Ehrlich R, Steiner G, Row VV.** 1984 Graves' disease in pregnancy years after hypothyroidism with recurrent passive-transfer neonatal Graves' disease in offspring. Therapeutic considerations. Am J Med. 77:572-578.

40. **Wenstrom KD, Weiner CP, Williamson RA, Grant SS.** 1990 Prenatal diagnosis of fetal hyperthyroidism using funipuncture. Obstet Gynecol. 76:513-517.

41. **Porreco RP, Bloch CA.** 1990 Fetal blood sampling in the management of intrauterine thyrotoxicosis. Obstet Gynecol. 76:509-512.

42. **Hadi HA, Strickland D.** 1995 Prenatal diagnosis and management of fetal goiter caused by maternal Graves' disease. Am J Perinat. 12:240-242.

43. **Watson WJ, Fiegen MM.** 1995 Fetal thyrotoxicosis associated with nonimmune hydrops. Am J Obstet Gynecol. 172:1039-1040.

44. **Wallace C, Couch R. Ginsberg J.** 1995 Fetal thyrotoxicosis: a case report and recommendations for prediction, diagnosis, and treatment. Thyroid 5:125-128.

45. **Rakover Y, Weiner E, Mosh N, Shalev E.** 1999 Fetal pituitary negative feedback at early gestational age. Clin Endocrinol. 50:809-814.

46. **Robinson PL, O'Mullane NM, Alderman B**. 1979 Prenatal treatment of fetal thyrotoxicosis. Br Med J. 1:383-384.
47. **Serup J, Petersen S**. 1979 Fetal thyrotoxicosis *in utero*. Biol Neonate. 35:175-179.
48. **Cove DH, Johnston P**. 1985 Fetal hyperthyroidism: experience of treatment in four siblings. Lancet. 1:430-432.
49. **Houck JA, Davis RE, Sharma HM**. 1988 Thyroid-stimulating immunoglobulin as a cause of recurrent intrauterine fetal death. Obstet Gynecol. 71:1018-1019.
50. **Treadwell MC, Sherer DM, Sacks AJ, Ghezzi F, Romero R**. 1996 Successful treatment of recurrent non-immune hydrops secondary to fetal hyperthyroidism. Obstet Gynecol. 87:838-840.
51. **Check JH, Rezvani I, Goodner D, Hopper B**. 1982 Prenatal treatment of thyrotoxicosis to prevent intrauterine growth retardation. Obstet Gynecol. 60:122-124.
52. **Zakarija M, McKenzie JM, Hoffman WH**. 1986 Prediction and therapy of intrauterine and late-onset neonatal hyperthyroidism. J Clin Endocrinol Metab. 62:368-371.
53. **Momotani N, Noh J, Oyanagi H, Ishikawa N, Ito K**. 1986 Antithyroid drug therapy for Graves' disease during pregnancy. Optimal regimen for fetal thyroid status. N Engl J Med. 315:24-28.
54. **Gardner DF, Cruikshank DP, Hays PM, Cooper DS**. 1986 Pharmacology of propylthiouracil (PTU) in pregnant hyperthyroid women: correlation of maternal PTU concentrations with cord serum thyroid function tests. J Clin Endocrinol Metab. 62:217-220.
55. **Davidson KM, Richards DS, Schatz DA, Fisher DA**. Successful in utero treatment of fetal goiter and hypothyroidism. 1991 N Engl J Med. 324:543-546.
56. **Van Loon AJ, Derksen JThM, Bos AF, Rouwe CW**. 1995 *In utero* diagnosis and treatment of fetal goitrous hypothyroidism, caused by maternal use of propylthiouracil. Prenat Diagn. 15:599-604.
57. **Cheron RG, Kaplan MM, Larsen PR, Selenkow HA, Crigler JF**. 1981 Neonatal thyroid function after propylthiouracil therapy for maternal Graves' disease. N Engl J Med. 304:525-528.
58. **Eisenstein Z, Weiss M, Katz Y, Bank H**. 1992 Intellectual capacity of subjects exposed to methimazole or propylthiouracil in utero. Eur J Pediatr. 151:558-559.
59. **McKenzie JM, Zakarija M**. 1989 Clinical review 3. The clinical use of thyrotropin receptor antibody measurements. J Clin Endocrinol Metab. 69:1093-1096.
60. **Tamaki H, Amino N, Iwatani Y, et al**. 1989 Evaluation of TSH receptor antibody by "natural in vivo human assay" in neonates born to mothers with Graves' disease. Clin Endocrinol. 30:493-503.
61. **Mortimer RH, Tyack SA, Galligan JP, Perry-Keene DA, Tan YM**. 1990 Graves' disease in pregnancy: TSH receptor binding inhibiting immunoglobulins and maternal and neonatal thyroid function. Clin Endocrinol. 32:141-152.
62. **Kohn LD, Suzuki K, Hoffman WH, et al**. 1997 Characterization of monoclonal thyroid-stimulating and thyrotropin binding-inhibiting autoantibodies from a Hashimoto's patient whose children had intrauterine and neonatal thyroid disease. j Clin Endocrinol Metab. 82:3998-4009.
63. **Zakarija M, McKenzie JM, Munro DS**. 1983 Immunoglobulin G inhibitor of thyroid-stimulating antibody is a cause of delay in the onset of neonatal Graves' disease. J Clin Invest. 72:1352-1356.
64. **Hoffman WH, Sahasrananan P, Ferandos SS, Burek CL, Rose NR**. 1982 Transient thyrotoxicosis in an infant delivered to a long-acting thyroid stimulator (LATS)- and LATS protector-negative, thyroid-stimulating antibody-positive women with Hashimoto's thyroiditis. 1982 J Clin Endocrinol Metab. 54:354-356.

65. **Dean HJ, Zakarija M**. 1986 Delayed onset of neonatal thyrotoxicosis may be caused by an inhibitor of thyroid stimulating antibody. Annual Meeting, Canadian Society for Clinical Investigation, Toronto, September.

16

THYROTOXICOSIS AND THE HEART

Wolfgang Dillman

INTRODUCTION

Cardiovascular signs and symptoms contribute in an important manner to the manifestations of thyrotoxicosis. This was first recognized over 200 years ago by the British physician Caleb Parry and was also noticed in the description of hyperthyroidism by Graves and Basedow (1,2). Patients with hyperthyroidism are usually well aware of their cardiovascular signs and symptoms. They frequently complain of a strong pounding heartbeat and of an increased heart rate. These features are frequently accompanied by increasing shortness of breath with vigorous exercise. The precise pathophysiological mechanisms which underlie the cardiovascular manifestations of hyperthyroidism are still, in part, unclear. I will first review the clinical manifestations of hyperthyroid cardiovascular disease and subsequently briefly discuss the pathophysiological basis of the clinical manifestations. In addition, more recent insights developed from transgenic and knockout mouse models in which different isoforms of thyroid hormone receptors are overexpressed or underexpressed will be considered. Some of these findings are providing novel insights into the molecular basis of thyroid hormone action in the cardiovascular system and can explain in more detail the cardiovascular manifestations of hyperthyroidism.

CLINICAL MANIFESTATIONS

The subjective complaint of an excessively vigorous and rapid heart rate can frequently be confirmed on physical examination in a significant number, but not all, patients with tachycardia (3). The blood pressure is generally normal but in some patients an elevated systolic blood pressure is noted which is in part due to accelerated emptying of the heart during systole (3a). Cardiac auscultation reveals a first heart sound which is frequently accentuated and an accentuated pulmonic component of the second heart sound (4). Systolic murmurs are frequently noted and are in part due to an increased amount of blood more rapidly expelled across the aortic valve. In addition systolic murmurs can be noted indicating mitral or tricuspid regurgitation and may result from papillary muscle dysfunction (4). These cardiac murmurs frequently disappear after the euthyroid status has been reestablished. Rarely the so-called Means-Lerman scratch is audible in the left second intercostal space. This is a systolic scratching sound which results from the rubbing of pleural and pericardial surfaces against each other during the hyperdynamic action of the heart. In patients with hyperthyroidism, the pulmonary artery is frequently dilated leading to a closer approximation of pleural and pericardial surfaces which also may contribute to the

Means-Lehrman scratch. In patients with Graves' disease a venous hum may be audible over the thyroid area consequent to a marked increase in blood supply to the hypertrophic thyroid gland. Only in a minority of patients are signs of true congestive heart failure noticeable (5), such as pulmonary congestion as evidenced by rales and a pulmonary effusion. Especially in older patients, worsening angina pectoris can occur due to pre-existing coronary artery disease and a hyperdynamic heart with increased metabolic demand outstripping its blood supply. Indeed, angina pectoris can occur even in the absence of underlying coronary artery disease (6,7). In the hyperthyroid heart, systolic function as well as diastolic function is enhanced. The circulation time is markedly shortened. In studies in hyperthyroid animals, increased relaxation of the smooth muscle cells of the arterial tree and increased venous constriction were noted which accelerate the return of blood to the heart (8).

The tachycardia found on physical examination is confirmed by obtaining an electrocardiogram. Many patients with hyperthyroidism have marked sinus tachycardia. In addition, 10 to 15 percent of these patients exhibit atrial fibrillation or flutter (9). Thyroid hormone enhances both chronotropic (impulse generating) and dromotropic (impulse conducting) events in the heart, leading to a rapid ventricular response rate. Tachycardia and atrial fibrillation can induce angina pectoris and myocardial ischemic events manifest by ST segment changes. Cardiac echography confirms the hyperdynamic action of the heart with accelerated left ventricular systolic contraction and diastolic relaxation(10). With long standing hyperthyroidism in both patients and in animal models, cardiac hypertrophy can develop. This hypertrophy is, in general, reversible after the thyroid status returns to normal (10). Cardiac hypertrophy is primarily mediated by myocyte hypertrophy without significant contribution by the interstitial tissue. Patients with Graves' disease have an increased incidence of mitral valve prolapse which can be diagnosed by cardiac echography (11). Mitral valve prolapse is especially common if hyperthyroidism is of an autoimmune origin. The basis for mitral valve prolapse may be increased mucopolysaccharide infiltration of the valve. Cardiac decompensation with congestive heart failure is more prevalent in thyrotoxic patients with advancing age, especially in patients with multiple toxic adenomas (Plummer's disease)(5,12). Atrial fibrillation and cardiomegaly are also more prevalent in the elderly.

AMIODARONE INDUCED CHANGES IN THYROID FUNCTION

Patients with cardiac arrhythmias are commonly treated with amiodarone, a molecule which contains two atoms of iodine (13). The compound has some structural similarities to thyroid hormone and may interact with the T_3 receptor (14). Amiodarone administration to patients living in areas of relative iodine deficiency, such as in some areas of Europe, leads more frequently to hyperthyroidism than to hypothyroidism. The reverse is true for patients living in areas of iodine excess. The pharmacological actions of amiodarone include inhibition of deiodination of T_4 leading to decreased conversion of T_4 to T_3 (13). This effect accounts for elevated serum T_4 and reverse T_3 levels, as well as a relative reduction in T_3 levels. Significant worsening of underlying cardiac arrthymias, especially supraventricular tachycardia, in patients taking amiodarone should raise suspicion for amiodarone induced hyperthyroidism. Amiodarone induced thyrotoxicosis can result from two different mechanisms. One relates to increased iodine released during the metabolism of the drug. Amiodarone can also induce a destructive thyroiditis with thyrotoxicosis consequent to increased thyroid hormone release from the thyroid gland (14). Treatment of amiodarone induced hyperthyroidism involves discontinuation of the medication and administration of propylthiouracil, preferred over methimazole because it reduces the conversion of T_4 to T_3. In addition, potassium perchlorate can be used at a dose of one gram per day (15). This medication inhibits iodine uptake and, at this dose, does not seem to have significant side effects such as leukopenia. In patients with the destructive form of thyrotoxicosis, large doses of glucocorticoids rapidly ameliorate the underlying thyroiditis (16).

HEART FAILURE IN THE THYROTOXIC PATIENTS

Thyrotoxicosis induced heart failure occurs with increased frequency in the older patients population, as indicated above (5). The main contributing factors are increased heart rate or cardiac arrthymias such as atrial fibrillation, as well as underlying cardiac diseases such as ischemic cardiomyopathy (17). The increased hemodynamic work load of the hyperthyroid heart cannot be accommodated and leads to relative ischemia. It should also be noted that some hyperthyroid patients complain of increased shortness of breath without evidence of heart failure. The thyrotoxic state leads to a marked weakness of proximal and distal skeletal muscles including the intercostal muscles required for respiration. Dyspnea may, therefore, result from weakness of the respiratory muscles rather than from a primary cardiac cause (18). Heart failure has also been described in younger patients or children without underlying heart disease (19). Thyrotoxicosis induced heart failure has been termed high output heart failure without providing a clear pathophysiological mechanism. Hyperthyroidism can lead to increased sodium retention and an expanded blood volume which then results in peripheral edema. It should also be noted that in animal studies, pacing-induced heart failure is well documented (20). The heart failure experienced by younger patients may, therefore, be precipitated by a very rapid heart rate which might not allow sufficient time for diastolic relaxation and cardiac muscle perfusion during diastole. Returning heart rate to the normal range quickly ameliorates this form of heart failure. In the older patients with an underlying cardiac abnormality, returning to a euthyroid status will markedly ameliorate the heart failure but a component of failure will remain.

TREATMENT OF HYPERTHYROID PATIENTS WITH CARDIOVASCULAR MANIFESTATIONS

The central treatment objective is to return the hyperthyroid patient to a euthyroid status as soon as possible. It is for this reason that antithyroid medication is preferred as the initial therapy. Treatment with radioactive iodine for hyperthyroidism is very effective but restoration of a euthyroid status may require several months. In severely hyperthyroid patients, we prefer to use propylthiouracil (PTU) rather than methimazole because the former inhibits, in addition, the peripheral conversion of T_4 to T_3. In hyperthyroid patients with severe cardiac manifestations, thyroidectomy is contra-indicated. Before a patient is submitted to such surgery a euthyroid status needs to be achieved and this surgery is not advisable if cardiac symptoms persist.

Because a significant part of cardiac manifestations result from tachycardia or atrial arrthymias, these manifestations can be ameliorated by β sympathetic blockade (21). Sympathetic blocking agents such as propranolol, therefore, present a good treatment option. propranolol also has a modest inhibitory effect on T_4 to T_3 conversion. Because the increased metabolic rate in hyperthyroidism increases drug metabolism, relatively high doses of propranolol, such as 40 to 60 mg 3 to 4 times a day, are used. Because β blockers such as propranolol increase smooth muscle contraction, these drugs are contraindicated in patients with asthma or with a history of obstructive pulmonary disease. Beta1-selective or cardio-selective β sympathetic blocking agents such as esmolol are also available for parental administration. Patients with heart failure consequent to a very rapid heart rate respond well to β sympathetic blockade. Recent evidence indicates that β sympathetic blockade may also be indicated in patients with other forms of heart failure (22).

In thyrotoxic patients with cardiac failure, digoxin treatment can also improve cardiac status. However, treatment should be undertaken with caution because patients have some degree of digoxin resistance and can develop digoxin toxicity (23). The reasons for this phenomenon is not completely clear but may relate to changes in the distribution volume of digoxin or shifts in the dose response curve. Development of digoxin toxicity occurs with doses that are effective and well tolerated in euthyroid patients because of the lower safety margin. The combination of digoxin and propranolol synergistically increases the atrial ventricular conduction time and prolongs the refractory period of the AV node. The ventricular response in patients with atrial fibrillation is therefore diminished. The main benefit of digoxin in the thyrotoxic patient is its chronotropic effect and marked increases in cardiac contractility frequently do not occur. The vascular bed is already dilated in thyrotoxic patients and vasodilators are therefore not indicated.

Anticoagulation therapy in thyrotoxic patients with atrial fibrillation is still controversial. It is my general practice to use anticoagulation in elderly patients with additional risk factors for systemic embolization and who are refractory to antiarrhythmic treatment. In younger patients with recent onset of atrial fibrillation and the likelihood that the cardiac arrhythmia will quickly return to normal, anticoagulation therapy is in general not chosen.

MECHANISMS UNDERLYING THYROTOXICOSIS INDUCED CARDIOVASCULAR MANIFESTATIONS

It has been postulated that three important mechanisms contribute to thyroid hormone influences on cardiac function:- 1) direct effects of thyroid hormones on cardiac myocytes; 2) interactions between thyroid hormones and the sympathoadrenal system; 3) indirect effects on the heart through changes in the peripheral circulation leading to alterations in hemodynamic loading of the heart and mediated by increases in peripheral oxygen consumption. Recent evidence from *ex vivo* approaches using cardiac myocytes in cell culture indicate direct thyroid hormone effects on the expression of cardiac genes, such as the genes for calcium ATPase in the sarcoplasmic reticulum and for myosin heavy chain isoforms (24,25). In addition, recent evidence from knockout mice in which either thyroid hormone receptor alpha or thyroid hormone receptor beta, or both, are eliminated indicates a direct, major effect of thyroid hormones on the cardiac myocyte (26,27).

Related to the second mechanism, the interaction of thyroid hormones and the sympathoadrenal system, the evidence is less strong. *Ex-vivo* studies indicate that thyroid hormones increase expression of the $\beta1$ sympathetic receptor which could potentially increase signaling by β sympathetic compounds (28). Demonstration of increased sensitivity to β sympathetic compounds in hyperthyroid patients or in animal models has not, however, been demonstrated in some carefully conducted studies (29). It is, therefore, possible that increases in thyroid hormone levels as well as increased β sympathetic stimulation both influence the same parameters, for example, an increase in heart rate. Tachycardia in hyperthyroid patients could therefore be an additive phenomena mediated by thyroid hormone action and β sympathetic action. The beneficial effects of β adrenergic blockade observed in hyperthyroid patients makes this explanation likely.

Indirect influences on cardiac function caused by peripheral hemodynamic changes are well documented, but are most likely only a modifying influence and not the primary mechanism for the cardiovascular changes in hyperthyroidism.. Most body organs participate in the increased oxygen consumption mediated by thyroid hormone excess. In order to meet this increased metabolic demand, cardiac output is augmented. The resistance of the arterial system decreases whereas constriction of venous vessels occurs (8). These changes result in increased mean circulatory filling pressure which promotes the flow of blood to the right atrium.

DIRECT EFFECTS OF THYROID HORMONE IN CARDIAC MYOCYTES

Very recently, knockout mice have been generated in which either the entire locus coding for the thyroid hormone receptor α gene or the thyroid hormone receptor β gene has been inactivated (26,29). In other knockout variants, mice expressed only the thyroid hormone $\alpha2$ receptor gene, which does not bind thyroid hormone, or the T_3 binding isoform thyroid hormone receptor $\alpha1$ receptor (26). Mice not lacking the thyroid hormone receptor $\alpha1$ (26), or with the entire α locus deleted, showed marked bradycardia. In contrast, no bradycardia occurred in mice in which the entire thyroid hormone receptor β locus was removed (29).

Recently, the genes coding for the hyperpolarization activated pacemaker ion channel I_f has been cloned (30). I_f function contributes significantly to generation of the heart rate in the sinus node. The genes coding for the I_f channel have been termed HCN2 and HCN4 (30). The ventricle of hypothyroid rats or thyroid hormone receptor α knockout mice shows a marked decrease in HCN2 (32) and HCN4 mRNA levels.(33). It should be noted that the HCN2 and HCN4 mRNA responses in the sinus node, present within the ventricular tissue used in these studies, may not necessarily be the same as in the ventricle itself, although a parallel response is likely. In addition, our preliminary studies indicate that thyroid hormone receptor α knockout mice have markedly decreased contractile function as determined by force development and force decay in papillary muscle (33). These data, therefore, indicate that thyroid hormone receptor α may be the isoform predominantly responsible for the cardiac actions of thyroid hormones. The tachycardia in hyperthyroid patients may result from a combination of β sympathetic effects and the direct influence of excess thyroid hormones on the expression of genes coding for pacemaker related ion channels, the latter predominantly mediated by the thyroid hormone receptor α gene.

It is also interesting to note that novel thyroid hormone analogs have recently been synthesized that bind preferentially to the thyroid hormone receptor β isoform as opposed to the thyroid hormone receptor α isoform.(34,35). One of these compounds has recently been administered to hypothyroid mice with bradycardia as well as elevated serum cholesterol and triglyceride levels. Administration of the GC1 compound, which preferentially binds to and activates the β1 receptor, normalizes the cholesterol and triglyceride levels without an increase in heart rate. In contrast administration of equimolar doses of T₃ to such mice also lowered lipid levels but markedly increased the heart rate. It may therefore be possible to develop novel thyroid hormone analogs with a cardiac sparing action. Using principles similar to those employed for the synthesis of GC1, it may be possible to synthesize thyroid hormone antagonists which may oppose general thyroid hormone action or specifically oppose thyroid hormone influences on cardiac function.

REFERENCES

1. **Parry CH.** 1825 Collections from the Unpublished Papers of the Late Caleb Hiliel Parry. London; vol. 2:111.
2. **Graves RJ.** 1835 Clinical Lectures. Lond Med Surg J. (Part II) 7:516.
3. **von Olshausen K, Bischoff S, Kahaly G, et al.** 1989 Cardiac arrhythmias and heart rate in hyperthyroidism. Am J Cardiol. 63:930-933.
3a. **Hurxthal LM.** 1931 Blood pressure before and after operation in hyperthyroidism. Arch Intern Med. 47:167.
4. **Skelton CL.** 1982 The heart and hyperthyroidism. N Engl J Med. 307:1206-1208.
5. **Sandler G, Wilson GM.** 1959 The nature and prognosis of heart disease in thyrotoxicosis. Q J Med. 28:347-369.
6. **Featherstone HJ, Stewart DK.** 1983 Angina in thyrotoxicosis: thyroid-related coronary artery spasm. Arch Intern Med. 143:554-555.
7. **Rowe GG, Huston JH, Weinstein AB, et al.** 1956 The hemodynamics of thyrotoxicosis in man with special reference to coronary blood flow and myocardial oxygen consumption. J Clin Invest. 35:272-276.
8. **Morkin E, Flink IL, Goldman S.** 1983 Biochemical and physiologic effects of thyroid hormone on cardiac performance. Prog Cardiovas Dis. 25:435-464.
9. **Nakazawa HK, Sakurai K, Hamada N. et al.** 1982 Management of atrial fibrillation in the post-thyrotoxic state. Am J Med. 72:903-906.
10. **Biondi B, Fazio S, Carella C, et al.** 1993 Cardiac effects of long-term thyrotropin-suppressive therapy with levothyroxine. J Clin Endocrinol Metab. 77:334-338.
11. **Kahaly G, Erbel R, Mohr-Kahaly S, et al.** 1987 Morbus basedow und mitraklappenprolaps. **Dtsch Med Wschr**. 112:248-253.
12. **Ikram H.** 1985 The nature and prognosis of thyrotoxic heart disease. Q J Med. 54:19-28.

13. **Nademanee K. Piwonka RW, Singh BN, Hershman JM.** 1989 Amiodarone and thyroid function. Prog Cardiovas Dis. 21:427-437.

14. **Smyrk TC, Goellner JR, Brennan MD, Carney JA.** 1987 Pathology of the thyroid in amiodarone-associated thyrotoxicosis. Am J Surg Pathol 11:197-204.

15. **Martino E, Aghini-Lombardi F, Mariotti S, et al.** 1986 Treatment of amiodarone associated thyrotoxicosis by simultaneous administration of potassium perchlorate and methimazole. J Endocrinol Invest. 9:201-207.

16. **Broussolle C, Ducottet X, Martin C, et al.** 1989 Rapid effectiveness of prednisone and thionamides combined therapy in severe amiodarone iodine-induced thyrotoxicosis: comparison of two groups of patients with apparently normal thyroid glands. J Endocrinol Invest 12:37-42.

17. **Graettinger JS, Muenster JJ, Selverstone LA, et al.** 1959 A correlation of clinical and hemodynamic studies in patients with hyperthyroidism with and without heart failure. J Clin Invest. 19:1316-1327.

18. **McElvaney GN, Wilcox PG, Fairbarn MS, et al.** 1990 Respiratory muscle weakness and dyspnea in thyrotoxic patients. Am Rev Respir Dis. 141:1221-1227.

19. **Cavallo A, Joseph CJ, Casta A.** 1984 Cardiac complications in juvenile hyperthyroidism. Am J Dis Child. 138:479.

20. **Perreault CL, Shannon RP, Komamura K, Vatner SF, Morgan JP.** 1992 Abnormalities in intracellular calcium regulation and contractile function in myocardium from dogs with pacing induced heart failure. J Clin Invest. 89:932-938.

21. **Ventrella S, Klein I.** 1994 Beta-adrenergic receptor blocking drugs in the management of hyperthyroidism. The Endocrinologist. 4:391.

22. **Waagstein F, Bristow MR, Swedberg K, et al.** 1993 Beneficial effects of metoprolol in idiopathic dilated cardiomyopathy. Lancet 342:1441-1446.

23. **Frye RL, Braunwald E.** 1961 Studies on digitalis. III. The influence of triiodothyronine on digitalis requirements. Circulation. 23:376-379.

24. **Gustafson TA, Bahl JJ, Markham BE, Roeske WR, Morkin E.** 1987 Hormonal regulation of myosin heavy chain and α-actin gene expression in cultured fetal rat heart myocytes. J Biol Chem. 262:13316-13322.

25. **Rohrer DK, Hartong R, Dillmann WH.** 1991 Influence of thyroid hormone and retinoic acid on slow sarcoplasmic reticulum Ca^{++} ATPase and myosin heavy chain alpha gene expression in cardiac myocytes: delineation of cis-active DNA elements that confer responsiveness to thyroid hormone but not to retinoic acid. J Biol Chem. 266:8638-8646.

26. **Wikstrom L, Johansson C, Salto C, et al.** 1998 Abnormal heart rate and body temperature in mice lacking thyroid hormone receptor $\alpha1$. EMBO J. 17:455-461.

27. **Fraichard A, Chassande O, Plateroti M, et al.** 1997 The T3Rα gene encoding a thyroid hormone receptor is essential for post-natal development and thyroid hormone production. EMBO J. 16:4412-4420.

28. **Bahouth SW.** 1991 Thyroid hormones transcriptionally regulate the $\beta1$-adrenergic receptor gene in cultured ventricular myocytes. J Biol Chem. 266:15863-15869.

29. **Weiss RE, Forrest D, Pohlenz J, Cua K, Curran T, Refetoff S.** 1997 Thyrotropin regulation by thyroid hormone in thyroid hormone receptor β-deficient mice. Endocrinology. 138:3624-3629.

30. **Ludwig A, Zong X, Stieber J, Hullin R, Hofmann F, Biel M.** 1999 Two pacemaker channels from human heart with profoundly different activation kinetics. EMBO J.. 18:2323-2329.

31. **DiFrancesco D.** 1993 pacemaker mechanisms in cardiac tissue. Annu Rev Physiol. 55:455-472.

32. **Pachucki J, Burmeister LA, Larsen PR.** 1999 Thyroid hormone regulates hyperpolarization activated cyclic nucleotide-gated channel (HCN2) mRNA in the rat heart.

Circ Res. 85:498-503.

33. **Gloss B, Swanson EA, Clark RB, et al.** 1999 Changes in cardiac ion channel expression induced by the lack of T3 receptor isoforms and alterations in thyroid status. 72nd Annual Meeting of the American Thyroid Association, Palm Beach, FL, p. 48.

34. **Chiellini G, Apriletti JW, al Yoshihara H, Baxter JD, Ribeiro RC, Scanlan TS.** 1998 A high affinity subtype selective agonist ligand for the thyroid hormone receptor. Chem Biol. 5:299-306.

35. **Taylor AH, Stephan ZF, Steele RE, Wong NC.** 1997 Beneficial effects of a novel thyromimetic on lipoprotein metabolism. Mol Pharmacol. 52:542-547.

17
IODINE AND GRAVES' DISEASE

Peter HK Eng and Lewis E Braverman

EFFECTS OF IODINE ON THYROID FUNCTION

The thyroid is able to adjust to available plasma iodide levels and maintain normal thyroid function by an intrinsic thyroidal mechanism that is independent of changes in thyroid stimulating hormone (TSH). This ability of the thyroid to regulate hormone synthesis is known as autoregulation. Iodide has two potentially adverse effects on the thyroid – inhibition of thyroid hormone synthesis and inhibition of thyroid hormone release.

Iodine is required for normal thyroid hormone synthesis and inadequate iodine intake can result in impaired thyroid hormone synthesis, iodine deficiency goiter and, if severe, hypothyroidism. Excess iodine can also paradoxically acutely decrease thyroid hormone synthesis in rats by blocking organification of iodine within the thyroid and decreasing subsequent thyroid hormone synthesis. This inhibition of thyroid hormone synthesis by excess iodide is known as the acute Wolff Chaikoff effect (1). It was found that above a certain level of plasma iodide, organification of iodide within the thyroid was inhibited and the majority of the iodide within the thyroid consisted of inorganic iodide. Raben (2) found that the intrathyroidal concentration of iodide was the important factor determining inhibition of hormone synthesis. Nagataki et al. (3) further refined the concept of the acute Wolff-Chaikoff effect and reported that small doses of excess iodide actually increased iodide organification, but with larger doses, there was a progressive decrease in total organification. This inhibition has been postulated to be due to an iodinated intermediary within the thyroid, either an iodolactone or iodoaldehyde (4). Wolff and Chaikoff subsequently reported that this acute inhibition of thyroid hormone formation by iodide excess was temporary and that with maintenance of high plasma iodide levels, the thyroid 'escaped' from this inhibition and resumed thyroid hormone synthesis (5). We subsequently showed that the cause of the escape was due to the ability of the thyroid to decrease transport of iodide into the gland (6). This would then lower the amount of intrathyroidal iodide below the critical inhibitory level and allow organification of iodide and thyroid hormone synthesis to resume. The epithelial cell surface protein responsible for iodide transport is called the sodium/iodide symporter (NIS). The cDNA encoding NIS was cloned by Dai et al. in 1996 (7). Recently, we have demonstrated that rats exposed to chronic iodide excess decreased thyroid NIS mRNA and protein (8). Thus, it is likely that the thyroid is able to escape from inhibition of thyroid hormone synthesis by down-regulating NIS, and thus decreasing the amount of intrathyroidal iodine necessary to inhibit organification and hormone synthesis.

The human response to excess iodide resembles that observed in rats. Acute administration of small doses of iodide does not affect the percentage uptake of iodide and thus leads to an increase in the absolute iodide uptake. The acute Wolff-Chaikoff effect in response to a large dose, however, has been more difficult to prove. Iodide administered in excess of 2 mg has been shown to proportionately decrease the organification of iodide, but it has not been demonstrated that total organification is decreased (9).

Iodide has been shown to decrease release of thyroid hormone from the gland. Excess iodide ingestion of up to 150 mg daily has been shown to decrease the release of T4 and T3 from the thyroid, resulting in small decreases in serum T4 and T3 concentrations with compensatory increases in basal and thyrotropin releasing hormone (TRH) stimulated TSH concentrations. These small changes in hormone concentrations all remain within the normal range (10-15). In addition, excess iodide caused small increases in thyroid volume as determined by echography (15), and decreases in blood flow as determined by Color Doppler Flow Imaging (16). The smallest quantity of excess iodide, in addition to that normally consumed with the diet, which does not affect thyroid function, was estimated to be approximately 500 μg per day (17). Higher amounts of iodide supplementation cause subtle changes in thyroid function (Table 1).

Table 1. Effect of small iodide supplements on serum TSH

I (μg/day)	Basal TSH (μU/ml)	TRH Δ TSH	Ambient I	Days	Reference
500	Increase	-------	Normal	28	Chow (18)
4500	Increase	Increase			
1500	Increase	Increase	Normal	14	
500	No change	Increase			
1500	Increase	Increase			
500	No change	No change	Normal	14	
250	No change	No change			
250 Hashimoto's	Elevated in 7 of 40; Low in 2	-------	Low	120	Reinhardt (20)

AMBIENT IODINE INTAKE AND GRAVES' DISEASE

Although still controversial, the ambient iodine intake may play a significant role in both the occurrence as well as the relapse rates of Graves' disease. Graves' disease has been reported to be more prevalent in countries with a higher iodine intake compared to countries with a lower intake. A recent study compared East-Jutland in Denmark and Iceland, two areas with a similar level of medical care, socio-economic background and similar genetic background. Iceland, which has a high iodine intake, had a significantly higher incidence of Graves' disease compared to East-Jutland, an area of low iodine intake (21), where toxic multinodular goiter was more prevalent. Iodination of salt and bread was instituted in many countries to eliminate endemic goiter caused by iodine deficiency. Iodine supplementation in endemic iodine deficient regions, while largely successful in eliminating endemic goiter and cretinism (22), has also resulted in an increase in iodide induced hyperthyroidism. Although the majority of patients with iodide induced hyperthyroidism have long-standing multinodular goiters with autonomous foci (23), some cases have been due to latent Graves' disease. An increase in dietary iodide may unmask patients with latent Graves' disease, whose hyperthyroidism had been previously suppressed by iodine deficiency (24). It has also been postulated that excess iodide can induce autoimmunity. Iodide given to hyperthyroid patients with Graves' disease significantly increased the levels of thyrotropin receptor antibody (25) and iodide has also been reported to promote IgG synthesis in lymphocytes (26).

The relapse rate of Graves' disease has also been linked to the ambient intake of iodine. The lower remission rates of Graves' Disease in the United States compared to Europe has been partially attributed to the higher iodine intake in the United States. The relapse rates of patients with Graves' disease treated with antithyroid drugs decreased from 1973 to 1985, in association with a decrease in iodine intake during the same period (27). A small study was performed to assess the effect of chronic iodine administration to euthyroid patients who were previously treated for Graves' disease with antithyroid drugs. It was found that after iodine withdrawal, two of ten patients developed recurrent hyperthyroidism (28). Contrary to this view, the remission rate of Graves' disease in Ireland, a country with a low iodide intake was reported to be similar to countries with adequate iodine intake (29). Similarly in the recently published long term prospective study of high and low dose methimazole regimens for the treatment of Graves' disease, urinary iodide excretion did not correlate with relapse rates (30).

THE USE OF EXCESS IODIDE IN GRAVES' DISEASE

Iodide has multiple effects on the thyroid, including inhibition of organification, inhibition of thyroid hormone release, reduction in thyroid size, and reduction in vascularity. All these effects are useful to a certain extent in the management of Graves' disease although one must be aware of certain caveats and potential drawbacks. High concentrations of iodide have also been shown to have immunomodulatory effects. Excess iodide possibly confers a benefit by reducing histocompatibility complex class I antigen expression on thyrocytes (31,32).

control of thyrotoxic symptoms

Iodide is extremely useful in the management of Graves' disease when rapid control of thyrotoxic symptoms is required. This is usually seen in the setting of thyroid storm or as rapid preparation for thyroid surgery as will be discussed in detail below. Iodine containing cholecystographic contrast agents have been proposed as alternatives to inorganic iodides and also rapidly reduce thyroid hormone levels. Two agents commonly used are ipodate (Oragraffin) and iopanoate (Telepaque). These drugs are potent inhibitors of type I 5'-deiodinase (33, 34) decreasing T4 to T3 conversion, and decrease T4 uptake into hepatic cells (35). In addition, they are deiodinated during their metabolism, liberating large quantities of free iodide (Table 2), which in turn decreases thyroid hormone secretion. Ipodate has been reported to induce a more rapid and greater fall in serum T3 levels compared to iodide administration. (36). In the patients treated with ipodate and methimazole, the marked decrease in serum T3 was associated with a lower heart rate compared to those patients treated with SSKI and methimazole or methimazole alone. This is similar to another study in which hyperthyroid patients treated with ipodate had a greater reduction in pulse rate compared to those treated with propylthiouracil alone (37). A loading dose of 2 to 3 g is given on the first day in 2 divided doses, followed by 500mg daily. In a group of hyperthyroid patients treated with sodium ipodate, the serum FT3 levels returned to normal by the second day compared to five days for those treated with iodide (38). Most studies find that ipodate decreases serum TT3 or FT3 rapidly and markedly whereas serum T4 concentrations, while showing a significant decline, do not reach normal levels

Table 2. Iodide content of commonly used iodide preparations

Drug	Iodide content
Lugol's solution	6.3 mg/drop
SSKI	38 mg/drop
Sodium iodide (recently withdrawn from US)	85 mg/ml
Iopanoic acid (Telepaque)	333 mg/tab
Ipodate (Oragrafin)	308 mg/tab

Thyroid storm

Thyroid storm is a life threatening form of severe thyrotoxicosis. It is a difficult diagnosis and is based entirely on the clinical presentation of fever, altered mental status, cardiac abnormalities, and a precipitating event such as infection or trauma. The patient may have a known history of thyrotoxicosis and an obvious goiter or ophthalmopathy, but may also present de novo after non-thyroid surgery or associated with non-thyroidal illness in an undiagnosed thyrotoxic patient. Thyroid function tests do not differentiate between severe but compensated hyperthyroidism and thyroid storm (39). There can be multiple organ decompensations and mortality rates range from 10% to 75%. (40-42). It is probably advisable to treat any severely ill thyrotoxic patient as a patient with thyroid storm. Management involves the use of multiple drugs to treat different pathogenic aspects of the illness. Therapy is first directed at inhibition of new thyroid hormone synthesis with the thionamide drugs. Subsequent therapy is directed at decreasing the release of T4 and T3 from the thyroid by inhibition of proteolysis of colloid. Two alternatives are available, iodide and lithium, but iodide is used much more extensively and has fewer adverse effects compared to lithium. Iodide causes rapid inhibition of thyroid hormone release from the thyroid and this property has made it a powerful pharmacologic agent in the management of thyroid storm. Finally, therapy is directed at antagonizing the peripheral effects of thyroid hormones with beta-adrenergic blocking agents. Additional measures that should be instituted involve specific therapy to treat any precipitating event like sepsis and also supportive therapy to treat associated hyperpyrexia and fluid imbalances. Corticosteroids are usually included in the treatment of thyroid storm, often empirically, to treat any relative adrenal insufficiency that may be present. Corticosteroids also decrease the peripheral deiodination of T4 to T3, the bioactive iodothyronine, and helps to alleviate the peripheral effects of the thyroid hormones.

Iodides primarily act by inhibiting the proteolysis of colloid, thus decreasing the release of T3 and T4. This action is rapid, and lasts for 2 to 3 weeks. The thyroid will later escape from these inhibitory effects of iodide on thyroid hormone secretion, and if iodides are used alone, the patient may have a severe relapse of thyrotoxicosis. Sodium or potassium iodide, 0.5-1 g in 500 ml of dextrose can be administered intravenously every 12 hours for the first few days. In certain countries, including the United States, it is no longer possible to obtain sterile intravenous iodide solutions. Oral iodide in the form of 10 drops of 'Lugol forte' or 10 drops of saturated solution of potassium iodide (SSKI) are alternatives to intravenous iodide. If oral or nasogastric routes of iodide administration are impossible, for example in patients with intestinal obstruction, rectal preparations of iodide have been used (43). In a patient who presented with duodenal obstruction and thyroid storm, treatment consisted of rectal propylthiouracil and 0.4ml of 5% SSKI sublingually (44). The absorption of sublingual SSKI was calculated to be 70% based on 24-hour free urinary iodide excretion indicating that this route of iodide administration is relatively efficient. The iodinated contrast agents, ipodate and iopanoate, are frequently used instead of iodides and are considered by some to be the treatment of choice in thyroid storm (45). As mentioned earlier, they act by inhibiting T4 to T3 conversion as well as by inhibiting thyroid hormone release.

There are two important caveats to remember when using iodides or iodinated contrast agents to treat thyroid storm. First, the sudden increase in iodine could theoretically increase thyroid hormone stores and, thus, increase the possibility of worsening thyrotoxicosis in 10 to 14 days. Thus, antithyroid drugs such as methimazole or propylthiouracil should be given prior to iodides or iodinated contrast agents to inhibit thyroid hormone synthesis. Second, iodides or iodinated contrast agents are never used as sole therapy for the treatment of thyroid storm and are not continued beyond 2 weeks, as the thyroid escapes from inhibition of thyroid hormone secretion after 2 weeks and severe and resistant hyperthyroidism can occur (46).

Sole Therapy in Graves' Disease

In 1923, Plummer reported that iodide administration was successful in the treatment of Graves' Disease (47). It was later observed that the utility of iodine in treating hyperthyroidism was temporary and that patients experienced a relapse or exacerbation after a few weeks of iodine administration. Since then, iodine has been primarily used for the short- term treatment of hyperthyroidism prior to thyroidectomy (see below). Antithyroid drugs are now used successfully in the long-term treatment of Graves' disease, as discussed elsewhere. However a few reports suggest that long-term administration of iodides could achieve a sustained remission in patients with Graves' disease. The advantages of iodide as sole therapy are that it is inexpensive, is easily administered as a single daily dose and, in small doses, is free from toxicity. The candidates for treatment with iodide as sole therapy tended to be patients with mild Graves' disease and small goiters (48). Hamburger selected a group of patients who had mild clinical features of hyperthyroidism, moderately elevated thyroid hormone concentrations, and who were compliant with this long-term treatment (49). They were given 3 drops of Lugol's solution daily for 8 to 18 months. In this group, 20 out of 46 patients remained in remission after iodide was discontinued. No differentiating characteristics were found between the patients who relapsed and those who remained euthyroid. Nagataki reported that in an unselected group of patients with Graves' disease, the use of inorganic iodide was associated with prolonged remission in 30% of patients (49). This compared well with the low remission rate in Japan of 25% after treatment with antithyroid drugs for 1 year. They found no difference between the group that remained in remission after iodide therapy and those that escaped from iodide in regard to clinical parameters of goiter size and degree of exophthalmos and laboratory tests such as the BMR and serum T4 and free T4 concentrations. However, those patients with a low 20 minute radioiodine uptake before treatment were less likely to escape iodide treatment suggesting that the 20-minute thyroid uptake might be useful in selecting patients who might respond to iodide therapy. Wood and Maloof reported that patients with mild disease, small firm thyroids and a positive iodide-perchlorate discharge test were most likely to respond to iodide as sole therapy (49).

Besides the obvious choice of more efficacious antithyroid drugs, there are significant disadvantages in using iodide as sole therapy for the management of Graves' disease. First, the effect of iodide on reducing thyroid hormone synthesis and release is often transient. Emerson et al. observed that thyroid function tests do not return to normal in most patients treated with iodide as sole therapy and that escape from the suppressive effects of iodide frequently occurs within 2-3 weeks (50). Second, in contrast to treatment with antithyroid drugs, iodide therapy results in a thyroid gland rich in hormone stores. Abrupt worsening of thyroid function can occur if there is sudden cessation of therapy, resulting in increased release of hormones form the iodine rich thyroid. Third, the use of iodides renders the thyroid more resistant to the action of the antithyroid drugs. (51) Fourth, there is a danger of iodide induced thyrotoxicosis in patients with functioning nodules in addition to Graves' disease. Finally, allergic reactions to iodide, though uncommon, may occur. Such reactions include hypocomplementemic vasculitis which can occur in patients with underlying autoimmune disease. Thus, the use of iodide as sole therapy in patients with mild disease and a small goiter may be considered but this must be carefully balanced against the disadvantages listed above. We have not used iodides alone and do not recommend such therapy.

Pre-operative preparation for thyroidectomy

The usual pre-operative preparation for thyroidectomy in patients with Graves' disease consists of the administration of antithyroid drugs to achieve a euthyroid state, followed by the use of iodide (Lugol's solution or saturated solution of potassium iodide (SSKI)) for 7-10 days prior to thyroidectomy. Preoperative treatment with Lugol's solution alone prior to thyroidectomy was introduced into the United States in the 1920s (47). Iodides were believed to reduce the vascularity and friability of the thyroid and therefor minimize blood loss during surgery. There was scant evidence regarding this effect of iodide until the 1980s. Marigold et al, using the thyroid uptake of thallium-201, demonstrated in an uncontrolled study that treatment with Lugol's solution for 10 days prior to surgery reduced thyroid blood flow in patients with Graves' disease (52). In a randomized, controlled clinical trial of iodine versus placebo, in which vascularity was assessed by weighing swabs as a measure of surgical blood loss, no benefit in terms of perioperative bleeding was observed in the patients receiving Lugol's solution (53). Thus the debate over the use of iodide pre-operatively remained unresolved. More recent studies using Duplex Doppler sonography have shown that iodides were effective in reducing thyroid blood flow, both in patients with Graves' disease (54) and in euthyroid subjects (16) and strongly argue for its use as preoperative preparation. In a controlled, double blind trial of 12 Graves' patients undergoing thyroidectomy, the patients were treated with antithyroid drugs prior to surgery, then randomized to receive either placebo or 0.3 ml of Lugol's solution thrice daily for 9 days prior to surgery (54). Patients were evaluated with a duplex ultrasound scanner before and after iodide treatment. Reduction in the diameter, time-averaged velocity, and volume flow of the superior thyroid artery was demonstrated in all patients in the treatment group, with no consistent changes in the placebo group. Arntzenius et al, using a Color Flow Doppler Imaging technique, demonstrated in euthyroid subjects that thyroid blood flow responded inversely to changes in iodide intake (16). These changes were independent of changes in TSH.

In addition to the standard method of preparation for thyroid surgery with antithyroid drugs with iodide, there have been alternative preoperative regimens. The β–adrenoreceptor blocking agent, propanolol, has been used as a sole drug preoperatively for patients undergoing thyroidectomy (55, 56). The advantages of propanolol compared to treatment with antithyroid drugs are that preparation time is shorter and the timing of the operation is more flexible. Unfortunately, thyroid storm has been reported to occur after surgery in patients treated with propanolol alone (57). In addition, there is difficulty titrating the dose of propanolol due to increased clearance in hyperthyroid patients and also a wide variability in plasma propanolol levels between individuals. Potassium iodide, 60 mg 3 times a day for 10 days has been successfully used in combination with propanolol to achieve euthyroidism prior to surgery (58, 59). In contrast to propanolol alone, the combination of propanolol and iodide is more likely to result in euthyroidism in patients with all grades of hyperthyroidism. These patients had a smoother clinical course compared to those treated with propanolol alone. The iodinated contrast agents have been successfully employed in the rapid preparation of patients requiring urgent thyroidectomy because they are non-compliant with antithyroid drugs or develop serious side effects. Berghout et al treated 7 patients with 500 mg sodium ipodate and low dose propanolol daily for 5 days prior to thyroid surgery (60). A control group undergoing thyroidectomy had conventional preparation with antithyroid drugs. All 7 patients given ipodate were clinically euthyroid and had normal serum T3 values on the day before surgery. Both groups had similar postoperative outcomes immediately after surgery and 12 months later, although the group given ipodate had a higher incidence of mild or subclinical post-operative hypothyroidism. Baeza et al used a combination of betamethasone (0.5 mg every 6 hours), iopanoic acid (500 mg every 8 hours) and propanolol (40 mg every 8 hours) for 5 days prior to thyroidectomy (61). Serum T3 concentrations normalized in all 14 patients by day 5 with no noted side effects and no post-operative complications.

The recommended preoperative preparation is still to restore the patient to a euthyroid state with antithyroid drugs for several months and add iodides for 10 days prior to surgery. However, when a more rapid pre-operative regimen is required, the combination of antithyroid drugs, iodide or iodinated contrast agents, corticosteroids and propanolol is a safe and efficacious alternative.

As adjunctive therapy following radioactive iodine or surgery

Treatment with ^{131}I has been associated with a high incidence of post-treatment permanent hypothyroidism. A study was designed to determine whether a lower dose of ^{131}I would lower the occurrence of permanent hypothyroidism (62). In patients given low dose ^{131}I, it was expected that a higher incidence of poorly controlled thyrotoxicosis would occur after treatment and that there might be a higher retreatment rate. To ameliorate this effect the patients were given 5 drops of SSKI 2 weeks after ^{131}I and continued for 4 months. SSKI was helpful in controlling the hyperthyroidism post ^{131}I treatment. In addition, fewer patients who received the low dose ^{131}I required re-treatment with [131]I. However, it was noted that 24% of the patients developed transient hypothyroidism during treatment with SSKI. Similar findings were reported by Ross et al, who retrospectively studied 119 patients with Graves' disease treated either with ^{131}I alone or ^{131}I followed by SSKI 1 week later. The patients who received the combination of ^{131}I and SSKI had a more rapid amelioration of hyperthyroidism, but also had a higher incidence of transient hypothyroidism. Sixty percent of the patients who received ^{131}I and SSKI were transiently hypothyroid. There was no difference in the rate of permanent hypothyroidism between the patients who had ^{131}I alone or ^{131}I followed by iodide. Schimmel and Utiger (63) found that if potassium iodide was given within 48 hours after ^{131}I, serum T4 and T3 concentrations transiently decreased and that the thyroid escaped after 2 weeks. In a randomized study of patients undergoing bilateral thyroidectomy, 1 mg iodide supplement given daily after the operation caused hypothyroidism in all patients at 6 months, whereas only 38% of patients given placebo were hypothyroid (64). Another study compared adjunctive treatment with propylthiouracil or iodine following radioiodine therapy for Graves' disease (65). Compared with the control group, patients receiving propylthiouracil or iodine had similar thyroid status at 6 weeks post radioiodine. They concluded that patients with mild or moderate hyperthyroidism do not benefit from either propylthiouracil or iodine after radioiodine therapy. We reported that euthyroid patients with Graves' disease previously treated with ^{131}I, surgery or antithyroid drugs are more susceptible to the induction of iodide myxedema than normal patients (28, 66). In summary, we do not recommend the use of iodide as adjunctive therapy either after ^{131}I or thyroidectomy.

In Pregnancy

Iodide readily crosses the placenta by 10-12 weeks of gestation and is avidly concentrated by the fetal thyroid for the duration of the pregnancy (67). Excess iodide increases the likelihood of fetal goiter and/or hypothyroidism possibly because the fetal thyroid is immature and may not be able to escape from the effects of iodide. Hence, iodide is generally avoided during pregnancy, and has no role in the routine management of Graves' disease in pregnancy (68). In contrast to this accepted view, a Japanese report showed that 6 to 40 mg of iodine alone was used successfully in pregnant patients with Graves' disease (69). Only 2 to the 35 newborns had mildly elevated serum TSH concentrations. These favorable results, however, may be largely influenced by the ambient dietary intake in Japan, which is several fold higher that in North America, perhaps resulting in earlier fetal adaptation to iodide. We suggest that the use of iodide in pregnancy should be restricted to treatment of thyroid storm in combination with other drugs or just prior to thyroidectomy, if necessary.

REFERENCES

1.   **Wolff J, Chaikoff IL** 1948 Plasma inorganic iodide as a homeostatic regulator of thyroid function. J Biol Chem 174:555-564
2.   **Raben MS** 1949 The paradoxical effects of thiocyanate and of thyroglobulin on the organic binding of iodine by the thyroid in the presence of large amounts of iodide. Endocrinology 45:296-304
3.   **Nagataki S, Ingbar SH** 1964 Relation between qualitative and quantitative alterations in thyroid hormone synthesis induced by varying doses of iodide. Endocrinol 74:731-736
4.   **Dugrillon A** 1996 Iodolactones and iodoaldehydes--mediators of iodine in thyroid autoregulation. Exp Clin Endocrinol Diabetes 104 Suppl 4:41-45
5.   **Wolff J, Chaikoff IL, Goldberg RC, Meier JR** 1949 The temporary nature of the inhibitory action of excess iodide on organic iodine synthesis in the normal thyroid. Endocrinol 45:504-513

6.   **Braverman LE, Ingbar SH** 1963 Changes in thyroidal function during adaptation to large doses of iodide. J Clin Invest 42:1216-1231

7.   **Dai G, Levy O, Carrasco N** 1996 Cloning and characterization of the thyroid iodide transporter. Nature 379:458-460

8.   **Eng PHK, Cardona GR, Fang S-L, Previti M, Alex S, Carrasco N, Chin WW, Braverman LE** 1999 Escape from the acute Wolff-Chaikoff effect is associated with a decrease in thyroid sodium/iodide symporter messenger ribonucleic acid and protein. Endocrinology 140:3404-3410

9.   **Nagataki S, Yokoyama N** 1990 Autoregulation: effects of iodine. Acta Med Austriaca 17 Suppl 1:4-8

10. **Vagenakis AG, Downs P, Braverman LE, Burger A, Ingbar SH** 1973 Control of thyroid hormone secretion in normal subjects receiving iodides. J Clin Invest 52:1010-1017

11. **Safran M, Braverman LE** 1982 Effect of chronic douching with polyvinylpyrrolidone-iodine on iodine absorption and thyroid function. Obstet Gynecol 60:35-40

12. **Ader AW, Paul TL, Reinhardt W, Safran M, Pino S, McArthur W, Braverman LE** 1988 Effect of mouth rinsing with two polyvinylpyrrolidone-iodine mixtures on iodine absorption and thyroid function. J Clin Endocrinol Metab 66:632-635

13. **Philippou G, Koutras DA, Piperingos G, Souvatzoglou A, Moulopoulos SD** 1992 The effect of iodide on serum thyroid hormone levels in normal persons, in hyperthyroid patients, and in hypothyroid patients on thyroxine replacement. Clin Endocrinol (Oxf) 36:573-578

14. **LeMar HJ, Georgitis WJ, McDermott MT** 1995 Thyroid adaptation to chronic tetraglycine hydroperiodide water purification tablet use. J Clin Endocrinol Metab 80:220-223

15. **Namba H, Yamashita S, Kimura H, Yokoyama N, Usa T, Otsuru A, Izumi M, Nagataki S** 1993 Evidence of thyroid volume increase in normal subjects receiving excess iodide. J Clin Endocrinol Metab 76:605-608

16. **Arntzenius AB, Smit LJ, Schipper J, van der Heide D, Meinders AE** 1991 Inverse relation between iodine intake and thyroid blood flow: color Doppler flow imaging in euthyroid humans. J Clin Endocrinol Metab 73:1051-1055

17. **Paul T, Meyers B, Witorsch RJ, Pino S, Chipkin S, Ingbar SH, Braverman LE** 1988 The effect of small increases in dietary iodine on thyroid function in euthyroid subjects. Metabolism 37:121-124

18. **Chow CC, Phillips DI, Lazarus JH, Parkes AB** 1991 Effect of low dose iodide supplementation on thyroid function in potentially susceptible subjects: are dietary iodide levels in Britain acceptable? Clin Endocrinol (Oxf) 34:413-416

19. **Gardner DF, Centor RM, Utiger RD** 1988 Effects of low dose oral iodide supplementation on thyroid function in normal men. Clin Endocrinol (Oxf) 28:283-288

20. **Reinhardt W, Luster M, Rudorff KH, Heckmann C, Petrasch S, Lederbogen S, Haase R, Saller B, Reiners C, Reinwein D, Mann K** 1998 Effect of small doses of iodine on thyroid function in patients with Hashimoto's thyroiditis residing in an area of mild iodine deficiency [see comments]. Eur J Endocrinol 139:23-28

21. **Laurberg P, Pedersen KM, Vestergaard H, Sigurdsson G** 1991 High incidence of multinodular toxic goitre in the elderly population in a low iodine intake area vs. high incidence of Graves' disease in the young in a high iodine intake area: comparative surveys of thyrotoxicosis epidemiology in East-Jutland Denmark and Iceland. J Intern Med 229:415-420

22. **Hetzel BS** 1989 The story of iodine deficiency-an international challenge in nutrition. Oxford: Oxford University Press; 1989.

23. **Stanbury JB, Ermans AE, Bourdoux P, Todd C, Oken E, Tonglet R, Vidor G, Braverman LE, Medeiros-Neto G** 1998 Iodine-induced hyperthyroidism: occurrence and epidemiology. Thyroid 8:83-100

24. **Adams DD, Kennedy TH, Stewart JC, Utiger RD, Vidor GI** 1975 Hyperthyroidism in Tasmania following iodide supplementation: measurements of thyroid-stimulating autoantibodies and thyrotropin. J Clin Endocrinol Metab 41:221-228

25. **Wilson R, McKillop JH, Thomson JA** 1990 The effect of pre-operative potassium iodide therapy on antibody production. Acta Endocrinol (Copenh) 123:531-534

26. **Weetman AP, McGregor AM, Campbell H, Lazarus JH, Ibbertson HK, Hall R** 1983 Iodide enhances IgG synthesis by human peripheral blood lymphocytes in vitro. Acta Endocrinol (Copenh) 103:210-215

27. **Solomon BL, Evaul JE, Burman KD, Wartofsky L** 1987 Remission rates with antithyroid drug therapy: continuing influence of iodine intake? Ann Intern Med 107:510-512

28. **Roti E, Gardini E, Minelli R, Bianconi L, Salvi M, Gavaruzzi G, Braverman LE** 1993 Effects of chronic iodine administration on thyroid status in euthyroid subjects previously treated with antithyroid drugs for Graves' hyperthyroidism. J Clin Endocrinol Metab 76:928-932

29. **Smith A, McKenna TJ** 1992 Management of patients with diffuse toxic goitre in Ireland, a country with low iodine intake. Ir J Med Sci 161:597-599

30. **Benker G, Reinwein D, Kahaly G, Tegler L, Alexander WD, Fassbinder J, Hirche H** 1998 Is there a methimazole dose effect on remission rate in Graves' disease? Results from a long-term prospective study. The European Multicentre Trial Group of the Treatment of Hyperthyroidism with Antithyroid Drugs. Clin Endocrinol (Oxf) 49:451-457

31. **Schuppert F, Taniguchi S, Schroder S, Dralle H, von zur Muhlen A, Kohn LD** 1996 In vivo and in vitro evidence for iodide regulation of major histocompatibility complex class I and class II expression in Graves' disease. J Clin Endocrinol Metab 81:3622-3628

32. **Taniguchi SI, Shong M, Giuliani C, Napolitano G, Saji M, Montani V, Suzuki K, Singer DS, Kohn LD** 1998 Iodide suppression of major histocompatibility class I gene expression in thyroid cells involves enhancer A and the transcription factor NF- kappa B. Mol Endocrinol 12:19-33

33. **Wu SY, Chopra IJ, Solomon DH, Bennett LR** 1978 Changes in circulating iodothyronines in euthyroid and hyperthyroid subjects given ipodate (Oragrafin), an agent for oral cholecystography. J Clin Endocrinol Metab 46:691-697

34. **Laurberg P, Boye N** 1987 Inhibitory effect of various radiographic contrast agents on secretion of thyroxine by the dog thyroid and on peripheral and thyroidal deiodination of thyroxine to tri-iodothyronine. J Endocrinol 112:387-390

35. **Felicetta JV, Green WL, Nelp WB** 1980 Inhibition of hepatic binding of thyroxine by cholecystographic agents. J Clin Invest 65:1032-1040

36. **Roti E, Robuschi G, Manfredi A, L DA, Gardini E, Salvi M, Montermini M, Barlli AL, Gnudi A, Braverman LE** 1985 Comparative effects of sodium ipodate and iodide on serum thyroid hormone concentrations in patients with Graves' disease. Clin Endocrinol (Oxf) 22:489-496

37. **Wu SY, Shyh TP, Chopra IJ, Solomon DH, Huang HW, Chu PC** 1982 Comparison sodium ipodate (oragrafin) and propylthiouracil in early treatment of hyperthyroidism. J Clin Endocrinol Metab 54:630-634

38. **Robuschi G, Manfredi A, Salvi M, Gardini E, Montermini M, d'Amato L, Borciani E, Negrotti L, Gnudi A, Roti E** 1986 Effect of sodium ipodate and iodide on free T4

and free T3 concentrations in patients with Graves' disease. J Endocrinol Invest 9:287-291

39. **Brooks MH, Waldstein SS, Bronsky D, Sterling K** 1975 Serum triiodothyronine concentration in thyroid storm. J Clin Endocrinol Metab 40:339-341

40. **Ingbar SH** 1966 Management of emergencies. IX. Thyrotoxic storm. N Engl J Med 274:1252-1254

41. **McDermott MT, Kidd GS, Dodson LF, Jr., Hofeldt FD** 1983 Radioiodine-induced thyroid storm. Case report and literature review. Am J Med 75:353-359

42. **Roth RN, McAuliffe MJ** 1989 Hyperthyroidism and thyroid storm. Emerg Med Clin North Am 7:873-883

43. **Yeung SC, Go R, Balasubramanyam A** 1995 Rectal administration of iodide and propylthiouracil in the treatment of thyroid storm. Thyroid 5:403-405

44. **Cansler CL, Latham JA, Brown PM, Jr., Chapman WH, Magner JA** 1997 Duodenal obstruction in thyroid storm. South Med J 90:1143-1146

45. **Burger AG, Philippe J** 1992 Thyroid emergencies. Baillieres Clin Endocrinol Metab 6:77-93

46. **Caldwell G, Errington M, Toft AD** 1989 Resistant hyperthyroidism induced by sodium iopodate used as treatment for Graves' disease. Acta Endocrinol (Copenh) 120:215-216

47. **Plummer HS** 1923 Results of administration of iodine to patients having exopthalmic goitre. JAMA 80:1955

48. **Hamburger JI** 1978 Clinical Exercises in Internal Medicine, Vol 1. Thyroid disease Philadelphia: Saunders; 1978.

49. **Hamburger JI** 1981 Is there a place for long-term stable iodine in the treatment of Graves' disease. In: Hamburger JI, Miller JM, eds. Controversies in clinical thyroidology. New York: Springer-Verlag; 1981:159-183.

50. **Emerson CH, Anderson AJ, Howard WJ, Utiger RD** 1975 Serum thyroxine and triiodothyronine concentrations during iodide treatment of hyperthyroidism. J Clin Endocrinol Metab 40:33-36

51. **Roti E, Gardini E, Minelli R, Bianconi L, Braverman LE** 1993 Sodium ipodate and methimazole in the long-term treatment of hyperthyroid Graves' disease. Metabolism 42:403-408

52. **Marigold JH, Morgan AK, Earle DJ, Young AE, Croft DN** 1985 Lugol's iodine: its effect on thyroid blood flow in patients with thyrotoxicosis. Br J Surg 72:45-47

53. **Coyle PJ, Mitchell JE** 1982 Thyroidectomy: is Lugol's iodine necessary? Ann R Coll Surg Engl 64:334-335

54. **Chang DC, Wheeler MH, Woodcock JP, Curley I, Lazarus JR, Fung H, John R, Hall R, McGregor AM** 1987 The effect of preoperative Lugol's iodine on thyroid blood flow in patients with Graves' hyperthyroidism. Surgery 102:1055-1061

55. **Michie W, Hammer-Hodges DW, Pegg CA, Orr FG, Bewsher PD** 1974 Beta-blockade and partial thyroidectomy for thyrotoxicosis. Lancet 1:1009-1011

56. **Toft AD, Irvine WJ, McIntosh D, MacLeod DA, Seth J, Cameron EH, Lidgard GP** 1976 Propranolol in the treatment of thyrotoxicosis by subtotal thyroidectomy. J Clin Endocrinol Metab 43:1312-1316

57. **Eriksson M, Rubenfeld S, Garber AJ, Kohler PO** 1977 Propranolol does not prevent thyroid storm. N Engl J Med 296:263-264

58. **Feek CM, Sawers JS, Irvine WJ, Beckett GJ, Ratcliffe WA, Toft AD** 1980 Combination of potassium iodide and propranolol in preparation of patients with Graves' disease for thyroid surgery. N Engl J Med 302:883-885

59. **Peden NR, Browning MC, Feely J, Forrest AL, Gunn A, Hamilton WF, Isles TE** 1985 The clinical and metabolic responses to early surgical treatment for hyperthyroid

Graves' disease: a comparison of three pre-operative treatment regimens. Q J Med 56:579-591

60. **Berghout A, Wiersinga WM, Brummelkamp WH** 1989 Sodium ipodate in the preparation of Graves' hyperthyroid patients for thyroidectomy. Horm Res 31:256-260

61. **Baeza A, Aguayo J, Barria M, Pineda G** 1991 Rapid preoperative preparation in hyperthyroidism. Clin Endocrinol (Oxf) 35:439-442

62. **Hagen GA, Ouellette RP, Chapman EM** 1967 Comparison of high and low dosage levels of 131-I in the treatment of thyrotoxicosis. N Engl J Med 277:559-562

63. **Schimmel M, Utiger RD** 1977 Acute effect of inorganic iodide after 131I therapy for hyperthyroidism. Clin Endocrinol (Oxf) 6:329-332

64. **Taylor JD, Radcliffe SN, Basu PK, Atkins P** 1993 Iodine therapy for thyroidectomy patients exhibiting high thyroid- stimulating hormone values: a randomised study. Ann R Coll Surg Engl 75:168-171

65. **Bazzi MN, Bagchi N** 1993 Adjunctive treatment with propylthiouracil or iodine following radioiodine therapy for Graves' disease. Thyroid 3:269-272

66. **Braverman LE, Woeber KA, Ingbar SH** 1969 Induction of myxedema by iodide in patients euthyroid after radioiodine or surgical treatment of diffuse toxic goiter. N Engl J Med 281:816-821

67. **Roti E, Gnudi A, Braverman LE** 1983 The placental transport, synthesis and metabolism of hormones and drugs which affect thyroid function. Endocr Rev 4:131-149

68. 1993 Thyroid disease in pregnancy. ACOG Technical Bulletin Number 181--June 1993. Int J Gynaecol Obstet 43:82-88

69. **Momotani N, Hisaoka T, Noh J, Ishikawa N, Ito K** 1992 Effects of iodine on thyroid status of fetus versus mother in treatment of Graves' disease complicated by pregnancy. J Clin Endocrinol Metab 75:738-744

18

PATHOGENESIS OF GRAVES' OPHTHALMOPATHY

Rebecca S. Bahn

INTRODUCTION

Graves' disease is a relatively common disorder occurring primarily in women with an incidence of 1/1000 population/year (1). In addition to hyperthyroidism, 25-50% of individuals with Graves' disease have clinical involvement of the eyes known as Graves' ophthalmopathy (GO)(2). While some patients with GO experience only mild ocular discomfort, 3-5% of patients suffer from intense pain and inflammation with diplopia or even loss of vision. At present, GO is not preventable and therapeutic options for severe disease are limited. Recent insights into the pathogenesis of GO, reviewed here, have the potential to lead to new preventive and treatment strategies for this debilitating condition.

HISTOLOGY

Many of the clinical symptoms and signs of GO may be explained on a mechanical basis by an increase in the volume of the orbital fatty connective tissues and extraocular muscle bodies. This expanded orbital tissue volume has been measured in CT scans taken of GO patients' orbits (3). Histologic examination of these tissues reveals excess adipose tissue and an accumulation of sulfated glycosaminoglycans (GAG)(4). These hydrophilic extracellular matrix components are produced by fibroblasts within the orbit (5). Their accumulation leads to gross edema of orbital tissues with resultant enlargement of the extraocular muscles and the fatty connective tissues. Proptosis, the forward displacement of the globe, stems from this increase in volume within the unyielding confines of the bony orbit. Chemosis and periorbital edema are caused primarily by decreased venous drainage from the orbit. Extraocular muscle enlargement and dysfunction are a consequence of GAG accumulation, edema, inflammation and fibrosis in the endomysial connective tissues. The muscle cells themselves are intact, but are widely separated by the edematous extracellular matrix components (6). Swelling of the extraocular muscles at the apex of the orbit may lead to compressive optic neuropathy and visual loss. In late stages of the disease, the extraocular muscles may become fibrotic and atrophic as a result of chronic compression of the muscle fibers.

Postmortem examination of GO orbital adipose tissues demonstrates an increase in both weight and volume compared to normal tissues. The degree of this increase correlates with the degree of exophthalmos present (7). While both the accumulation of hydrated GAG and the expansion of the adipose tissues contribute to the overall increase in orbital tissue volume, the latter likely accounts for the majority of the observed change. The density of fat seen in GO orbital CT scans is indistinguishable from that seen in normal scans, suggesting that hydrated GAG contribute little to the mass of the non-muscle tissue compartment (8).

A diffuse infiltration of lymphocytes, with sparse lymphoid aggregates, is present in the extraocular muscle interstitial tissue and in the orbital fatty connective tissues of patients with GO (9,10). The majority of these cells are T-lymphocytes (CD2+/CD3+), with the minority being B-lymphocytes (Leu26+). Both helper/inducer (CD4+) and suppressor/cytotoxic (CD8+) T-lymphocytes are present, with a slight predominance of the latter. A substantial proportion of the T cells, frequently detected around blood vessels, are activated memory cells (CD45RO). Immunoreactivity for interferon-gamma (IFN-γ), tumor necrosis factor-α (TNF-α), and interleukin-1α (IL-1α) is demonstrable both in the cytoplasm of infiltrating mononuclear cells and in adjacent connective tissue (9).

ROLE OF CYTOKINES

Several recent studies have attempted to characterize the profile of cytokines secreted by orbital-infiltrating T helper (CD4+) cells in GO in order to determine whether these cells are involved primarily in a cell-mediated (Th1) or a humoral-mediated (Th2) immune response. Two groups of investigators reported that the majority of Graves' retroocular T cell clones produce Th1-type cytokines (IL-2, IFN-γ, and TNF-α, but not IL-4 or IL-5) (11,12). A third group detected the presence of mRNA encoding a Th2 dominant profile (IL-4, IL-5 and IL-10)(13), while another group of investigators identified clones secreting cytokines characteristic of both subtypes (IFN-γ, IL-4 and IL-10) (14). These studies suggest that T helper cells of both subtypes may be represented in the retroocular infiltrates in GO. It is possible that the predominant T-helper cell subset changes over the course of the disease and that the reported findings reflect the "activity" or stage of disease represented in the tissue samples. Our demonstration of abundant IFN-γ in surgical tissues obtained from patients with early, active GO supports the concept that T_H1 cells may be involved in the initial stages of the disease (9,15).

The initial host response to an abnormal immune process includes the synthesis of various cytokines. These mediators contribute to the T-cell response, propagation of the disease process, and further production of cytokines. Particular cytokines have "effector" functions in the pathogenesis of some autoimmune diseases. For example, IL-1 participates in the selective destruction of pancreatic beta cells in early type I diabetes mellitus (16). In contrast, rather than causing tissue destruction, cytokines within the orbit in GO (including IL-1α, transforming growth factor-β, IFN-γ, and leukoregulin) are thought to stimulate orbital fibroblasts to produce excessive quantities of GAG (5,17). As described above, the accumulation of GAG in the orbital tissues contributes to the development of the clinical signs and symptoms of the disease. Particular cytokines are also capable of inducing the expression of immunomodulatory proteins, including human leukocyte antigen-DR, intercellular adhesion molecule-1 and heat shock protein-72, in cultured orbital fibroblasts (5). The expression of these molecules within the orbit in GO would be expected to aid in the propagation of the autoimmune response.

Another effect of cytokines relevant to GO is their ability to stimulate the proliferation of orbital fibroblasts. Significantly increased proliferation of orbital fibroblasts from patients with GO was observed following treatment with IL-1α, IL-4, insulin-like growth factor-1, and transforming growth factor-β (TGF-β), but not with IL-2 or IL-6 (18). This effect of cytokines may be especially relevant in the later stages of GO when fibrosis of the extraocular muscles may develop and lead to constant and debilitating diplopia.

SITE-SPECIFIC DISEASE INVOLVEMENT

The extrathyroidal manifestations of Graves' disease are generally restricted to the orbit and pretibial skin, although other areas of skin may rarely be affected. This apparent restriction of disease involvement to two anatomic regions, with the orbit being the more severely affected, can be partially explained by phenotypic differences and similarities that have been described between fibroblasts from various sites. Leukoregulin, a lymphokine derived from activated T lymphocytes, induces dramatic increases in the synthesis of GAG (hyaluronan) and prostaglandin-endoperoxidase H synthetase 2 (an inflammatory cyclo-oxygenase) in cultured orbital, but not skin fibroblasts (17,19). However, studies using two-dimensional gel electrophoresis demonstrate that leukoregulin treatment up-regulates a unique set of proteins in both orbital and pretibial skin cultures (20). IFN-γ appears to be selective in its stimulation of GAG production by orbital fibroblasts, as fibroblasts from skin sites are not stimulated by this cytokine (5). Other studies have shown rapid changes in the morphology of orbital fibroblasts treated with agents that elevate cyclic AMP levels, while dermal fibroblasts fail to respond in this manner (21).

THE ORBITAL AUTOANTIGEN

The autoantigen involved in the hyperthyroidism of Graves' disease is known to be the thyrotropin receptor (TSHR). However, whether this antigen plays a role in the pathogenesis of GO is unclear. Certainly, TSHR is a prime candidate to be the orbital autoantigen because its involvement would help to explain the close clinical and laboratory associations between GO and hyperthyroidism. Reports by several laboratories have identified TSHR mRNA, or a variant TSHR transcript, in human GO orbital tissues and cell cultures using the reverse-transcriptase polymerase chain reaction (22-24). However, RNA transcripts detected only by PCR-based amplification of cDNA may have little physiologic relevance. In order to clarify this issue, we performed studies using a ribonuclease protection assay for semiquantitative detection of this low abundance mRNA. The presence of mRNA corresponding to TSHR extracellular domain was clearly demonstrated in uncultured GO orbital adipose/connective tissue specimens (25). In contrast, TSHR mRNA was absent (or just barely detectable) in normal orbital fatty connective tissue samples. We interpreted these results to suggest that TSHR expression is induced in the orbit in GO, making this receptor available to act as an autoantigen.

While these studies support the concept that TSHR mRNA and protein is expressed in the orbit in GO, direct evidence that this receptor acts as the orbital autoantigen in GO is lacking. A limited number of studies, with conflicting results, have assessed antigenic reactivity of orbital lymphocytes in GO (14,26). Differences in cloning protocols, limitations in the assays, and the use of poorly-defined antigen preparations may have contributed to the disparate results. Future studies will better define the reactivity of the orbital-infiltrating T cells in GO and determine whether they recognize TSHR epitopes.

Studies concerning the pathogenesis of Graves' disease and GO have long been hampered by the lack of a useful animal model (see chapter 9). Recently, a novel animal model was developed in which thyroiditis was transferred to naïve BALB/c mice with human splenocytes that were primed either with TSHR fusion protein or the cDNA for the human TSHR (27). Thyroiditis was induced in 60-100% of these animals and was associated with the production of TSH binding inhibiting IgGs. Examination of the orbits in 17/25 of these animals revealed lymphocytic and mast cell infiltration, accumulation of adipose tissue and edema with periodic acid Schiff-positive material (putative GAG), dissociation of muscle fibers, and the presence of TSHR immunoreactivity (28). Whether this particular animal model accurately reflects the autoimmune processes involved in the development of Graves' disease with ophthalmopathy is unclear. However, these studies will lead to further refinements of the model and to new approaches to the study of GO etiology.

ADIPOGENESIS AND TSHR EXPRESSION IN HUMAN ORBITAL CELLS

The finding of TSH-stimulated lipolysis in rat epididymal adipose cells was the first suggestion that TSHR might be expressed in tissues other than the thyroid (29). Subsequently, specific TSH binding to guinea pig adipose and retro-orbital tissues (30) or to porcine orbital connective tissue membranes was reported (31), and lipolysis of rat adipose cells incubated with long-acting thyroid stimulator was demonstrated (32). TSHR protein, purified from guinea pig fat cell membranes, was shown to be functional with an M_r of approximately 50,000 (33). Following the cloning of TSHR, both guinea pig brown and white adipose tissues were shown to express TSHR (34), and the expression and function of this gene in rat adipocytes was found to parallel the process of adipocyte differentiation in these cells (35).

Determining whether TSHR is expressed in human fat tissues has been more problematic. Some investigators reported low-affinity TSH binding to human fat cell membrane preparations (36), while others found no specific TSH-binding to human adult fat cells (30). Later studies demonstrated lipolysis at physiologic TSH doses in neonatal, but not in adult, human fat cells (37). These effects declined rapidly with age, suggesting a role for TSH in human neonatal thermogenesis. Further studies in neonatal adipocytes showed that the lipolytic effect of TSH could be reproduced by treating cells with stimulatory TSHR autoantibodies, and inhibited with TSHR blocking autoantibodies (38).

Adipocyte precursor cells, called preadipocytes, have been isolated from the stromal-vascular fraction of neonatal and adult human adipose/connective tissues from various regions of the body (39). These cells appear to be a subpopulation of fibroblasts with the potential to undergo adipocyte differentiation when exposed to appropriate tissue culture conditions (40). A recent report by Sorisky and colleagues demonstrated that cultures derived from orbital connective tissue contain such adipocyte precursor cells (comprising 5-10% of the total) capable of responding to adipogenic stimuli *in vitro* (41). These cells may represent an orbital cell subpopulation that can differentiate *in vivo* into mature adipocytes, given appropriate stimuli.

Our recent studies explored the link between adipogenesis and the expression of TSHR in orbital preadipocyte fibroblasts. In these studies, confluent GO and normal preadipocyte fibroblasts were exposed for 7-10 days to *in vitro* conditions shown to stimulate adipogenesis in these cells (41). Mature adipose cells staining with antibodies directed against leptin (an adipocyte-specific gene product) were apparent in the differentiated cultures. The majority of cells in control undifferentiated cultures appeared fibroblast-like in morphology. A significant increase in cAMP production (96-183 fold) following rhTSH stimulation was demonstrated in the differentiated cultures (42). In contrast, there was no significant rhTSH-dependent cAMP production in the undifferentiated cultures. We interpreted these results to suggest that, while cultured orbital preadipocyte fibroblasts do not express measurable functional TSHR, these cells

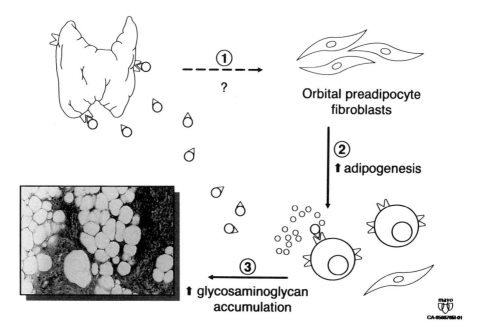

Figure 1. Proposed sequence of events leading to the development of Graves' ophthalmopathy. 1) Unknown Graves' disease-specific factors circulate to the orbit; 2) Adipogenesis and TSH receptor expression is stimulated within the orbital tissues. As a consequence, TSH receptor-directed T cells infiltrate the orbit and release cytokines; 3) Glycosaminoglycan synthesis increases, as does the expression of immunomodulatory proteins within the orbit. These changes, along with the expanded orbital adipose tissue volume, lead to development of the clinical disease.

can be stimulated *in vitro* to differentiate into TSHR-bearing adipocytes. These finding suggest that a stimulus for adipogenesis with accompanying adipocyte TSHR expression may be present in the orbit in GO. It would seem logical that Graves' disease-specific factors, such as particular TSHR-directed autoantibodies, might function in this manner.

SUMMARY

In light of the studies reviewed above, we propose the following scheme for the pathogenesis of GO (Figure 1). Preadipocyte fibroblasts within the orbit may be stimulated in the setting of Graves' disease to differentiate into mature adipocytes that express TSHR. Factors responsible for this stimulation are unknown, but are likely disease-specific. This process results in an increase in the volume of the fatty connective tissues within the orbit. The accompanying up-regulation of TSHR expression in the differentiated cells leads to orbital infiltration by TSHR-reactive T cells. The local release of cytokines by these activated T cells and resident macrophages/dendritic cells stimulates glycosaminoglycan synthesis and the expression of immunomodulatory proteins within the orbit. These changes further increase the volume of the orbital fatty connective tissues and extraocular muscle bodies. As a result of these mechanical and inflammatory processes occurring within the confines of the bony orbit, patients develop clinical eye disease including proptosis, extraocular muscle dysfunction, periorbital congestion and pain.

REFERENCES

1.   **Vanderpump M, Turnbridge W, French J, et al.** 1995 The incidence of thyroid disorders in the community: a twenty-year follow-up of the Whickham Survey. Clin Endocrinol. 43:55-68.
2.   **Bahn RS.** 1995 Assessment and management of the patient with Graves' ophthalmopathy. Endocr Pract. 1:172-178.
3.   **Forbes G, Gorman CA, Brennan MD, Gehring DG, Ilstrup DM, Earnest F.** 1986 Ophthalmopathy of Graves' disease: computerized volume measurements of the orbital fat and muscle. AJNR. 7:651-656.
4.   **Kahaly G, Forester G, Hansen C.** 1998 Glycosaminoglycans in thyroid eye disease. Thyroid 8:429-432.
5.   **Bahn RS, Heufelder AE.** 1993 Mechanisms of disease: Pathogenesis of Graves' ophthalmopathy. N Engl J Med. 329:1468-1475.
6.   **Tallstedt L, Norberg R.** 1988 Immunohistochemical staining of normal and Graves' extraocular muscle. Invest Ophthalmol Vis Sci. 29:175-184.
7.   **Rundle FF, Pochin EE.** 1973 The orbital tissues in thyrotoxicosis: a quantitative analysis relating to exophthalmos. Clin Sci. 5:51-74.
8.   **Peyster RG, Ginsberg F, Silber JH, Adler LP.** 1986 Exophthalmos caused by excessive fat: CT volumetric analysis and differential diagnosis. AJNR. 7:35-40.
9.   **Heufelder AE, Bahn RS.** 1993 Detection and localization of cytokine immunoreactivity in retro-ocular connective tissue in Graves' ophthalmopathy. Eur J Clin Invest. 23: 10-17.
10.   **Weetman AP.** 1991 Thyroid-associated eye disease: pathophysiology. Lancet 338:25-28.
11.   **DeCarli M, D'Elios MM, Mariotti S, et al.** 1993 Cytolytic T cells with Th-1-like cytokine profile predominate in retroorbital lymphocytic infiltrates in Graves' ophthalmopathy. J Clin Endocrinol Metab. 77:1120-1124.

12. **Yang D, Hiromatsu Y, Hoshino T, Inoue Y, Itoh K, Nonaka K.** 1999 Dominant infiltration of T_H 1-type CD4+ cells at the retrobulbar space of patients with thyroid-associated ophthalmopathy. Thyroid 9:305-310.

13. **McLachlan SM, Prummel MF, Rapoport B.** 1994 Cell-mediated or humoral immunity in Graves' ophthalmopathy? Profiles of T-cell cytokines amplified by polymerase chain reaction from orbital tissue. J Clin Endocrinol Metab. 78:1070-1074.

14. **Grubeck-Loebenstein B, Trieb K, Sztankay A, Holter W, Anderl H, Wick G.** 1994 Retrobulbar T cells from patients with Graves' ophthalmopathy are CD8+ and specifically recognize autologous fibroblasts. J Clin Invest. 93:2738-2743.

15. **Natt N, Bahn RS.** 1997 Cytokines in the evolution of Graves' ophthalmopathy. Autoimmunity 26:129-136.

16. **Dinarello CA.** 1991 Inflammatory cytokines: Interleukin-1 and tumor necrosis factor as effector molecules in autoimmune diseases. Curr Opin Immunol. 4:941-951.

17. **Smith TJ, Wang HS, Evans CH.** 1995 Leukoregulin is a potent inducer of hyaluronan synthesis in cultured human orbital fibroblasts. Am J Physiol. 268:C382-C388.

18. **Heufelder AE, Bahn RS.** 1994 Modulation of orbital fibroblast proliferation by cytokines and glucocorticoid receptor agonists. Invest Ophthalmol Vis Sci. 35:120-127.

19. **Wang HS, Cao HJ, Winn VD, et al.** 1996 Leukoregulin induction of prostaglandin-endoperoxide H synthase-2 in human orbital fibroblasts. An in vitro model for connective tissue inflammation. J Biol Chem. 271:22718-22728.

20. **Young DA, Evans CH, Smith TJ.** 1998 Leukoregulin induction of protein expression in human orbital fibroblasts: evidence for anatomical site-restricted cytokine-target cell interactions. Proc Natl Acad Sci USA. 95:8904-8909.

21. **Reddy L, Wang HS, Keese CR, Giaever I, Smith TJ.** 1998 Assessment of rapid morphological changes associated with elevated cAMP levels in human orbital fibroblasts. Exp Cell Res. 245:360-367.

22. **Heufelder AE, Dutton CM, Sarkar G, Donovan KA, Bahn RS.** 1993 Detection of TSH receptor RNA in cultured fibroblasts from patients with Graves' ophthalmopathy and pretibial dermopathy. Thyroid 3:297-300.

23. **Feliciello A, Porcellini A, Ciullo, Bonavolonta G, Avvedimento EV, Fenzi G.** 1993 Expression of thyrotropin-receptor mRNA in healthy and Graves' retro-orbital tissue. Lancet 342:337-338.

24. **Mengistu M, Lukes YG, Nagy EV, Burch HB, Carr FE, Lahiri S, Burman KD.** 1994 TSH receptor expression in retroocular fibroblasts. J Endocrinol Invest. 17:437-441.

25. **Bahn RS, Dutton CM, Natt N, Joba W, Spitzweg C, Heufelder AE.** 1998 Thyrotropin receptor expression in Graves' orbital adipose/connective tissues: Potential autoantigen in Graves' ophthalmopathy. J Clin Endocrinol Metab. 83:998-1002.

26. **Förster G, Otto E, Hansen C, Ochs K, Kahaly G.** 1998 Analysis of orbital T cells in thyroid-associated ophthalmopathy. Clin Exp Immunol. 112:427-434.

27. **Costagliola S, Rodien P, Many MC, Ludgate M, Vassart G.** 1998 Genetic immunization against the human thyrotropin receptor causes thyroiditis and allows production of monoclonal antibodies recognizing the native receptor. J Immunol. 160:1458-1465.

28. **Many MC, Costagliola S, Detrout M, Denef F, Vassart G, Ludgate MC.** 1999 Development of an animal model of autoimmune thyroid eye disease. J Immunol. 162:4966-4974.

29. **Rodbell M.** 1964 Metabolism of isolated fat cells. I. Effects of hormones on glucose metabolism and lipolysis. J Biol Chem. 239:375-380.

30. **Davies TF, Teng CS, McLachlan SM, Smith BR, Hall R.** 1978 Thyrotropin receptors in adipose tissue, retro-orbital tissue and lymphocytes. Mol Cell Endocrinol. 9:303-310.

31. **Perros P, Kendall-Taylor P**. 1994 Demonstration of thyrotropin binding sites in orbital connective tissue: Possible role in the pathogenesis of thyroid-associated ophthalmopathy. J Endocrinol Invest. 17:163-170.

32. **Kendall-Taylor P, Munro DS.** 1971 The lipolytic activity of long-acting thyroid stimulator. Biochem Biophys Acta. 231:314-319.

33. **Iida Y, Amir, S, Ingbar SH.** 1987 Stabilization, partial purification, and characterization of thyrotropin receptors in solubilized guinea pig fat cell membranes. Endocrinology 121:1627-1636.

34. **Roselli-Rehfuss L, Robbins LS, Cone RD.** 1992 Thyrotropin receptor messenger ribonucleic acid is expressed in most brown and white adipose tissues in the guinea pig. Endocrinology 130:1857-1861.

35. **Haraguchi K, Shimura H, Ling Lin, Saito T, Endo T, Onaya T**. 1996 Differentiation of rat preadipocytes is accompanied by expression of thyrotropin receptors. Endocrinology 137: 3200-3205,.

36. **Mullin BR, Lee G, Ledley FD, Winand RJ, Kohn LD.** 1976 Thyrotropin interactions with human fat cell membrane preparations and the finding of a soluble thyrotropin binding component. Biochem Biophys Res Comm. 69:55-62.

37. **Marcus C, Ehren H, Bolme P, Arner P**. 1988 Regulation of lipolysis during the neonatal period: Importance of thyrotropin. J Clin Invest. 82:1793-1797.

38. **Janson A, Karlsson FA, Micha-Johansson G, Bolme P, Bronnegard M, Marcus C**. 1995 Effects of stimulatory and inhibitory thyrotropin receptor antibodies on lipolysis in infant adipocytes. J Clin Endocrinol Metab. 80:1712-1716.

39. **Poznanski W, Waheed I, Van R**. 1973 Human fat cell precursors. Morphologic and metabolic differentiation in culture. J Lab Invest. 29: 570-576.

40. **Smas CM, Sul HS.** 1995 Control of adipocyte differentiation. Biochem. 309:697-710.

41. **Sorisky A, Pardasani D, Gagnon A, Smith TJ.** 1996 Evidence of adipocyte differentiation in human orbital fibroblasts in primary culture. J Clin Endocrinol Metab. 81:3428-3431.

42. **Valyasevi RW, Erickson DZ, Harteneck DA, et al.** 1999 Differentiation of human orbital preadipocyte fibroblasts induces expression of functional thyrotropin receptor. J Clin Endocrinol Metab. 84:2557-2562.

19

THERAPY OF GRAVES' OPHTHALMOPATHY

Leonard Wartofsky, Matthew D. Ringel, and Kenneth D. Burman

GENERAL PRINCIPLES

As described in Chapter 18, the characteristic ophthalmopathy of Graves' disease is marked by impaired eye muscle movement, periorbital edema, with or without actual proptosis. The exophthalmos may be unilateral early but usually becomes bilateral with time. With moderate to advancing severity, the proptosis will be accompanied by varying degrees of ophthalmoplegia and congestive oculopathy characterized by chemosis, conjunctivitis, and periorbital swelling. The most dreaded potential complications are corneal ulceration, optic neuritis, and optic atrophy. When exophthalmos becomes more severe and progresses rapidly to this point, it has been termed "malignant exophthalmos". The term exophthalmic ophthalmoplegia refers to the ocular muscle weakness that results in impaired upward gaze and convergence and strabismus with varying degrees of diplopia. Progressive ophthalmopathy is the most difficult component of Graves' disease to treat successfully. Given four fixed bony orbital walls, the increased intraorbital contents (enlarged external ocular muscles due to lymphocytic infiltration and edema, increased retrobulbar fat) cause the globe to protrude outward causing proptosis. With limits to outward proptosis, pressure can be directed posteriorly on the optic nerve in its course between the bodies of the eye muscles causing ischemia and blindness. In its later stages, the external eye muscles and the levator palpebrae become fibrotic with resultant restricted movement leading to blurred vision, diplopia, and lid retraction. A consequence of lid retraction may be corneal drying and exposure keratitis and ulceration.

Fortunately, even eye disease which is moderately severe may eventually improve with time and with only symptomatic therapy. Initial therapy may consist of reducing periorbital edema and congestive symptoms by elevation of the head of the bed at night, diuretics, use of an eye patch for sleep and a 1% solution of methylcellulose eye drops to prevent corneal drying in patients unable to close the lids during sleep. Prisms may be employed to correct diplopia, as well as tinted lenses for protection from sun and wind. In more severe cases with progressive exophthalmos, chemosis, ophthalmo-plegia, or loss of vision, high dose prednisone (100 to 120 mg per day) may be effective in reducing edematous and infiltrative components. However, an observed reduction of visual acuity is an ophthalmologic emergency which will often require orbital decompression - i.e., removal of one or more walls of the bony orbit to relieve intraorbital pressure on the optic nerve. Orbital radiation (usually 2000 R given as 10 x 200 R treatments) may be helpful in some patients with acute, severe infiltrative manifestations, particularly when administered concomitantly with glucocorticoids. Even after relatively successful therapy of these manifestations, patients may be left with defects in muscle function or unsatisfactory cosmesis due to upper or lower lid retraction. Assuming that the ophthalmopathy is no longer active and the residua are stable, these problems can be corrected by a skilled ophthalmologic surgeon experienced in thyroid eye disease. The management must always be conducted in concert with an ophthalmologist. Several recent general reviews on management of ophthalmopathy can be recommended (1-3).

TREATMENT OF THE UNDERLYING HYPERTHYROIDISM

The fact that most patients develop their ophthalmopathy either simultaneously or within a year or so of their thyrotoxicosis has led to theories of pathogenesis linking the ophthalmopathy to the underlying hyperthyroidism (see previous Chapter). While the course of ophthalmopathy on occasion may be independent of that of the hyperthyroidism, the eye disease in general will tend to improve as the thyroid disease is brought under control in the majority of patients. Hence, most authorities believe the first step in management of ophthalmopathy is to rapidly bring the thyrotoxicosis under control. The issue as to which therapy (surgery, antithyroid drugs, or radioiodine) may be best to do so, and whether radioiodine treatment may actually worsen or precipitate ophthalmopathy remains highly controversial and is dealt with briefly at the close of this chapter and by Bartalena et al. in the next chapter. Until the controversy is resolved by future well-controlled, prospective studies, the authors' view is to avoid radioiodine therapy in those patients who may be most predisposed to worsening ophthalmopathy. Patients at risk of worsening eye disease could include those who smoke, have more severe thyrotoxicosis, have pre-existent ophthalmopathy, or high titers of TSH receptor antibodies.

LOCAL MEASURES

Most patients with Graves' disease have only mild ophthalmopathy which requires local measures for symptomatic relief primarily to preclude corneal drying. Artificial tears (methylcellulose) is prescribed for instillation three times per day and at bed time, along with wearing an eye patch during sleep. Gravity drainage may tend to reduce periorbital edema, and patients should be encouraged to sleep supine (rather than prone, face-down). Blocks to raise the head of the bed and low doses of diuretics have also been employed. The eyes are often easily irritated by wind and dust, and eyeglasses (wraparounds are particularly useful) offer protection, with tinted lenses to reduce photophobia if present. Topical guanethidine eye drops were used in the past but are no longer readily available. For mild degrees of diplopia, non-operative management may include prisms which can be fastened to eye lenses and changed as required with time.

IMMUNOSUPPRESSIVE THERAPY

Corticosteroids

In those patients whose symptoms do not respond sufficiently to simple local measures, the anti-inflammatory effects of immunosuppressive corticosteroids represent the next line of treatment. Steroids have been shown to have a salutary effect on soft tissue swelling, periorbital edema, subconjunctival edema and suffusion, with reduction of sensations of grittiness, orbital ache, and often improved muscle function with diminution in diplopia and improvement in visual acuity. The mechanism of the beneficial effect may relate in part to reduction in glycosaminoglycan (GAG) synthesis and release by intraorbital fibroblasts. Unfortunately, the improvement in muscle function is only minimal, and there is usually variable improvement in proptosis. In spite of the absence of any apparent clinical improvement in muscle function, reduced extraocular muscle volume has been noted on computed tomography during treatment with corticosteroids (4,5).

Many clinicians with experience treating these patients state that high doses of corticosteroid are required, in the range of 120 to 160 mg of prednisone daily. However, Brown et al. (6) noted significantly improved proptosis in 13/19 patients, 4 of whom had papilledema, with the administration of only 40-80 mg prednisone daily for up to 8 weeks. Dosage was tapered after that, and continued for an average interval of 10 months. Soft tissue swelling was reduced in all patients, and 8 patients with optic nerve involvement had improved visual fields and visual acuity and reduced papilledema. Another 8 patients who improved on steroid therapy had an exacerbation of signs and symptoms as the steroids were being tapered. Responses can be seen in 24-48 hours with dramatic improvement in periorbital edema and congestive symptoms. Indeed, it often appears that patients will either respond reasonably quickly (within the first 7-10 days) or very little at all. This belief has prompted the recommendation that the steroids be rapidly tapered and discontinued if there is no clear response within that time frame, in order to avoid the adverse effects of such high doses. The one caveat to this practice relates to those patients with optic nerve involvement who may take as long as two weeks to demonstrate improvement. In particular, lower doses of corticosteroid will take longer to demonstrate benefit. Thus, Day and Carroll (7) did not see benefit until after two weeks of therapy in 10 patients with optic neuropathy who they treated with only 20-40 mg of prednisone daily, and they indicated that peak effectiveness was not reached until almost two months of treatment.

Some groups have attempted to identify laboratory or clinical parameters predictive of responsiveness to corticosteroids (8-11). One approach has been to take advantage of the fact that inflamed tissues with somatostatin-expressing cells in autoimmune disorders will take up octreotide. Scanning with [^{111}In-DTPA-D-phe^1]-octreotide has permitted distinction between acutely inflamed versus fibrotic eye muscles, and positive uptake has been suggested as a marker of disease activity (12). Higher octreotide uptake was subsequently shown by Colao et al. (9) to correlate with clinical responses to corticosteroid therapy. The same distinction between fibrotic and inflamed tissues can be inferred from T2 relaxation times on magnetic resonance imaging (MRI) and has been suggested as a means to select patients for immunosuppressive therapy with corticosteroids (8). Similarly, Sergott et al. observed that patients with suppressed T-cell levels as determined with rosette formation assays were more likely to respond to corticosteroid therapy (11).

Pulse therapy with intravenous methylprednisolone has been advocated by some workers on the grounds that it allows delivery of an immunosuppressive dose with fewer adverse effects than with traditional high-dose prednisone (4,5,13). Kendall-Taylor et al. (5) have reported salutary results in patients with severe ophthalmopathy after administration of two 0.5 g infusions of methylprednisolone over 3 days followed by 40 mg daily of oral methylprednisolone which is then tapered to 10 mg per day over four weeks (5). After 6 months, there was noted improvement in visual acuity, extraocular muscle size, proptosis, and intraocular pressure. Improvement was most marked in patients with disease of shorter duration. A more recent study has shown similar results (14).

Some years ago, a number of ophthalmologists attempted direct local retrobulbar injection of corticosteroids (15,16). This approach was not shown to provide any greater benefit than systemic steroids which can obviously be administered with much less patient discomfort (16,17). Rather, systemic administration is recommended with starting doses of 60-80 mg prednisone daily (18-20). If there is no therapeutic benefit in one week and the medication is being tolerated, the dose can be increased to 120 mg per day. High doses may be required in thyrotoxic individuals, in part because of accelerated metabolism in hyperthyroidism (21). With no apparent benefit in another 1-2 weeks, we would discontinue the steroids after a rapid taper. Just as with cyclosporin (see below), the best response to corticosteroids is seen in those patients with disease of the shortest duration (4-7,13). In addition to their use as single therapy, corticosteroids may act synergistically with other treatment modalities such as external orbital radiation therapy and cyclosporine (discussed below).

Cyclosporine

Weetman et al. 1983 were the first to apply cyclosporine A therapy to Graves' ophthalmopathy based on its selective inhibition of both T-helper cell proliferation and cytotoxic T-cell activation, while allowing T-suppressor cell activation (22). The dramatic salutary effects seen in their first two patients were not reproduced with subsequent patients (23,24), or in more controlled studies on cyclosporin vs. corticosteroids (25,26). Interpretation of the responses was often complicated by the fact that many patients included in these series had also received orbital radiotherapy or prior courses of corticosteroid therapy. For example, in the series of 10 patients reported by Utech et al. (25) 10/10 had previously received corticosteroids and 9/10 had received orbital radiation. However, 7/10 had reduced symptomatology within 1-4 weeks of starting cyclosporine.

Two prospective randomized controlled trials have examined efficacy of cyclosporin vs. corticosteroids (27,28). In one study of 40 patients treated with steroids alone vs. steroids plus cyclosporin, Kahaly et al. (28) concluded that cyclosporin could be useful therapy for Graves' ophthalmopathy in cases where other measures have

Table 1. Management of Graves' ophthalmopathy

Mild pressure discomfort	Methylcellulose drops (Liquid tears)
Dryness (gritty sensation)	Lacrilube ointment
Photophobia	-Eye patch at night
Exposure keratitis	-Tinted lenses
	-Tarsorrhaphy
Congestive symptoms	Methylcellulose drops
-Conjunctival injection	Diuretics
-Periorbital puffiness	Elevate head of bed
-Chemosis	Orbital radiation ± corticosteroids
Diplopia	Ascertain euthyroidism
	Block out one lens of eyeglasses
	Eyeglass prisms
	a) Fresnel prism: paste-on
	b) Ground-in lens
	Extraocular muscle surgery
Proptosis (severe)	Corticosteroids; Immunotherapy
	Decompressive surgery
	Eyelid surgery
Decreasing visual acuity	Decompressive surgery; urgent
	Orbital radiation
	Corticosteroids
Post-decompression	
-Diplopia	Prisms
-Cosmesis	Extraocular muscle recession
-Lid retraction	Cosmetic repair
	-Blepharoplasty
	-Recession of Muller's muscle
	-Tenotomy of levator palpebrae

failed, particularly for Class IV-VI eye disease of brief duration. Patients receiving cyclosporine with prednisone were found to have a greater decrease in muscle thickness by CT, and disease activity did not tend to flare up when steroids were tapered if cyclosporin was continued. They suggested that the initial high dose steroid therapy served to lyse existent activated T-lymphocytes, and continuing cyclosporine dosage served to permit expansion of suppressor T-lymphocyte subsets. These results are largely in accord with those seen in a controlled trial of cyclosporin vs. high dose prednisone in 36 patients by Prummel et al. (27). With monotherapy, these workers observed a response rate of 61% in the steroid group but only 22% in the cyclosporin group. However, in a second phase of the study in which patients who had failed either prednisone or cyclosporin alone were treated with both agents in combination, 59% of patients improved. We would conclude that corticosteroids are more effective as single agent therapy, but that addition of cyclosporin could allow reduction in steroid dosage and avoidance of adverse effects of higher dose steroid. Careful drug level monitoring of cyclosporin is necessary to avoid the drug's numerous potential side effects. Maximal daily doses should not exceed 5.0 mg/kg, with the dose titrated down should significant (>30%) increases in baseline serum creatinine be observed (29). Consideration should be given to adding cyclosporin in patients failing to respond to the regimen for corticosteroids described above.

Intravenous immunoglobulin

High dose intravenous immunoglobulin (IV IgG) therapy has been attempted for Graves' ophthalmopathy because of some success with this therapy for other autoimmune disorders. Some initial success with this therapy (30) led to a larger trial comparing effectiveness of IV IgG in 35 patients to corticosteroids in another 30 patients (31). Improvement in soft tissue swelling, diplopia, orbital CT findings, and proptosis were comparable in the two groups. Similar results were obtained in a randomized controlled trial comparing IV IgG to oral prednisone by Kahaly et al. (32). Given the potential adverse side effects of prolonged high dosage corticosteroids, IV IgG appears to be an effective alternative, although the cost of treatment is high, and its safety, vis á vis freedom of transmission of HIV or hepatitis virus, remains to be determined.

Other immunosuppressive agents

A number of studies have assessed the potential benefit of anti-immune therapy for Graves' ophthalmopathy with a variety of agents (33). The potential efficacy of *azathioprine* was first studied almost 30 years ago (34) and the initial results and those of a more recent, larger, and controlled study by Perros et al. (35) of 10 patients given azathioprine for one year were disappointing. Although antithyroid antibodies and TBII activity fell during therapy, there was no effect on their ophthalmopathy. Small uncontrolled studies have suggested some benefit from *cyclophosphamide* therapy (36,37), but the absence of well controlled clinical trials mitigates against recommending either its use or that of *methotrexate.* Another immunomodulatory drug, *ciamexone*, which may add to the efficacy of other agents in a combined approach (38), was without benefit over placebo in 26 patients given a single daily dose of 300 mg (39,40).

There has been considerable recent interest in the role of local cytokines in the pathogenesis of ophthalmopathy (41), and the possible benefit of therapy with IL-1 antagonists. This interest is based on reports of inhibition of glycosaminoglycans (GAG) synthesis by orbital fibroblasts in vitro by IL-1 receptor antagonists (42); and by a second report of correlation between benefits of orbital radiation therapy and serum levels of IL-1 receptor inhibitor (43). In one clinical trial of 10 patients with moderately severe ophthalmopathy, therapy with *pentoxifylline*, an inhibitor of HLA-

DR expression and GAG synthesis, was found to be associated with improved soft tissue swelling and falling serum levels of GAG and TNF-α (44).

Somatostatin

Trials of somatostatin therapy for ophthalmopathy were undertaken based upon the detection of somatostatin receptors in orbital fibroblasts and lymphocytes. The mechanism of action is presumed to be based upon reduction of IGF-1 mediated edema and reduction of autoreactivity of T cells via inhibition by somatostatin of proliferation of activated T cells. Octreotide has also been shown to reduce circulating levels of intercellular adhesion molecule-1 (sICAM-1), thought to be a marker for orbital fibroblast activation which correlates with inflammatory changes (45). In the latter study, 8/10 patients demonstrated improvement in soft tissue swelling and proptosis which appeared to correlate with reduction in sICAM-1 levels.

Various analogues of somatostatin including Indium-labeled octreotide and pentetreotide have been effectively employed with single photon emission computed tomography (SPECT) to scintigraphically image active ophthalmopathy (12,46-50). Moreover, there may be a correlation between intensity of octreotide uptake on scintiscan and clinical responsiveness to corticosteroids (9). A drawback of somato-statin therapy is the need to give multiple daily subcutaneous injections due to its brief half life, but longer lived analogues will soon be available in the USA. One such analogue, lanreotide, is given only once every two weeks and has been associated with comparable clinical benefit in preliminary trials. Krassas et al. (51) observed clinical improvement in 4/5 patients treated with lanreotide for 3 months, by which time all had disappearance of orbital octreotide uptake. This same phenomenon was seen in an extension of their study with 5 additional patients treated with octreotide (52). The authors believe the mechanism of reduced octreoscan uptake to be due to a reduction in proliferation of activated T cells rather than just a reduction in somatostatin receptors. This concept appears likely because reduced octreoscan uptake is also seen after steroid therapy (46,47) or orbital irradiation (12). In one comparative study with steroids (53), 8 patients with mild ophthalmopathy treated with somatostatin (200 μg subcutaneously every 8 hours) were compared to 10 patients treated with prednisone (1 mg per kg per day). Somatostatin was as effective for relief of symptoms and soft tissue inflammation but not as effective as steroids in reducing muscle size and intraocular pressure.

Plasmapheresis

Based upon the hypothetical benefit of removing circulating immunoglobulins in Graves' disease, plasma exchange for ophthalmopathy has been attempted intermittently since 1979. The failure of this therapeutic modality to attain popularity is testimony to the results of the trials (54-57). The scope of management that is typically required includes 3-11 exchanges averaging 2.5 liters per exchange over a period of several weeks (54). In spite of concomitant administration of azathioprine to most patients in one study, no significant improvement was noted in proptosis, CT or ultrasound appearance of muscles or muscle dysfunction, visual acuity, or intraocular pressure (54). Ten of 13 patients treated by Berlin et al. (6 exchanges over two weeks) were symptomatically improved, and 9/13 had an improved ophthalmopathy index score (57). Eight patients of their patients also had received concurrent therapy with azathioprine. Glinoer and Schrooyen treated 11 patients with severe ophthalmopathy with plasma exchange followed by immunosuppressive therapy with azathioprine and prednisolone, and noted significant improvement in proptosis and soft tissue swelling immediately following exchange (55). The mean reduction in ophthalmopathy index score was 40%. CT measurement of extraocular muscle thickness improved in 4 of 6 patients tested. Follow-up examination six months after plasma exchange indicated persistent benefit in 7 patients but recurrence in four. There is a prospective, controlled trial which examined plasma exchange with immunotherapy (azathiaprine and prednisone) to plasma exchange alone. In the 10 patients studied, there was some marginally positive benefit from the addition of plasma exchange (58). Other reports in the literature have provided variable results with either some (56,59,60) or little improvement (61,62). Specific evaluation of the efficacy of plasma exchange is rendered difficult by the fact that most studies employed concomitant adjunctive immunosuppressive therapy. Until we have the benefit of randomized, controlled studies examining the efficacy of plasmapheresis, we believe that this therapy should be considered only in patients with ophthalmopathy refractory to steroids and other conventional treatments.

ORBITAL RADIATION THERAPY

Whether or not orbital irradiation can be considered a well-established and effective therapeutic approach has been recently debated (63). The reader is referred to the more extensive reviews of the numerous studies which suggest that this treatment is effective (2,3,64,65). The presumed efficacy of this therapy rests upon the radiosensitivity of lymphocytes infiltrating the orbit as well as on radiation-induced reduction of proliferation of orbital fibroblasts and their production of glycosaminoglycans (GAG). Modern megavoltage linear accelerators allow delivery of collimated high-energy therapy to the involved retroorbital structures without scatter damage to adjacent structures such as the lens. The therapy to the orbits is generally given by administering 10 fractions of 2 Gy (total of 20 Gy or 2000 rads) over two weeks. In some reports, dramatic improvement has been seen in soft tissue inflammation and swelling with some reduction in proptosis within a few months to a year after treatment. Not infrequently, a transient worsening of conjunctival inflammation may be seen in the first 5-10 days following initiation of radiation treatment, but improvement should be seen with a few weeks after that. Little benefit is usually seen in external ocular muscle function or diplopia. It has been possible for approximately 75% of patients on corticosteroids to discontinue drug therapy within a few months of their radiation treatment. Results of treatment in one of the larger, earlier studies employing megavoltage irradiation in 311 patients indicated improvement in soft tissues in 80%, proptosis in 51%, and visual acuity in 67% (66). About a third of the patients were taking concomitant corticosteroids, and 76% of them were able to stop the drugs within a few months of completing orbital irradiation.

Prognostic factors indicating a less favorable response included male gender, older age, more severe thyrotoxicosis or the need for concurrent antithyroid therapy, and no history of prior hyperthyroidism (66). Sixty-nine patients received 30 Gy rather than 20 Gy but experienced no appreciable benefit from the higher dosage, notwithstanding a potentially greater risk of radiation retinopathy. Somewhat better results have been observed when corticosteroids are administered along with radiation therapy, and the best responses are seen in patients whose ophthalmopathy is of recent duration.

Bartalena et al. compared the results of treatment of 36 patients with Graves' ophthalmopathy with combined orbital radiation and systemic corticosteroids versus their results in 12 patients treated with corticosteroids alone (67). Steroids were given as methylprednisolone, initially as 70-80 mg daily for three weeks which was then tapered and discontinued over 5-6 months. Orbital radiation (20 Gy over two weeks) with steroids was associated with improvement in soft tissue changes in 35/36 (97%) whereas all 12 (100%) of the patients treated with methylprednisolone alone were improved. Proptosis decreased by >2 mm in 19/34 (56%) of patients treated with combination therapy and in 5/11 (45%) of patients given steroids alone. Extraocular muscle dysfunction improved in 26/28 (93%) affected patients receiving radiation plus steroids, compared to 5/9 (56%) on steroids alone. Using the Kriss/Donaldson criteria or ophthalmopathy index, 72% of patients in the combination therapy group experienced an 'excellent' or 'good' response, compared to only 25% in the steroid only group of 12 patients. As with other therapeutic modalities described above, the best responses were seen in patients with disease of shorter duration. Other favorable reports have appeared (68-71) more recently.

The Bartalena study (66) has been criticized for being uncontrolled, leading Prummel et al. to perform a randomized, double blind trial of 56 patients with moderately severe ophthalmopathy who were treated with either orbital radiation and placebo or corticosteroids and placebo (sham) radiation (72). Given the propensity for spontaneous improvement in Graves' ophthalmopathy, it would have been of value to have had a true control (sham/sham) group. The results were comparable in that improvement was seen in 13/28 radiation-treated and 14/28 steroid-treated patients. However, the high frequency of adverse side effects with corticosteroids led the authors to propose that orbital radiation should be considered as preferable.

In summary, radiation therapy for Graves' ophthalmopathy appears to be safe when performed at a center with modern equipment and extensive experience with the technique. Orbital radiation has little benefit to offer to patients with long-standing disease with stable proptosis and eye muscle dysfunction due to fibrosis and tethering of the muscles. When improvement is seen, it is most impressive in patients with disease of recent onset, particularly on soft-tissue inflammatory changes with less dramatic effects upon proptosis and ophthalmoplegia. Therapy may be as effective as corticosteroids, but definitive judgement on this issue remains uncertain, absent carefully controlled large trials. Given the proven safety of radiation therapy, we believe it reasonable to continue employing this therapy for selected patients, particularly as an alternative to steroids, until the results of more definitive studies dictate otherwise.

SURGICAL THERAPY

There are multiple surgical approaches to the treatment of Graves' ophthalmopathy which range from relatively minor, cosmetic corrections of the eyelids to more dramatic removal of walls of the bony orbit in order to increase the intraorbital capacity for its soft tissue contents and thereby reduce proptosis or the risk of threatened blindness. The ophthalmologic literature includes excellent detailed procedural reviews on orbital decompression (73-76) and surgery on the extraocular muscles (77-79) or eyelids (80-83), all of which will be only briefly summarized below.

Surgical decompression of orbit

An often effective yet conservative orbital decompression can be achieved with minimal invasiveness by removal of orbital fat (84,85). Should fat removal and medical therapy with corticosteroids fail, a more aggressive surgical approach to allow expansion of the existing orbital contents into a more capacious volume may need to be undertaken. The indications for orbital decompression vary considerably among different institutions, but generally include one or more of the following: 1) severe proptosis with corneal exposure, exposure keratitis or ulceration; 2) presence of rapidly progressive optic neuropathy unresponsive to steroid or orbital radiation therapy ; 3) severe orbital inflammation or pain; 4) dependency on corticosteroids or adverse steroid-related complications; 5) as a preliminary procedure to eye muscle surgery if eventual decompression is deemed likely (such as for persistent severe proptosis); and 6) for cosmetic or rehabilitative purposes.

Historically, there have been several approaches to decompression of the orbit, which have differed on the basis of which regions of the bony orbit have been removed. The inferior approach uses either a transantral or transorbital (anterior) technique for removal of the inferior (antral) and medial walls, and is probably the most frequently used technique (86,87). Ophthalmologists tend to prefer a *transorbital approach*, removing three walls of the orbit - the lateral wall, the floor, and the medial wall. Otolaryngologists may perform decompression preferably by a *transantral approach,* removing the floor and medial wall (75). Both these approaches decompress the orbital contents into the paranasal sinuses. The transantral route allows better decompression of the orbital apex than does the transorbital procedure. Advantages of the transantral approach for the patient include absence of an external scar, a short (1-2 day) hospitalization; for the surgeon, this approach offers good visualization of the operative field, a shorter operating time, and good access to the posterior ethmoids which is a benefit in patients with optic neuropathy. Complications of the transantral approach include diplopia, lip numbness, cerebrospinal fluid leak, meningitis, sinusitis, nasolacrimal duct obstruction, and entropion (eyelid inversion) (75).

In contrast, neurosurgeons may decompress the orbit by *transcranial or coronal approach* (88) involving removal of the roof. Restoration of visual acuity is comparable after either transantral or transcranial decompression, whereas the transorbital technique may require adjunctive orbital radiotherapy. All are equally effective in diminishing proptosis. If warranted, it is possible to decompress both orbits in one stage by either the transcranial or transantral technique. The superior or transfrontal approach allows removal of the roof of the orbit through a transfrontal craniotomy. Effective volume expansion is readily achieved via this approach, but it is not generally popular due to the risks associated with craniotomy, which include cerebrospinal fluid leak, frontal lobe damage, meningitis, and intracerebral hemorrhage. When the transorbital approach is employed, most surgeons will decompress only one orbit, and then do the other orbit if indicated after a week's interval.   A *transnasal* endoscopic technique (89) has also been used with success in achieving a comparable degree of decompression. Chronic sinusitis constitutes a contraindication to decompression into the paranasal sinuses. The highest morbidity is seen with the transcranial approach.

Table 2. Indications for decompression

Optic neuropathy

Severe inflammatory changes

Severe proptosis with exposure keratitis

Proptosis prior to EOM recession

Severe pain

Dependency on high dose corticosteroids

Cosmetic considerations

An increase in diplopia may be a consequence of transantral decompression as a result of entrapment of the medial rectus muscles into the ethmoid sinuses, a complication that will require additional corrective surgery (77,90). Cerebrospinal fluid leaks are reported in a small percentage of patients undergoing transantral decompression resulting from penetration of the cribriform plate. Damage to the infraorbital sensory nerve may occur with either the transantral or orbital approach, resulting in permanent anesthesia of the upper lip and gum. Jaw pain on chewing will occur if the temporalis muscle is severed when performing a lateral wall resection via the transorbital approach. Transcranial decompression may result in pulsation of the orbital structures. Pneumoproptosis may occur with either transorbital or transantral decompression if an ethmoid air cell ruptures into the orbital tissues after removal of the medial wall. To avoid this frightening experience, these patients should be warned not to blow their noses forcefully. However, the air rapidly absorbs, and the proptosis subsides. A history of sudden proptosis and crepitation with confirmation by CT scan confirms this diagnosis. Patients with optic neuropathy may require either a medial or superior wall procedure to adequately decompress the orbital apex. Patients without baseline diplopia may be better served by an approach other than a transantral decompression because of the risk of a postoperative strabismus with diplopia. Patients with extreme proptosis may require removal of three or four-walls of the orbit. In general, the reduction in proptosis is proportional to the number of walls removed, ranging from an average of 2-3 mm reduction for a single wall decompression to as much as 14 to 16 mm of globe recession for decompression of all four walls (73,90, 92)(Table 3). Patients with optic neuropathy who fail to improve after transantral decompression may be salvaged by a second transfrontal procedure (93,94).

Table 3. Orbital decompression

Advantages	Adverse sequelae
Transantral approach (floor + medial wall removed)	
No external scar	Postoperative facial swelling
Good visualization	Diplopia, numb lip
Good control of bleeding	Sinusitis; CSF leak
Anterior approach (1,2,3 or 4 walls)	
Less postoperative diplopia	Poor sinus bleeding control
Anatomy better visualized	Numb lip
Transfrontal approach (lateral wall + roof)	
Less postoperative diplopia	External scar with burr holes
No lip numbness	Possible paresis of frontalis
Effective after failure of other approaches	Postoperative pulsation of eyeball

Adapted from Garrity, J.A., Thyroid Today XV: Jan-Mar 1992.

The outcome of orbital decompression surgery is generally favorable. In their large experience of over 450 patients operated via the transantral approach, the Mayo Clinic group (75,86,90,95,96) report improvement in visual acuity in 94% of 84 patients in whom orbital decompression was performed because of a threat to vision (86). A reduction in proptosis averaged 5.5 mm and all patients with corneal ulceration had complete resolution. In their review of 305 patients who underwent transantral decompression, Warren et al. (97) observed preserved or improved visual acuity in over 95% of patients, although 5 patients progressed to total blindness.

Results of orbital decompression by either a two or three-wall procedure were reported by Mourits et al. (98) in 60 patients for whom the indications for surgery were optic neuropathy in 42% and cosmetic in nature for the remaining 58%. Proptosis was reduced from 2.0 to 4.7 mm in the former group and from 3.0 to 4.6 mm in the latter patients. Vision improved in 76% of patients with optic neuropathy after the procedure.

Improvement in extraocular muscle function was seen in only 4 patients developing new onset of diplopia. A necessity for corrective eye muscle surgery post-decompression is not unusual. In a series of 104 patients undergoing transantral decompression, Calcaterra and Thompson (99) found that 30% required extraocular muscle surgery following decompression and 12% required lid surgery. Thus, it appears that the transantral approach to decompressive surgery successfully provides improvement in all aspects of ophthalmopathy except for extraocular muscle dysfunction.

Extraocular Muscle Surgery

Surgery to correct dysfunction of the extraocular muscles is also known as strabismus surgery. The intent of strabismus surgery is to improve ocular alignment and eliminate diplopia by repositioning of the attachments of the extraocular muscles

Table 4. Proptosis regression after decompression.

Walls removed	Number of walls	Degree of regression (mm)
Medial	1	0-4
Lateral + floor	2	3-6
Medial + floor	2	3-6
Medial + floor + lateral	3	6-10
All	4	10-17

Adapted from Kennerdell et al., Orbit 6:153, 1987

onto the globe of the eye. Next to proptosis, extraocular muscle dysfunction may be the aspect of Graves' ophthalmopathy that is least likely to resolve spontaneously or improve with medical therapy alone. As already described above, diplopia is the principal problem which can be worsened after orbital decompression surgery (100). As a result, approximately 30-60% of patients undergoing decompression will subsequently require strabismus surgery (90,96,98, 101). Thus, the indication for strabismus surgery is diplopia in primary gaze, and the goal of therapy is single vision on looking straight ahead and in the reading position. Some postoperative persistence of diplopia on lateral gaze is acceptable, rather than performing additional muscle surgery which may threaten primary gaze, and the patient learns to move their head when looking to the side.

Timing of strabismus surgery is critical in that eye muscle function needs to be stable without corticosteroids for 3-6 months prior to surgery (102,103). In order to avoid the risk of worsening proptosis after strabismus surgery, it is often advisable for patients with significant proptosis to first have decompressive surgery (77), followed by strabismus surgery three months later. To assess which muscles to operate upon, the ophthalmologist will determine if the diplopia is vertical, horizontal, or torsional. The most frequent eye muscles requiring corrective surgery are the inferior rectus, followed by the medial rectus, the superior rectus, and only rarely the lateral rectus muscle (77). Restriction of movement of the medial rectus will cause inward deviation or esotropia. Restriction in movement of several muscles may be contributing to the strabismus, and this can be determined by measuring the degree of deviation in different gaze positions. Generally, because of the risk of damaging the vasculature in recessing muscles, no more than two or three muscles will be operated at one time, and as a consequence, several strabismus surgeries may be required for a successful outcome.

In the Mayo Clinic series of 428 patients (75), 70% of the patients required strabismus surgery after decompression, and single vision on primary gaze and in the reading position was achieved in 77% of them. For the failures, additional attempts at corrective strabismus surgery is not attempted for 6-10 weeks, but the salvage rate in these patients is extremely low, and corrective measures such as prisms are required. A common postoperative complication is lower lid retraction following recession of the inferior rectus, and additional corrective surgery is required. Patients need to be advised early on that the attainment of satisfactory results will likely require several procedures.

Eyelid Surgery

Eyelid surgery is directed at correction of retraction and cosmetic reduction of soft tissue swelling. Eyelid retraction in Graves' disease is the result of increased adrenergic tone of Muller's muscle and the levator palpebrae superioris. The goal of corrective surgery is to prevent corneal exposure, keratitis and ulceration which might lead to perforation. Since extraocular muscle surgery and decompression may both affect position of the eyelids, surgery on the eyelids should not be done until at least 6-12 weeks after these procedures (90,104).

Surgical procedures on the upper eyelid include excision or recession of Muller's muscle (83), transection or recession of the levator aponeurosis with or without interposition of scleral grafts (105,106), levator myotomy (107,108), and a temporary tarsorrhaphy or permanent lateral tarsorrhaphy for lateral fissure reduction (109) which surgically fuses the upper and lower eyelids temporally for greater globe protection. Lower lid entropion is a common problem following transantral decompression, and surgical approaches to its correction are well described (80,81). The most effective lower lid techniques involve recession of the lid retractors usually via a transconjunctival approach, followed by insertion of a spacer material such as a scleral or hard palate mucosal graft to maintain tissue separation (80,106). In order to reduce the risk of an unsatisfactory cosmetic outcome, the timing of eyelid surgery, like that of strabismus surgery, must be considered in relation to the overall strategy for surgical rehabilitation in the individual patient. With the exception of urgent tarsorrhaphy, eyelid surgeries should be postponed until patients have been euthyroid with no further requirement for antithyroid agents for at least one year and the extent of their eye disease should be stable and non-progressive for six months prior to lid surgery in patients not undergoing strabismus or decompression surgery (82).

PREVENTION: DOES CHOICE OF MEDICAL THERAPY AFFECT OPHTHALMOPATHY?

Clearly, it would be preferable to prevent development of ophthalmopathy rather than have patients suffer the consequences and morbidity of this problem and that of its medical or surgical management. Whether or not our choice of treatment for the thyrotoxicosis may influence the course of ophthalmopathy is an issue which is discussed at length by Bartalena et al. in the next chapter, and the relevant prior literature has been previously reviewed (2) and debated (63). The basis for worsening ophthalmopathy is believed to be the release of thyroid antigen secondary to the radiation thyroiditis, which in turn generate TSH-receptor (or other) antibodies which fuel activation of orbital T cells and release of local cytokines. The controversy regarding radioiodine treatment is based largely upon the only prospective study to date, that of Tallstedt et al. (110), which demonstrated that ^{131}I treated patients were more likely to develop new or worsening ophthalmopathy than those treated with thioureas or by surgery. In that study, risk of progressive ophthalmopathy was associated with more severe thyrotoxicosis as indicated by higher basal serum T3 concentrations. Whether or not concomitant L-thyroxine was given early on in the Tallstedt study (as in their patients treated with thioureas or surgery) or only after hypothyroidism appeared in the radioiodine-treated group may or may not be relevant (111). This is so because the initial report of an improved therapeutic outcome due to concomitant thyroxine treatment as reported by Hashizume et al. (112) was not confirmed by several other investigators.

Other studies have continued to incriminate radioiodine in the pathogenesis of worsening ophthalmopathy (113-117). In a study of Fernandez-Sanchez et al. (118), improvement in ophthalmopathy occurred after either radioiodine or surgical treatment, but improvement was greater in the surgical group. In fact, improvement was noted in 34 orbits of 21 patients treated by surgery and only in 8 orbits of 24 patients treated with [131]I. Moreover, deterioration of ophthalmopathy was more common after ^{131}I, and surgical treatment was associated with greater improvement in proptosis and a greater decrease in extraocular muscle size as estimated by CT scan. An earlier report by Sridama and DeGroot (119) reflected a large number of patients and supported the position that exacerbation of ophthalmopathy was no greater after radioiodine than the other therapies, but it was not a prospectively controlled study. Additional evidence incriminating radioiodine as an aggravating factor is provided by the prospective studies of Bartalena and coworkers. In their first report (120), patients with little or no baseline ophthalmopathy received radioiodine alone or radioiodine plus prednisone. In those patients without baseline ophthalmopathy, no new eye involvement occurred in either group. However, during an 18 month follow-up period, worsening of pre-existing ophthalmopathy occurred in 9/16 (56%) of patients with baseline eye involvement in group 1, compared to no worsening in 21 patients given corticosteroids. In a second prospective follow-up study (121) of 443 patients, these workers monitored ophthalmopathy after radioiodine alone, radioiodine plus prednisone, or methimazole alone. Again, worsening ophthalmopathy was noted after radioiodine which could be blunted or prevented by prednisone therapy, whereas worsening ophthalmopathy only very rarely followed methimazole therapy.

Since our ability to predict which patients will get worsening ophthalmopathy is poor at best, we would urge clinicians to be sensitive to a possible worsening of ophthalmopathy after radioiodine, and to counsel their patients on the risk and to document that counseling had been given. Based upon many reports of rising TSH receptor antibody titers after ^{131}I as important to the underlying pathophysiology, and upon the weight of the only randomized prospective studies (110,120,121), there exists some basis to believe that Graves' ophthalmopathy may be worsened by radioiodine until proven otherwise. A history of prior ^{131}I or multiple ^{131}I therapies also has been suggested as associated with worsening ophthalmopathy (122), although the critical factor may be the more severe Graves' disease requiring multiple therapies. In general, we should attempt to identify those patients who may be at greater risk of worsening ophthalmopathy, such as those with pre-existent ophthalmopathy, smokers, and those with very large goiters and more severe thyrotoxicosis. Either thyroidectomy or continuing antithyroid drug therapy may be preferable in such patients. When these therapies are not an option in a patient at higher potential risk for worsening ophthalmopathy, strong consideration should be given to concomitant corticosteroid administration as advocated by Bartalena et al. (121,123), and possibly to early replacement with thyroxine.

REFERENCES

1. **Bartalena L, Marcocci C, Pinchera A**. 1997 Treating severe Graves' ophthalmopathy. Baillieres Clin Endocr Metab. 11:521-36.
2. **Burch HB, Wartofsky L**. 1993 Graves' ophthalmopathy: Current concepts regarding pathogenesis and management. Endocr Rev. 14:747-93.
3. **Wiersinga WM**. 1996 Advances in medical therapy of thyroid-associated ophthalmopathy. Orbit.15:177-186.
4. **Nagayama Y, Izumi M, Kiriyama T, Yokoyama N, Morita S, et al.** 1987 Treatment of Graves' ophthalmopathy with high-dose intravenous methylpred-nisolone pulse therapy. Act Endocrinol. 116:513-518.
5. **Kendall-Taylor P, Crombie AL, Stephenson AM, Hardwick M, Hall K.** 1988 Intravenous methylprednisolone in the treatment of Graves' ophthalmopathy. Brit Med J. 297:1574-1578.
6. **Brown J, Coburn JW, Wigod RA, Hiss JM, Dowling JT.** 1963 Adrenal steroid therapy of severe infiltrative ophthalmopathy of Graves' disease. Amer J Med. 34:786-794
7. **Day RM, Carroll FD.** 1968 Corticosteroids in the treatment of optic nerve involvement associated with thyroid dysfunction. Arch Ophthal.79:279-282.
8. **Utech CI, Khatibnia U, Winter PF, Wulle KG.** 1995 MR T2 relaxation time for the assessment of retrobulbar inflammation in Graves' ophthalmopathy. Thyroid 5:185-193.
9. **Colao A, Lastoria S, Ferone D, et al.** 1998 Orbital scintigraphy with ^{111}In-diethylenetriamine pentaacetic acid-D-phe1]-Octreotide predicts the clinical response to corticosteroid therapy in patients with Graves' ophthalmopathy. J Clin Endocrinol Metab.83:3790-3794.
10. **Mourits MP, Koornneef L, Wiersinga WM, Prummel MF, Berghout A, van der Gaag R.** 1989 Clinical criteria for the assessment of disease activity in Graves' ophthalmopathy: A novel approach. Brit J Ophthal.73:639-644.

11. **Sergott RC, Felberg NT, Savino PJ, Blizzard JJ, Schatz NJ.** 1981 Graves' ophthalmopathy - immunologic parameters related to corticosteroid therapy. Investig Ophthal Vis Sci. 20:173-181.

12. **Postema PTE, Krenning EP, Wijngaarde R, et al.** 1994 [^{111}In-DTPA-D-phe^1]-Octreotide scintigraphy in thyroidal and orbital Graves' disease: a parameter for disease activity. J Clin Endocrinol Metab.79:1845-1851.

13. **Guy JR, Fagien S, Donavan JP, Rubin ML.** 1989 Methylprednisolone pulse therapy in severe dysthyroid optic neuropathy. Ophthalmol. 96:1048-1053.

14. **Matejka G, Verges B, Vaillant G, et al.** 1998 Intravenous methylprednisolone pulse therapy in the treatment of Graves' ophthalmopathy. Horm Metab Res. 30:93-98.

15. **Trobe JD, Glaser JS, LaFlamme P.** 1978 Dysthyroid optic neuropathy. Clinical profile and rationale for managment. Arch Ophthal. 96:1199-1209.

16. **Marcocci C, Bartalena L, Panicucci M, Marconcini C, Cartei F, et al.** 1987 Orbital cobalt irradiation combined with retrobulbar or systemic corticosteroids for Graves' ophthalmopathy: a comparative study. Clin Endocrinol. 27:33-42.

17. **Kahaly G, Beyer J.** 1988 Immunosuppressant therapy of thyroid eye disease. Klin Wochenschr. 66:1049-1059.

18. **Bahn RS, Gorman CA.** 1987 Choice of therapy and criteria for assessing treatment outcome in thyroid-associated ophthalmopathy. Endocrinol Metab Clin N Amer. 16:391-407.

19. **Burman KD.** 1991 Treatment of autoimmune ophthalmopathy. The Endocrinologist. 1:102-110.

20. **Wiersinga WM.** 1990 Immunosuppressive treatment of Graves' ophthalmopathy. Trends in Endocrinol Metab. 1:377-381.

21. **Frey FJ, Horber FF, Frey BM.** 1988 Altered metabolism and decreased efficacy of prednisolone and prednisone in patients with hyperthyroidism. Clin Pharmacol Ther. 44:510-521.

22. **Weetman AP, Ludgate M, Mills PV, McGregor AM, Beck L, et al.** 1983 Cyclosporin improves Graves' ophthalmopathy. Lancet. 2:486-489.

23. **Brabant G, Peter H, Becker H, Schwarzrock R, Wonigeit K, Hesch RD.** 1984 Cyclosporin in infiltrative eye disease. Lancet. 1:515-516.

24. **Howlett TA, Lawton NF, Fells P.** 1984 Deterioration of severe Graves' ophthalmopathy during cyclosporine treatment. Lancet.2:1101.

25. **Utech C, Wulle KG, Panitz N, Kiefer H.** 1985 Immunosuppressive treatment of Graves' ophthalmopathy with cyclosporin A. Acta Endocrinol.110:493-498.

26. **McGregor AM, Beck L, Hall R.** 1985 Cyclosporin A in management of Graves' disease. J Roy Soc Med. 78:511-512.

27. **Prummel MF, Mourits MP, Berghout A, Krenning EP, van der Gaag R, et al.** 1989 Prednisone and cyclosporine in the treatment of severe Graves' ophthal-mopathy. N Engl J Med. 321:1353-1359.

28. **Kahaly G, Schrezenmeir J, Krause U, et al.** 1986. Cyclosporine and prednisone in treatment of Graves' ophthalmopathy: a controlled, randomized and prospective study. Eur J Clin Invest 16:415-422.

29. **Feutren G, Mihatsch MJ.** 1992 Risk factors for cyclosporine-induced nephro-pathy in patients with autoimmune diseases. N Engl J Med. 326:1654-1660.

30. **Antonelli A, Saracino A, Alberti B, Canapicchi R, Cartei F, et al.** 1992 High-dose intravenous immunoglobulin treatment in Graves' ophthalmopathy. Acta Endocrinol. 126:13-23.

31. **Baschieri L, Antonelli A, Nardi S, et al.** 1997 Intravenous immunoglobulin ver-sus corticosteroid in treatment of Graves' ophthalmopathy. Thyroid. 7:579-585.

32. **Kahaly GJ, Pitz S, Muller-Forell W, Hommel G.** 1996 Randomized trial of intravenous

immunoglobulins versus prednisolone in Graves' ophthalmopathy. Clin Exper Immun. 106:197-202.

33. **Prummel MF, Wiersinga WM.** 1998 Immunomodulatory treatment of Graves' ophthalmopathy. Thyroid. 8:545-548.

34. **Burrow GN, Mitchell MS, Howard RO, Morrow LB.** 1970 Immuno- suppressive therapy for the eye changes of Graves' disease. J Clin Endocrinol. 31:307-311.

35. **Perros P, Weightman DR, Crombie AL, Kendall-Taylor P.** 1990 Azathioprine in the treatment of thyroid-associated ophthalmopathy. Acta Endocrinol. 122:8- 12.

36. **Wall JR, Strakosch CR, Fang SL, Ingbar SH, Braverman LE.** 1979 Thyroid binding antibodies and other immunological abnormalities in patients with Graves' ophthalmopathy: Effect of treatment with cyclophosphamide. Clin Endocrinol. 10:79-91.

37. **Bigos ST, Nisula BC, Daniels GH, Eastman RC, Johnston HH, Kohler PO.** 1979 Cyclophosphamide in the managment of advanced Graves' ophthalmopathy. A preliminary report. Ann Intern Med. 90:921-0923.

38. **Utech C, Wulle KG, Panitz N, Kiefer H.** 1989 Treatment of Graves' ophthalmopathy with new immunosuppressive agents. Devel Ophthal. 20:94-99.

39. **Kahaly G.** 1989 Endocrine exophthalmos and ciamexone. Acta Endocrinol. 121:142-144.

40. **Kahaly G, Lieb W, Muller-Forell W, Mainberger M, Beyer J, et al.** 1990 Ciamexone in endocrine orbitopathy. A randomized double-blind, placebo-controlled study. Acta Endocrinol. 122:13-21.

41. **Bartalena L, Marcocci C, Pinchera A.** 1996 Editorial:Cytokine antagonists: new ideas for the management of Graves' ophthalmopathy. J Clin Endocrinol Metab. 81:446-448.

42. **Tan GH, Dutton CM, Bahn RS.** 1996 Interleukin-1 receptor antagonist and soluble interleukin-1 receptor inhibit interleukin-1-induced glycosaminoglycan production in cultured human orbital fibroblasts from patients with Graves' ophthalmopathy. J Clin Endocrinol Metab. 81:449-452.

43. **Hofbauer LC, Muhlberg T, Konig A, et al.** 1997 Soluble IL-1 receptor antagonist serum levels in smokers and nonsmokers with Graves' ophthalmopathy undergoing orbital radiotherapy. J Clin Endocrinol Metab. 82:2244-2247.

44. **Balazs C, Kiss E, Vamos A, Molnar I, Farid NR.** 1997 Beneficial effect of pentoxifylline on thyroid associated ophthalmopathy: a pilot study. J Clin Endocr Metab. 82:1999-2002.

45. **Ozata m, Bolu E, Sengul A, Tasar M, Beyhan Z, et al.** 1996 Effects of Octreotide treatment on Graves' ophthalmopathy and circulating sICAM-1 levels. Thyroid. 6:283-288.

46. **Kahaly GJ, Diaz M, Just M, Beyer J, Lieb W.** 1995 Role of octreoscan and correlation with MR imaging in Graves' ophthalmopathy. Thyroid. 5:107- 111.

47. **Kahaly GJ, Gorges R, Diaz M, et al.** 1998 Indium-111-pentreotide in Graves' disease. J Nucl Med. 39:533-536.

48. **Wiersinga WM, Gerding MN, Prummel MF, Krenning EP.** 1998 Octreotide scintigraphy in thyroidal and orbital Graves' disease. Thyroid. 8:433-436.

49. **Kahaly GJ, Forster GJ.** 1998 Somatostatin receptor scintigraphy in thyroid eye disease. Thyroid. 8:549-552.

50. **Krassas GE.** 1998 Somatostatin analogues in the treatment of thyroid eye disease. Thyroid. 8:443-446.

51. **Krassas GE, Kaltsas T, Dumas A, Pontikides N, Tolis G.** 1997 Lanreotide in the treatment of patients with thyroid eye disease. Eur J Endocrinol. 136:416-422.

52. **Krassas GE, Doumas A, Kaltsas T, Halkias A, Pontikides N.** 1999 Somatostatin receptor scintigraphy before and after treatment with somatostatin analogues in patients with thyroid eye disease. Thyroid. 9:47-52.

53. **Kung AWC, Michon J, Tai KS, Chan FL.** 1996 The effect of somatostatin versus

corticosteroid in the treatment of Graves' ophthalmopathy. Thyroid. 6:381-384, and p. 489.

54. **Kelly W, Longson D, Smithard D, Fawcitt R, Wensley R, et al.** 1983 An evaluation of plasma exchange for Graves' ophthalmopathy. Clin Endocrinol. 18:485-493.

55. **Glinoer D, Schrooyen M.** 1987 Plasma exchange therapy for severe Graves' ophthalmopathy. Horm Res. 26:184-189.

56. **Zielinski CC, Weissel M, Muller C, Till P, Hofer R.** 1989 Long-term follow- up patients with Graves' orbitopathy treated by plasmapheresis and immuno- suppression. Devel Ophthal. 20:130-138.

57. **Berlin G, Hjelm H, Lieden G, Tegler L.** 1990 Plasma exchange in endocrine ophthalmopathy. J Clin Apheresis. 5:192-196.

58. **DeRosa G, Menichella G, Della S, Rossi PL, Testa A, et al.** 1990 Plasma exchange in Graves' ophthalmopathy. Progr Clin Biol Res. 337:321-325.

59. **Yamamoto K, Saito K, Takai T, Yoshida S.** 1982 Treatment of Graves' ophthalmopathy by steroid therapy, orbital radiation therapy, plasmapheresis, and thyroxine replacement. Endocrinol Jpn. 29:495-501.

60. **Dandona P, Marshall NJ, Bidey SP, Nathan A, Havard CWH.** 1979 Successful treatment of exophthalmos and pretibial myxedema with plasmapheresis. Brit Med J. 1:374-376.

61. **Lewis RA, Slater N, Croft DN.** 1979 Exophthalmos and pretibial myxedema not responding to plasmapheresis. Brit Med J. 2:390-391.

62. **Dandona P, Marshall NJ, Bidey SP, Nathan A, Havard CWH.** 1979 Exophthalmos and pretibial myxedema not responding to plasmapheresis. Brit Med J. 2:667-668.

63. **DeGroot LJ, Gorman CA, Pinchera A, Bartalena L, Marcocci C, et al.** 1995 Therapeutic controversies: Radiation and Graves' ophthalmopathy. J Clin Endocrinol Metab. 80:339-349.

64. **Kao SCS, Kendler DL, Nugent RA, Adler JS, Rootman J.** 1993 Radiotherapy in the management of thyroid orbitopathy. Arch Ophthalmol. 111:819-823.

65. **Bartalena L, Marcocci C, Manetti L, et al.** 1998 Orbital radiotherapy for Graves' ophthalmopathy. Thyroid. 8:439-442.

66. **Peterson IA, Kriss JP, McDougall IR, Donaldson SS.** 1990 Prognostic factors in the radiotherapy of Graves' ophthalmopathy. Int J Radiat Oncol Biol Phys. 19:259-264.

67. **Bartalena L, Marcocci C, Chiovato L, et al.** 1983 Orbital cobalt irradiation combined with systemic corticosteroids for Graves' ophthalmopathy: comparison with systemic corticosteroids alone. J Clin Endocrinol Metab. 56:1139-1144.

68. **Hurbli T, Char DH, Harris J, Weaver K, Greenspan F, Sheline G.** 1985 Radiation therapy for thyroid eye disease. Amer J Ophthal. 99:633-637.

69. **Sakata K, Hareyama M, Oouchi A, et al.** 1998 Radiotherapy in the management of Graves' ophthalmopathy. Japan J Clin Oncol. 28:364-367.

70. **Claridge KG, Ghabrial R, Davis G, et al.** 1997 Combined radiotherapy and medical immunosuppression in the management of thyroid eye disease. Eye.11:717-722 and 581-582.

71. **Wiersinga WM, Smit T, Schuster-Uittenhoeve ALJ, van der Gaag R, Koornneef L.** 1988 Therapeutic outcome of prednisone medication and of orbital irradiation in patients with Graves' ophthalmopathy. Ophthalmologica. 197:75-84.

72. **Prummel MF, Mourits MP, Blank L, et al.** 1993 Randomized double-blind trial of prednisone versus radiotherapy in Graves' ophthalmopathy. Lancet.342:949-954.

73. **Kennerdell JS.** 1990 Orbital decompression: an overview. In: Graves' ophthalmopathy, Wall JR and How J (eds), Blackwell Scientific Publ., Cambridge, Mass,. pp. 159-170.

74. **Tallstedt L.** 1998 Surgical treatment of thyroid eye disease. Thyroid. 8:447-452.

75. **Garrity JA, Fatourechi V, Bergstralh EJ, Bartley GB, Beatty CW, et al.** 1993 Results

of transantral orbital decompression in 428 patients with severe Graves' ophthalmopathy. Amer J Ophthal. 116:533-547.

76. **Fells P.** 1987 Orbital decompression for severe dysthyroid eye disease. Brit J Ophthal. 71:107-111.

77. **Dyer JA.** 1984 Ocular muscle surgery. In: The Eye and Orbit in Thyroid Disease. Gorman, CA, Campbell RJ, Dyer JA (Eds), Raven Press, New York,.pp. 253-262.

78. **Ellis FD.** 1979 Strabismus surgery for endocrine ophthalmopathy. Ophthalmol. 86:2059-2063.

79. **Boergen KP.** 1989. Surgical repair of motility impairment in Graves' orbitopathy. Devel Ophthal 20:159-168.

80. **Waller RR, Samples JR, Yeatts RP.** 1984 Eyelid malpositions in Graves' ophthalmopathy. In: The Eye and Orbit in Thyroid Disease. Gorman, CA, Campbell RJ, Dyer JA (Eds), Raven Press, New York,. pp. 263-300.

81. **Beyer-Machule C-K.** 1989 Surgical management of eye lid retractions. Devel Ophthal. 20:192-212.

82. **Codére FC.** 1990 Cosmetic and corrective eye surgery. In: Graves' Ophthalmo-pathy. Wall JR and How J (eds), Blackwell Scientific Publ., Cambridge, Mass,. pp. 183-188.

83. **Putterman AM.** 1981 Surgical treatment of thyroid-related upper eylid retraction. Graded Müller's muscle excision and levator recession. Ophthalmol. 88:507-512.

84. **Adenis JP, Robert PY, Lasudry JG, Dalloul Z.** 1998 Treatment of proptosis with fat removal for orbital decompression in Graves' ophthalmopathy. Europ J Ophthal. 8:246-252.

85. **Trokel S, Kazim M, Moore S.** 1993 Orbital fat removal: Decompression for Graves' ophthalmopathy. Ophthalmol. 100:674-682.

86. **DeSanto LW.** 1984 Transantral orbital decompression. In: The Eye and Orbit in Thyroid Disease. Gorman, CA, Campbell RJ, Dyer JA (Eds), Raven Press, New York,. pp. 2312-2352.

87. **Ogura JH, Tawley SE.** 1980 Orbital decompression for exophthalmos. Otolaryngol Clin N Amer. 13:29-38.

88. **Kalmann R, Mourits MP, van der Pol JP, Koornneef L.** 1997 Coronal approach for rehabilitative orbital decompression in Graves' ophthalmopathy. Brit J Ophthal. 81:41-45.

89. **Lund VJ, Larkin G, Fells P, Adams G.** 1997 Orbital decompression for thyroid eye disease: a comparison of external and endoscopic techniques. J Laryngol Otol. 111:1051-1055.

90. **DeSanto LW.** 1980 The total rehabilitation of Graves' ophthalmopathy. Laryngoscope. 90:1652-1678.

91. **McCord CD.** 1985 Current trends in orbital decompression. Ophthalmol. 92:21-33.

92. **Garrity JA, McCaffrey TV, Gorman CA.** 1989 Compression and decompression of orbital contents in Graves' ophthalmopathy. Acta Endocrinol. 121 (Suppl 2):160-168.

93. **Fatourechi V, Bartley GB, Garrity JA, Bergstralh EJ, Ebersold MJ, Gorman CA.** 1993 Transfrontal orbital decompression after failure of transantral decom-pression in optic neuropathy of Graves' disease. Mayo Clin Proc. 68:552-555.

94. **Feldon SE.** 1993 Management of Graves' ophthalmopathy with optic nerve involvement. Mayo Clin Proc. 68:616-617.

95. **Gorman CA, DeSanto LW, MacCarthy CS, Riley FC.** 1974 Optic neuropathy of Graves' disease. Treatment by transantral or transfrontal orbital decompression. N Engl J Med. 290:70-75.

96. **Garrity JA, Bartley GB, DeSanto LW, Offord KP, Gorman CA.** 1990 Orbital decompression: Long-term results. In: Graves' Ophthalmopathy. Wall JR and How J (eds), Blackwell Scientific Publ., Cambridge, Mass,. pp. 171-82.

97. **Warren JD, Spector G, Burde R.** 1989 Long-term follow-up and recent observations on

305 cases of orbital decompression for dysthyroid orbitopathy. Laryngoscope. 99:35-40.

98. **Mourits MP, Koornneef L, Wiersinga WM, Prummel MF, Berghout, van der Gaag R.** 1990 Orbital decompression for Graves' ophthalmopathy by inferomedial, by infermedial plus lateral, and by coronal approach. Ophthalmol. 97:636-641.

99. **Calcaterra TC, Thompson JW.** 1980 Antral-ethmoidal decompression of the orbit in Graves' disease; ten-year experience. Laryngoscope. 90:1941-1949.

100. **Shorr N, Neuhaus RW, Baylis HI.** 1982 Ocular motility problems after orbital decompression for dysthyroid ophthalmopathy. Ophthalmol. 89:323-328.

101. **Garrity JA, Saggau DD, Gorman CA, Bartley GB, Fatourechi V, et al.** 1992 Torsional diplopia after transantral orbital decompression and extraocular muscle surgery associated with Graves' orbitopathy. Amer J Ophthal. 113:363-373.

102. **Fells P.** 1991 Management of dysthyroid eye disease. Brit J Ophthalmol. 75:245-246.

103. **Burch HB, Gorman CA, Bahn RS, Garrity JA.** 1996 Ophthalmopathy In: Werner and Ingbar's The Thyroid, Braverman LE and Utiger RD (Eds), Lippincott- Raven, Philadelphia, 7th Edition,. pp. 536-553.

104. **Schimek RA.** 1972 Surgical management of ocular complications of Graves' disease. Arch Ophthalmol. 87:655-664.

105. **Harvey JT, Corin S, Nixon D, Veloudios A.** 1991 Modified levator aponeurosis recession for upper eyelid retraction in Graves' disease. Ophthalmol Surg. 22:313-317.

106. **Mourits MP, Koorneef L.** 1991 Lid lengthening by sclera interposition for eyelid retraction in Graves' ophthalmopathy. Brit J Ophthal. 75:344-347.

107. **Grove AS.** 1980 Eyelid retraction treated by levator marginal myotomy. Ophthalmol. 87:1013-1018.

108. **Grove AS.** Upper eyelid retraction and Graves' disease. 1981 Ophthalmol. 88:499-506.

109. **Leone CR.** 1984 The management of ophthalmic Graves' disease. Ophthalmol. 91:770-779.

110. **Tallstedt L, Lundell G, Torring O, et al.** 1992 Occurrence of ophthalmopathy after treatment for Graves' hyperthyroidism. N Engl J Med. 326:1733-1738.

111. **Tallstedt L, Lundell G, Blomgren H, Bring J.** 1994 Does early administration of thyroxine reduce the development of Graves' ophthalmopathy after radioiodine treatment? Europ J Endocrinol. 130:494-497.

112. **Hashizume K, Ichikawa K, Sakurai A, et al.** 1991 Administration of thyroxine in treated Graves' disease: Effects of the level of antibodies to thyroid stimulating hormone receptor and on the risk of recurrence of hyperthyroidism. N Engl J Med. 324:947-953.

113. **Kung AWC, Yau CC, Cheng A.** 1994 The incidence of ophthalmopathy after radioiodine therapy for Graves' disease: Prognostic factors and the role of methimazole. J Clin Endocrinol Metab. 79:542-546.

114. **Marcocci C, Bartalena L, Bogazzi F, Bruno-Bossio G, Pinchera A.** 1992 Relationship between Graves' ophthalmopathy and type of treatment of Graves' hyperthyroidism. Thyroid. 2:171-178.

115. **Lazarus JH.** 1998 Relation between thyroid eye disease and type of treatment of Graves' hyperthyroidism. Thyroid. 8:437.

116. **Manso PG, Furlanetto RP, Wolosker AMB, et al.** 1998 Prospective and controlled study of ophthalmopathy after radioiodine therapy for Graves' hyperthyroidism. Thyroid. 8:49-52.

117. **Burmeister LA, Beatty RL, Wall JR.** 1999 Malignant ophthalmopathy presenting one week after radioiodine treatment of hyperthyroidism. Thyroid. 9:189-192.

118. **Fernandez-Sanchez JR, Pradas JR, Martinez OC et al.** 1993 Graves' ophthalmopathy after subtotal thyroidectomy and radioiodine therapy. Brit J Surg. 80:1134-1136.

119. **Sridama V, DeGroot LJ.** 1989 Treatment of Graves' disease and the course of ophthalmopathy. Amer J Med. 87:70-73.

120. **Bartalena L, Marcocci C, Bogazzi F, Panicucci M, Lepri A, et al.** 1989 Use of corticosteroids to prevent progression of Graves' ophthalmopathy after radioiodine therapy for hyperthyroidism. N Engl J Med. 321:349-352.
121. **Bartalena L, Marcocci C, Bogazzi F, et al.** 1998   Relation between therapy for hyperthyroidism and the course of Graves' ophthalmopathy. N Engl J Med. 338:73-78 and 1546-1547.
122. **DeGroot LJ, Mangklabruks A, McCormick M.** 1990 Comparison of RA ^{131}I treatment protocols for Graves' disease. J Endocrinol Invest. 13:111-118.
123. **Bartalena L, Marcocci C, Pinchera A.** 1998 On the effects of radioiodine therapy on Graves' ophthalmopathy. Thyroid. 8:533-534.

20

RADIOIODINE THERAPY AND GRAVES' OPHTHALMOPATHY

Luigi Bartalena, Claudio Marcocci and Aldo Pinchera

INTRODUCTION

A close temporal relationship has clearly been demonstrated between the onset of Graves' ophthalmopathy and that of hyperthyroidism (1,2). In more than three quarters of cases, hyperthyroidism and ophthalmopathy occur within 18 months of each other (1,2). When ophthalmopathy follows hyperthyroidism it may be difficult to establish whether changes in ocular conditions reflect the natural history of the disease or are etiologically related to the treatment of hyperthyroidism. This uncertainty may explain why results reported in the literature, mostly derived from retrospective, uncontrolled and non-randomized studies, are often contradictory (3).

In spite of these limitations, it is widely recognized that treatment of hyperthyroidism with thionamides is not associated with significant progression of ophthalmopathy (3). We contributed to this notion by observing that among 148 patients receiving methimazole treatment, 3 of 74 patients with preexisting ophthalmopathy (4%) showed an amelioration of eye disease and 4 patients in the entire group (3%) had progression of the ophthalmopathy (4). Although thionamide treatment is usually not related to exacerbation of the ophthalmopathy, it is frequently followed by relapse of hyperthyroidism (5). The latter is associated with a reactivation of thyroid autoimmunity that, in view of the purported relationship between thyroid and orbit autoimmune phenomena (6), may negatively influence the course of the ophthalmopathy (3). For these reasons, at variance with the view that in patients with ophthalmopathy hyperthyroidism should preferably be treated with antithyroid drugs (7,8), we believe that, under most circumstances, patients with relevant ocular manifestations should receive definitive treatment for their hyperthyroidism by either radioiodine therapy or thyroidectomy (9). These treatments would bear the advantage of leading to the deprivation of thyroid-orbit shared antigen(s) and to removal of autoreactive intrathyroidal T lymphocytes possibly involved in the pathogenesis of Graves' ophthalmopathy (9).

As far as thyroidectomy is concerned, both progression, improvement and no change of Graves' ophthalmopathy following thyroid surgery have been reported in mostly retrospective and uncontrolled studies (see 3,6 for reviews). In a recent prospective, case-control study involving 30 patients with mild or no ophthalmopathy we documented that near-total thyroidectomy has no relevant role in the progression of the ophthalmopathy, since exacerbation of eye disease occurred only in one patient (who had preexisting ophthalmopathy), a proportion was similar to that observed with antithyroid drug treatment (10). It seems, therefore, unlikely that thyroidectomy carries the risk of causing progression of eye disease.

RADIOIODINE THERAPY AND GRAVES' OPHTHALMOPATHY

The information concerning the influence of radioiodine on Graves' ophthalmopathy is far less straightforward. Reports addressing this issue have produced controversial information supporting both the idea that radioiodine therapy does not aggravate the ophthalmopathy (11) and the view that this treatment may indeed be bad for eye disease (12)(Table 1). It is conceivable that conflicting results are, at least in part, attributable to the retrospective and non-randomized features of most studies, the lack of appropriate control groups and of standardized methods for the assessment of ocular changes, and the inclusion in different series of patients with variable degrees of disease severity, duration and activity (12).

Non-randomized Studies

Werner et al. (13) observed that after radioiodine therapy development or progression of the ophthalmopathy occurred, over a 10-year follow-up period, in only 15 of 433 patients (3%), an overall outcome that appeared to be more favorable than with antithyroid drugs or thyroidectomy. Hamilton et al. (14,15) reported that new ophthalmopathy occurred in 8% of patients without preexisting eye involvement and progressed in 18% of those with ophthalmopathy clinically evident prior to radio-iodine, indicating that worsening of ophthalmopathy after radioiodine administration might take place in about one quarter of cases. Pequegnat et al. (16), after administration of large doses of radioiodine (20-100 mCi), observed progression of ophthalmopathy in 16 of 57 patients (28%), more frequently in those with eye disease clinically evident before radioiodine therapy. Kriss et al. (17) reported increased exophthalmometer readings in 8 of 24 patients (33%) after radioiodine therapy. Hetzel et al. (18) found a progression of ophthalmopathy after radioiodine in 9 of 17 patients (53%). Aron-Rosa et al. (19) documented only 22 cases (4%) of development or progression of eye disease among 604 patients after radioiodine therapy. Calissendorf et al. (20) reported no case of deterioration of eye disease among 17 patients treated with radioiodine. In a large retrospective study, Sridama and DeGroot (21) evaluated 537 patients with Graves' disease and found that there was no difference in the occurrence of new ophthalmopathy after radioiodine therapy (5%), thyroidectomy (7%) or thionamide treatment (7%), nor in the deterioration of preexisting ophthalmopathy, which was more frequent but apparently unrelated to the modality of treatment of hyperthyroidism (radioiodine, 23%; thyroidectomy, 19%; antithyroid drugs, 19%). Vestergaard et al. (22) in a series of 50 patients given radioiodine therapy observed that new ophthalmopathy developed only in 1 of 28 patients (4%) without preexisting ocular disease, but

Table 1. Radioiodine therapy and development or progression of Graves' ophthalmopathy

Author	Year	Patient number	Development or Progression	
			number	%
Non-randomized Studies				
Werner	1957	433	15	3
Hamilton	1960	165	30	18
Pequenat	1967	57	16	28
Kriss	1967	24	8	33
Hetzel	1967	17	9	53
Hamilton	1967	158	12	8
Aron-Rosa	1973	604	22	4
Calissendorf	1986	17	0	0
Sridama	1989	385	88	23
Vestergard	1989	50	6	12
Barth	1989	89	17	19
Fernandez-Sanchez	1993	24	6	25
Kung	1994	114	27	24
Abe	1998	67	7	10
Manso	1998	22	0	0
Spitzweg	1998	48	2	4
Total		2274	265	12
Randomized Studies				
Bartalena	1989	26	9	35
Tallstedt	1992	39	13	33
Vazquez-Chavez	1993	24	9	37
Bartalena	1998	150	23	15
Total		239	54	23

worsened in 5 of 22 (23%) patients with pre-radioiodine eye disease. Barth et al. (23) retrospectively evaluated the records of 89 radioiodine-treated patients with Graves' disease, and found that radioiodine therapy was followed by an exacerbation of the ophthalmopathy in 17 cases (17%); also in this report progression was more likely in patients with preexisting eye disease. In Fernàndez-Sanchez et al.'s series (24), worsening of the ophthalmopathy occurred in 6 of 24 patients (25%) treated with radioiodine, while there was no case of progression of the disease following subtotal thyroidectomy. Kung et al. (25) reported that 27 of 114 patients (24%)

given radioiodine showed the occurrence or progression of eye disease; the risk of progression of eye disease was higher in patients who had an increase in serum TSH levels after radioiodine, and was not decreased by the use of a combined regime of high-dose methimazole and levothyroxine after radioiodine therapy (25). Abe et al. (26) reported that ophthalmopathy progressed in 7 (10%), improved in 2 (3%), remained unchanged in 62 (87%) of 67 patients receiving radioiodine therapy: the course of the ophthalmopathy was worse after radioiodine than after subtotal thyroidectomy. Recently, Manso et al. (27) prospectively evaluated, in a non-randomized study, 22 patients treated with radioiodine and found no worsening of ophthalmopathy. However, ocular control measurements were made quite late, so that transient exacerbation of eye disease, which may occur as early as few days after radioiodine (28), might have been missed. Furthermore, most of the patients had little, if any, pre-radioiodine ocular involvement and none of them smoked (27), making progression of the ophthalmopathy less likely. Most of the above limitations apply to a retrospective and uncontrolled study by Spitzweg et al. (29), who reported no case of ophthalmopathy progression in 68 patients with no pre-radioiodine ophthalmopathy and observed deterioration of eye disease in only 2 of 48 (4%) with preexisting ophthalmopathy. In addition, in this study the evaluation of outcome was based only on the subjective self-assessment assessed by a questionnaire and not on objective measures (29).

Randomized Studies

Few randomized and controlled studies addressing the problem of the relationship between radioiodine therapy and the course of Graves' ophthalmopathy are available. We randomly treated a relatively small group of patients with Graves' hyperthyroidism and mild or no ophthalmopathy with either radioiodine alone or radioiodine associated with a 3-month course of oral prednisone (0.4-0.5 mg/Kg/day, initial dose) (30). Worsening of ophthalmopathy occurred in 9 of 26 patients (35%) with eye involvement prior to radioiodine therapy, whereas in the group receiving also prednisone, progression did not occur and preexisting ophthalmopathy improved in most cases (30). This study did not include a control group of patients receiving methimazole treatment. In a subsequent randomized, controlled study Tallstedt et al. (31) reported that the rate of development or progression of eye disease was superimposable in patients treated with antithyroid drugs (4 of 38 patients, 10%) or thyroidectomy (6 of 37 patients, 16%), but was significantly higher in those given radioiodine (13 of 39 patients, 33%). This study was criticized (11) because the prevalence of smokers was higher in the radioiodine group than in the other groups and because the radioiodine-treated group was given levothyroxine replacement therapy only after a variable period of hypothyroidism that might have contributed to the progression of eye disease. As a matter of fact, the same group subsequently reported that prompt administration of levothyroxine and avoidance of untreated post-radioiodine hypothyroidism was associated with a decreased risk of ophthalmopathy progression after radioiodine (45 of the 248 patients, 18%, receiving levothyroxine when hypothyroid; 27 of the 244 patients,

11%, treated with levothyroxine 2 weeks after radioiodine)(32,33). Vàzquez-Chàvez et al. (34) randomly assigned 40 Graves' patients to treatment with either radioiodine or thyroidectomy, and found no differences in the ocular conditions between these two groups, based, however, only on exophthalmometer readings.

In a prospective, randomized study we assigned 450 patients with Graves' hyperthyroidism and mild or no ophthalmopathy to treatment with either radioiodine alone, methimazole, or radioiodine followed by treatment with oral prednisone (4). Among the 150 patients receiving radioiodine alone, progression of eye disease occurred in 23 cases (15%), and this was persistent only in 8 (5%) who subsequently required treatment for ophthalmopathy. Progression of eye disease was not observed in the group treated also with prednisone, in which preexisting eye disease improved in about two thirds of cases. Treatment with methimazole did not affect the course of the ophthalmopathy (4). It should be noted that radioiodine only rarely caused appearance of new ophthalmopathy (4), confirming previous data of the literature that treatment-associated changes in ocular conditions are more frequent in patients with preexisting ocular involvement. In our study thyroid status did not affect the outcome of the ophthalmopathy, because post-radioiodine hyper- or hypothyroidism was promptly and appropriately corrected.

It has been argued that the prospective study described above (4) does not definitively support a relationship between radioiodine therapy and ophthalmopathy because progression of ophthalmopathy after radioiodine administration might simply be coincidental and reflect the natural history of the disease (11,35), while the different outcome in the methimazole group might reflect a beneficial effect of thionamide treatment, which would then be the true eye disease-modifying treatment (7). However, although patients in both radioiodine and methimazole groups were pretreated with methimazole, progression occurred only in the former group. Admittedly, progression of ophthalmopathy after radioiodine does not occur in the majority of patients, implying that other risk factors or cofactors for the progression of eye disease likely contribute to this outcome. These factors include smoking (36), high pretreatment T3 values (31), high serum TSH-receptor antibody (25) and thyrotropin (37,38) levels and preexisting ophthalmopathy (4, 30). Identification of other risk factors should also allow better coordinate treatment of high-risk patients (37). Such patients should receive a 3-month course of intermediate-dose oral prednisone concomitantly with radioiodine therapy in order to prevent possible progression of ophthalmopathy and to improve preexisting ophthalmopathy (4,30).

The development or progression of Graves' ophthalmopathy following radioiodine administration might be related to the release of thyroid antigens from the radiation-damaged thyroid (Table 2), with subsequent enhancement of the autoimmune response towards antigens shared by the thyroid and the orbit (6), as suggested also for the occurrence of eye disease after irradiation of the neck for nonthyroidal disorders (38,39) or after thyroid-destructive processes (40). Radioiodine therapy for differentiated thyroid carcinoma is followed by the release of thyroperoxidase in the circulation (41), but demonstration of this phenomenon in Graves' disease is hampered by the interfering presence of autoantibodies. Radioiodine therapy is followed by an increase in concentration and activity of

TSH-receptor antibodies (42,43) and by peripheral blood T cell activation (44); a prolonged increase (lasting more than two years) in thyroid autoantibody production has been described after radioiodine therapy (45).

Table 2. Putative effects of radioiodine on Graves' ophthalmopathy.

Lag period after radioiodine	Effect on ophthalmopathy	Mechanism
Short	Progression*	- Release of thyroid-orbit shared antigens - Exacerbation of autoimmune response
Long	Beneficial**	- Antigen deprivation - Removal of intrathyroidal T-lymphocytes

* Occurs more frequently in patients with preexisting ophthalmopathy and can be prevented by concomitant glucocorticoid administration.
** Remains to be proven

It must be noted that our large study (4) included only patients with non-severe ophthalmopathy. It is unknown what effect radioiodine *per se* might have in the minority of patients with severe eye disease. This question will be difficult to assess because patients with severe ophthalmopathy require prompt therapeutic measures (orbital radiotherapy, high-dose glucocorticoids, orbital decompression) which obscure possible radioiodine-related ocular changes.

CONCLUDING REMARKS

In a recent survey of European endocrinologists, the selected modality of treatment of recurrent hyperthyroidism after antithyroid drug therapy was thyroidectomy in 43% of cases, a second course of antithyroid drugs in 32%, and radioiodine in only 25% (46). In other words, when ablative therapy was selected, the preference was surgery rather than radioiodine therapy, suggesting that the possible negative effects of radioiodine might modify the attitude of many endocrinologists as to the use of radioiodine therapy in patients with clinically evident eye disease. We do not share the view that radioiodine therapy should be avoided in patients with ophthalmopathy, because progression of the ophthalmopathy does not occur in the majority of cases and can easily be prevented by concomitant prednisone therapy (30,47) (Table 2). In addition, ablation of the thyroid might in the long run prove useful for the long-term outcome of eye disease, as a consequence of antigen deprivation and removal of intrathyroidal autoreactive T lymphocytes (9,48).

To summarize, radioiodine treatment seems to be associated with possible progression of preexisting ophthalmopathy (4,30,31); this is more likely in smokers (36). Progression does not occur in the majority of patients and, most important, can easily be prevented by concomitant glucocorticoid treatment (4,30). Therefore, this risk of progression should not be taken as an argument to avoid or postpone radioiodine treatment in hyperthyroid patients for whom such a treatment is indicated. On the contrary, we favor such a treatment, because, even though this remains to be proven, radioiodine thyroid ablation might in the long term be beneficial for eye disease. Accordingly, in patients with non-severe ophthalmopathy the use of antithyroid drugs or thyroidectomy for hyperthyroidism does not require anything but local measures for the ophthalmopathy, whereas selection of radioiodine for the management of thyroid hyperfunction should be accompanied by administration of intermediate-dose glucocorticoids (Table 3). In patients with severe Graves' ophthalmopathy, appropriate therapeutic approaches for eye disease should promptly be taken independently of the treatment selected for hyperthyroidism (Table 3).

Table 3. Coordinate treatment of Graves' hyperthyroidism and ophthalmopathy.

Hyperthyroidism	Ophthalmopathy	
	Mild or Moderate	Severe
Antithyroid drugs	Local measures	Specific treatments*
Radioiodine	Intermediate dose	Specific treatments*
Thyroidectomy	Local measures	Specific treatments*

* High-dose glucocorticoids, orbital radiotherapy, orbital decompression.

REFERENCES

1. **Marcocci C, Bartalena L, Bogazzi F, Panicucci M, Pinchera A** 1989 Studies on the occurrence of ophthalmopathy in Graves' disease. Acta Endocrinol. (Copenh) 120: 473-478

2. **Gorman CA** 1983 Temporal relationship between onset of Graves' ophthalmopathy and diagnosis of thyrotoxicosis. Mayo Clin Proc. 58: 515-519

3. **Marcocci C, Bartalena L, Bogazzi F, Bruno-Bossio G, Pinchera A** 1992 Relationship between Graves' ophthalmopathy and type of treatment of Graves' hyperthyroidism. Thyroid 2: 171-178

4. **Bartalena L, Marcocci C, Bogazzi F, et al.** 1998 Relation between therapy for hyperthyroidism and the course of Graves' ophthalmopathy. N Engl J Med. 338: 73-78

5. **Vitti P, Rago T, Chiovato L, et al.** 1997 Clinical features of patients with Graves' disease undergoing remission after antithyroid drug treatment. Thyroid 7: 369-375

6. **Burch HB, Wartofsky L** 1993 Graves' ophthalmopathy: current concepts regarding pathogenesis and management. Endocr Rev. 14: 747-793

7. **Wiersinga WM** 1998 Preventing Graves' ophthalmopathy. N Engl J Med 338: 121-122

8. **Weetman AP, Harrison BJ** 1998 Ablative or non-ablative therapy for Graves' hyperthyroidism in patients with ophthalmopathy? J Endocrinol Invest. 21: 472-475

9. **Marcocci C, Bartalena L, Pinchera A** 1998 Ablative or non-ablative therapy for Graves' hyperthyroidism in patients with ophthalmopathy? J Endocrinol Invest. 21: 468-471

10. **Marcocci C, Bruno-Bossio G, Manetti L, et al.** 1999 The course of Graves' ophthalmopathy is not influenced by near total thyroidectomy: a case-control study. Clin Endocrinol. (Oxf), in press.

11. **Gorman CA** 1995 Radioiodine therapy does not aggravate Graves' ophthalmopathy. J Clin Endocrinol Metab. 80: 340-342

12. **Pinchera A, Bartalena L, Marcocci C** 1995 Radioiodine may be bad for Graves' ophthalmopathy, but..... J Clin Endocrinol Metab. 80: 342-345

13. **Werner SC, Coelho B, Quimby EH** 1957 Ten year results of I-131 therapy in hbyperthyroidism. Bull NY Acad Med. 33: 783-806

14. **Hamilton HE, Schutz RO, De Gowil EL** 1960 The endocrine eye lesion in hyperthyroidism. Arch Intern Med. 105: 675-685

15. **Hamilton RD, Mayberry VE, McConahey WM, Hanson KC** 1967 Ophthalmopathy of Graves' disease: a comparison between patients treated surgically and patients treated with radioiodine. Mayo Clin Proc. 42: 812-818

16. **Pequegnat EP, Mayberry WE, McConahey WM, Wyse EP** 1967 Large doses of radioiodine in Graves' disease: effects on ophthalmopathy and long-acting thyroid stimulator. Mayo Clin Proc. 42: 802-811

17. **Kriss JP, Pleshakov V, Rosenblum AL, Holderness M, Sharp G, Utiger R** 1967 Studies on the pathogenesis of the ophthalmopathy of Graves' disease. J Clin Endocrinol Metab. 27: 582-593

18. **Hetzel BS, Mason EK, Kwan WH** 1967 Studies of serum long-acting thyroid stimulator (LATS) in relation to exophthalmos after therapy for thyrotoxicosis. Australas Ann Med. 17: 307-311

19. **Aron-Rosa D, Pérez R, Abitbol Y** 1973 Malignant exophthalmos after iodine-131 treatment. Mod Probl Ophthalmol. 14: 432-434

20. **Calissendorf BM, Soderstrom M, Alveryd A** 1986 Ophthalmopathy and hyperthyroidism, a comparison between patients receiving different antithyroid treatments. Acta Ophthalmol. 64: 698-703

21. **Sridama V, DeGroot LJ** 1989 Treatment of Graves' disease and the course of ophthalmopathy. Am J Med. 87: 70-73

22. **Vestergaard H, Laurberg P** 1989 Radioiodine and aggravation of Graves' ophthalmopathy. Lancet 2: 47

23. **Barth A, Probst P, Burgi H** 1989 Identification of a subgroup of Graves' disease patients at higher risk for severe ophthalmopathy after radioiodine. J Endocrinol Invest. 14: 209-212

24. **Fernàndez Sànchez JR, Rosell Pradas J, Carazo Martinez O, et al.** 1993 Graves' ophthalmopathy after subtotal thyroidectomy and radioiodine therapy. Br J Surg. 80: 1134-1136

25. **Kung AWC, Yau CC, Cheng A** 1994 The incidence of ophthalmopathy after radioiodine therapy for Graves' disease: prognostic factors and the role of methimazole. J Clin Endocrinol Metab. 79: 542-546

26. **Abe Y, Sato H, Noguchi M, et al.** 1998 Effect of subtotal thyroidectomy on natural history of ophthalmopathy in Graves' disease. World J Surg. 22: 714-717

27. **Manso PG, Furlanetto RP, Wolosker AMB, Paiva ER, de Abreu MT, Maciel RMB** 1998 Prospective and controlled study of ophthalmopathy after radioiodine therapy for Graves' hyperthyroidism. Thyroid 8: 49-52

28. **Burmeister LA, Beatty RL, Wall JP** 1999 Malignant ophthalmopathy presenting one week after radioiodine treatment of hyperthyroidism. Thyroid 9: 189-192

29. **Spitzweg C, Rossmuller B, Heufelder AE** 1998 Radioiodine therapy and Graves' ophthalmopathy. Thyroid 8: 1193 (Letter)

30. **Bartalena L, Marcocci C, Bogazzi F, Panicucci M, Lepri A, Pinchera A** 1989 Use of corticosteroids to prevent progression of Graves' ophthalmopathy after radioiodine therapy for hyperthyroidism. N Engl J Med. 321: 1349-1352

31. **Tallstedt L, Lundell G, Torring O, et al.** 1992 Occurrence of ophthalmopathy after treatment for Graves' hyperthyroidism. N Engl J Med. 326: 1733-1738

32. **Tallstedt L, Lundell G, Blomgren H, Bring J** 1994 Does early administration of thyroxine reduce the development of Graves' ophthalmopathy after radioiodine treatment? Eur J Endocrino.l 130: 494-497

33. **Tallstedt L, Lundell G** 1997 Radioiodine treatment, ablation, and ophthalmopathy: a balanced perspective. Thyroid 7: 241-245

34. **Vàzquez-Chàvez C, Nishimura Megura E, Espinosa Said L, Delgado Falfari A, Sàinz de Viteri M** 1992 influencia del tratamento del hipertiroidismo en el curso del exoftalmos. Rev Invest Clin. 44: 241-247

35. **Gorman CA, Offord KP** 1998 Therapy for hyperthyroidism and Graves' ophthalmopathy. N Engl J Med. 338: 1546 (Letter)

36. **Bartalena L Marcocci C, Tanda ML, et al.** 1998 Cigarette smoking and treatment outcomes in Graves ophthalmopathy. Ann Intern Med. 129: 632-635

37. **Karlsson AF, Dahlberg PA, Jansson R, Westermark K, Enoksson P** 1989 Importance of TSH receptor activation in the development of severe endocrine ophthalmopathy. Acta Endocrinol. (Copenh) 121 (Suppl 2): 132-141

38. **Karlsson AF, Wetermark K, Dahlberg PA, Jansson R, Enoksson P** 1989 Ophthalmopathy and thyroid stimulation. Lancet 2: 691

38. **Wasnich RD, Grumet FC, Payne RO, Kriss JP** 1973 Graves' ophthlmopathy following external neck irradiation for nonthyroidal neoplastic disease. J Clin Endocrinol Metab. 37: 703-713

39. **Jackson R, Rosenberg C, Kleinmann R, Vagenakis AG, Braverman LE** 1979 Ophthalmopathy after neck irradiation therapy for Hodgkin's disease. Cancer Treat Rep. 63: 1393-1395

40. **Bartalena L, Bogazzi F, Pecori F, Martino E** 1996 Graves' disease occurring after subacute thyroiditis: report of a case and review of the literature. Thyroid 6: 345-348

41. **Ozata M, Bayhau H, Bingol N, et al.** 1995 Sequential changes in serum thyroid peroxidase following radioiodine therapy of patients with differentiated thyroid carcinoma. J Clin Endocrinol Metab. 80: 3634-3638

42. **Pinchera A, Liberti P, Martino E, et al.** 1969 Effects of antithyroid therapy on the long-acting thyroid stimulator and the antithyroglobulin antibodies. J Clin Endocrinol Metab. 29: 231-238

43. **Fenzi GF, Hashizume K, Roudebush C, DeGroot LJ** 1979 Changes in thyroid-stimulating immunoglobulins during antithyroid therapy. J Clin Endocrinol Metab. 48: 572-578

44. **Teng W-P, Stark R, Munro AJ, Young SM, Borysiewicz LK, Weetman AP** 1990 Peripheral blood T cell activation after radioiodine treatment for Graves' disease. Acta Endocrinol. (Copenh) 122: 233-240

45. **Aizawa Y, Yoshida K, Kaise N, Fukazawa H, Kiso Y, Mori K, Sayama N, Kikuchi K, Abe K** 1995 Long-term effects of radioiodine on thyrotrophin receptor antibodies in Graves' disease. Clin Endocrinol. (Oxf) 4: 517-522
46. **Weetman A, Wiersinga WM** 1998 Current management of thyroid-associated ophthalmopathy in Europe. Results of an international survey. Clin Endocrinol. (Oxf) 49: 21-28
47. **Bartalena L, Marcocci C, Pinchera A** 1998 Therapy for hyperthyroidism and Graves' ophthalmopathy. N Engl J Med. 338: 1546-1547 (Letter)
48. **DeGroot LJ** 1997 Radioiodine and the immune system. Thyroid 7: 259-264

21
GRAVES' DERMOPATHY

Terry J. Smith

INTRODUCTION

The dermopathy associated with Graves' disease, sometimes referred to as circumscribed myxedema, represents a curious process of tissue remodeling that is both unusual and characteristic. While dermopathy occurs most commonly in the skin of the anterior shin, involvement of a wide variety of other anatomic regions has been documented. Often the lesions found in unusual places have been preceded by trauma. Depending upon the particular series, dermopathy has been found to occur in approximately 3% of individuals with Graves' disease and almost invariably is seen in those patients who also manifest ophthalmopathy (TAO). This relationship between involvement of the two distant anatomic regions in Graves' disease implies that a common etiologic factor might be driving the orbital and dermal processes. Certainly the two manifestations share common histochemical features. But the tissue changes in both remain ill defined with regard to the early cellular and molecular events that initiate and sustain them and no therapeutic strategy has proven consistently effective and safe in either. In this chapter, I will attempt to review our current understanding of the pathogenesis of Graves' dermopathy and the treatment options currently available.

DESCRIPTION OF DERMOPATHY

It is believed that Von Basedow was the first to describe the dermopathy associated with Graves' disease (1). He wrote in 1840 that:

'the legs became, from the lower third of the thighs to extremities, very fat, however not edematous, the cellular tissues seemed rather brawny, such as often found in chlorosis, on pressure leaves no dent and often acupuncture [sic] produces no falling out of serum'.

This presentation of myxedema we now refer to as the elephantiasic form of the disease.

Nearly 60 years later, Osler described an apparently different presentation of the same process and thus provided documentation that the presentation of the disease can be diverse. The classification system proposed for pretibial myxedema by Cairns includes three types 1) sharply circumscribed with both nodular and tuberous lesions appearing on the shins and toes 2) diffuse with solid, nonpitting edema of the shins and feet and 3) a form resembling elephantiasis in which both edema and nodular lesions can occur. Examples of dermopathy are pictured in Fig. 1.

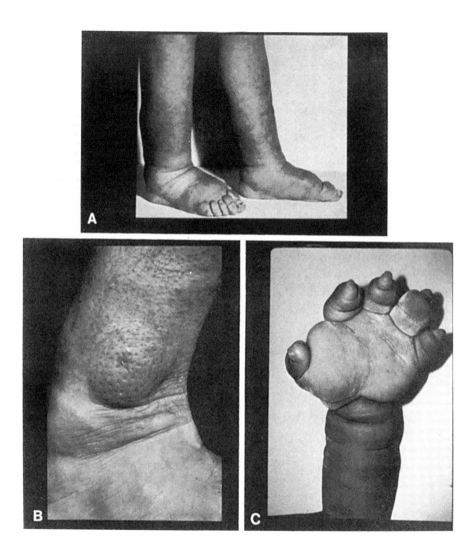

Figure 1. Types of myxedema. (A) Elephantiasic form. (B) Nodular form. Notice the thickened, orange-peel appearance of the dermis. The prominence of hair follicles is caused by interfollicular edema. © Severe localized myxedema of the hand and arm in a patient who had self-administered multiple intravenous injections. (Reproduced with permission from Smith TJ, Bahn RS, Gorman CA. Connective tissue, glycosaminoglycans and diseases of the thyroid. Endocr Rev. 10:366-391)

The factors governing the emergence of one pattern of myxedema lesion as opposed to another in a given patient are uncertain but the different forms are thought to share common etiologies. The timing of onset of ophthalmopathy and dermopathy often does not coincide but the tight association between the two is unmistakable. It is stated that onset of ophthalmopathy occurs within 18 months before or after the onset of hyperthyroidism in 80% of patients. Virtually all individuals with clinically significant dermopathy manifest substantial eye disease. The most unusual aspects of the tissue remodeling shared by these dermal and orbital lesions in Graves' disease relate to the disordered accumulation of hyaluronan, an abundant glycosaminoglycan or complex carbohydrate (2). With regard to the skin of the leg, the increase in tissue volume accounts for the edema. Lesions of dermopathy resist deformation, usually allowing the distinction with cardiogenic edema to be made on clinical grounds. Dermopathy has been reviewed by several investigators. Among the earliest and most comprehensive is that of Trotter and Eden in 1942 containing 73 previously reported cases and 4 cases of their own (3). They appreciated the common features shared by hypothyroid and Graves' disease associated myxedema, including the accumulation of a "mucin"-like substance which we now know is largely composed of glycosamino-glycan. A much larger and more comprehensive review has appeared (4). It contained a 20 year experience with dermopathy and contained 150 cases, 33 of whom were men. Pretibial dermopathy occurred most frequently in the sixth decade of life. All patients save one had ophthalmopathy with the mean proptosis of 22.2 mm in the right eye and 22.6 mm in the left. The study concluded that dermopathy occurred late in Graves' disease and that complete remission, even after long term follow-up, was not common.

HISTOLOGY

The histological appearance of dermopathy includes edema and the deposition of metachromatic-staining material that is digested with hyaluronidase. This material separates frayed, swollen collagen fibers (2,5,6). Features of inflammation are characteristically absent, although a single case involved extensive numbers of eosinophils (7). In a study by Matsuoka and colleagues (8), elastic fibers were reported to be sparse and fragmented in 5 patients with dermopathy, including three who were hypothyroid. This histological picture was also evident in 6 of 7 patients with primary hypothyroidism. In contrast, the histology associated with ophthalmopathy includes the infiltration of numerous lymphocytes which have been found to include both CD4[+] and CD8[+] cells (9,10). However, the predominant population is a topic of some debate. In addition to the lymphocytes, mast cells can be found abundantly in the affected orbital tissue (11).

PATHOGENESIS OF THE EXTRA-THYROIDAL MANIFESTATIONS of GRAVES' DISEASE

The proposed role of the fibroblast

Several investigators have suggested that the fibroblast might play a central role in the pathogenesis of the extrathyroidal manifestations of Graves' disease, including ophthalmopathy and dermopathy. The well-recognized, diverse biosynthetic activities ascribed to fibroblasts make such a role plausible (12). For instance, fibroblasts are known to produce large amounts of glycosaminoglycan and collagen, two abundant and important components of the extracellular matrix that figure prominently in the histopathological picture of both pretibial and orbital disease. But there is currently very little direct evidence that the fibroblast is the key cellular figure in either of the disease processes. Rather, circumstantial evidence points to the fibroblasts as critical to at least some of the discreet processes in tissue remodeling found in Graves' disease. The fibroblasts from the orbit and pretibial skin have been examined and are found to possess phenotypic attributes that set them apart from other fibroblasts. However, they differ substantially from each other. Thus, we hypothesize that it is these peculiar cellular features that are exhibited by orbital and pretibial fibroblasts that underlie the propensity of these two anatomic regions for involvement in Graves' disease. A recent report from Young *et al* suggested that the protein phenotype of cytokine-treated orbital and pre-tibial dermal fibroblasts differed from that observed in fibroblasts from an area of the body (abdominal skin) that is ordinarily not involved in the manifestations of Graves' disease (13). In particular, a set of proteins was found to be inducible by the lymphocyte-derived cytokine, leukoregulin. These proteins are induced in orbital and pretibial fibroblasts but not in the abdominal wall fibroblasts. While the identities of these proteins are as yet uncertain, they remain attractive candidates as factors that potentially tie together the involvement in the orbit and pretibial skin.

The factor(s) responsible for the trafficking of immunocompetent cells, including lymphocytes and mast cells, to the orbit and pretibial skin has not been found. Recently, a number of investigators have provided evidence that orbital connective tissue, particularly the fibroblast, expresses thyrotropin receptor (TSHR) mRNA and protein (14-16). The finding of TSHR expressed by orbital and pretibial fibroblasts has suggested to some that the receptor might represent an autoantigen potentially linking together the thyroid gland and these tissues. They have contended that the expression of the TSHR is anatomically restricted to fibroblasts derived from the areas manifesting Graves' disease but not from those areas of the body where myxedema does not occur. Seeming to contradict this hypothesis is the finding of TSHR in fibroblasts from areas of the body seemingly irrelevant to Graves' disease, including the omentum and subcutaneous abdominal wall fat (17). Thus while the TSHR may well play an important role in the pathogenesis of TAO and pretibial myxedema, it is unlikely that site restricted expression of the receptor can account for the peculiar disease distribution. Rather, the substantial differences in phenotype exhibited by orbital and pretibial fibroblasts compared with other fibroblasts, especially in the setting of activation by cytokines, suggests that their respective biosynthetic repertoires might account for the anatomical distribution of the disease.

Hyaluronan accumulation is a key component of both TAO and pretibial myxedema

Hyaluronan, a non-sulfated glycosaminoglycan, is synthesized by a wide-array of cell types. The disordered accumulation of this polymer in Graves' disease has not been convincingly ascribed to a particular cell but it is presumed that the fibroblast is the most important source. When the tissue from the orbit or dermopathic skin is stained with alcian blue or toluidine blue, abundant extracellular material stains with a metachromatic quality. This is abolished with hyaluronidase treatment, suggesting that the material is hyaluronan. However, because of the uncertainty of the type of hyaluronidase used in these studies, the specificity of the enzyme cannot be ascertained. The hydrophilic nature hyaluronan molecules and the dramatic volumes they assume when hydrated are thought to account for the substantial increases in volume that propel orbital contents anteriorly in TAO. Hyaluronan differs from the other abundant glycosaminoglycans by virtue of an absence of a core protein backbone. However, the rheological properties of hyaluronan are very similar to the other glycosaminoglycans and the hydrated molecule is extremely bulky. Watson and Pearse characterized the mucin-like material accumulating in the skin of two patients with dermopathy and confirmed that acid glycosaminoglycans were predominant components (18). They found that much of the material reacted with hyaluronidase. A subsequent study conducted by Sisson determined that the glycosaminoglycan content of the dermopathic skin, consisting mainly of hyaluronan, was 6 to 16 fold increased above normal controls (19). A more recent study by Shishiba *et al* (20) examined and characterized the proteoglycans accumulating in dermopathic skin. While an important biological result of hyaluronan accumulation relates to the increase in water-binding and attendant expansion of tissue volume, another biological consequence of such a deposition has only recently been recognized. Noble and colleagues have reported that short-chain hyaluronan is capable of inducing a number of macrophage genes that are relevant to inflammation (21,22). At least some of these immunological effects might be mediated through surface CD44, a putative hyaluronan receptor. While the profile of hyaluronan chains occurring in dermopathy and ophthalmopathy remain uncertain, it is possible that the macromolecule may amplify the inflammatory response through this newly identified mechanism.

Orbital fibroblasts have been shown to exhibit an enormous capacity to produce hyaluronan in response to pro-inflammatory cytokines such as leukoregulin, a 50 kDa product of activated T lymphocytes and IL-1 (23). Hyaluronan synthesis in irrelevant fibroblasts, such as those from the abdominal wall is substantially less and the effects on pretibial fibroblasts are intermediate. It would appear that the regulation of hyaluronan accumulation by cytokines in fibroblasts is mediated at the level of macromolecular synthesis since hyaluronan degradation is nil in human fibroblast cultures (24). It would also seem that the exaggerated responses to pro-inflammatory cytokines with regard to hyaluronan synthesis found in the orbital fibroblasts are not shared with those cells from the pretibial skin (23,25). This may relate more to the degree of the hyaluronan accumulation in the two anatomic sites rather than to qualitative differences in the disease mechanism. It should be remembered that those studies involved fibroblasts from skin that was not grossly dermatopathic. Clearly, more detailed studies examining the expression and regulation of the hyaluronan biosynthetic cascade are warranted. The relationship between the circulating immunoglobulins found in Graves' disease and the pathogenesis of dermopathy are uncertain but some early reports had suggested that these antibodies could enhance glycosaminoglycan and proteoglycan production in fibroblasts (26-28).

Progress into defining the molecular control of hyaluronan synthesis in normal tissues and under pathological situations, such as exists in TAO and dermopathy, had languished for many years because of our inability to clone and characterize the synthetic enzymes. Insight into the mechanisms related to biosynthesis of hyaluronan has been enhanced by the recent identification and cloning of three members of a family of mammalian hyaluronan synthase genes (29-31) and a UDP glucose dehydrogenase gene (32). The three hyaluronan synthase genes exhibit substantial sequence identity. The question of why there should be three closely related HAS proteins, each encoded by a separate gene, is as yet unanswered but could relate to differences in tissue distribution of enzyme expression, subcellular location, substrate utilization or variations in size or fate of the enzyme products. In any event, the recent identification of several important components of the hyaluronan synthetic cascade and the recognition that several of these are regulatable should help invigorate investigation into the molecular pathogenesis of dermopathy. Relevant to the pathogenesis of Graves' disease, a report has emerged demonstrating that IL-1ß can induce in orbital fibroblasts the mRNAs encoding all three of these hyaluronan synthases (33). Moreover, the induction could be attenuated by glucocorticoids. Another study demonstrated that IL-1ß could induce UDP glucose dehydrogenase mRNA in orbital fibroblasts (32). Thus, it is possible that an increase hyaluronan synthase and UDP glucose dehydrogenase expression is at least partially responsible for the accumulation of hyaluronan seen in the manifestations of Graves' disease.

Several genes are differentially regulated in orbital and pretibial fibroblasts

One gene that appears to be particularly inducible in orbital fibroblasts is prostaglandin endoperoxide H synthase (PGHS-2 or COX-2), the inflammatory cyclo-oxygenase (34). This bifunctional enzyme is expressed at extremely low levels in most normal tissue and cell types but when the tissues are inflamed or cells exposed to mitogens, growth factors or cytokines, PGHS-2 expression is dramatically up-regulated (34). In contrast to PGHS-2, the isoform designated PGHS-1 is constitutively expressed in most cell and tissue types. Moreover, PGHS-1 unlike PGHS-2, is poorly regulated but seems to be expressed at more or less constant levels in health and disease. PGHS-1 is currently felt to produce the vast majority of prostanoids involved in housekeeping functions such as the maintenance of the epithelium of the gastrointestinal tissues (34). From recent studies, it would seem that in some tissues, such as thyroid epithelium, PGHS-2 is expressed at high levels under physiological conditions (35). When orbital fibroblasts, particularly those from individuals with TAO, are treated with IL-1ß or leukoregulin, PGHS-2 mRNA and protein expression, and PGE_2 production, are dramatically up-regulated (36). The vast majority of the increase in prostanoid production can be blocked with SC 58125, a PGHS-2 selective inhibitor (36). In contrast to orbital fibroblasts, PGHS-2 expression in abdominal wall dermal fibroblasts is modestly increased while in pretibial dermal fibroblast cultures, PGHS-2 expression is decreased by the pro-inflammatory cytokines (36). These fibroblasts actually express higher levels of constitutive PGHS-2 than that observed in most other fibroblast types.

Pretibial fibroblasts exhibit a pattern of PGHS-2 induction that is different from orbital and abdominal wall (irrelevant) fibroblasts. They appear to express low levels of basal PGHS-2 but when treated with cytokines that up-regulate the cyclooxgenase in other fibroblasts, the levels of PGHS-2 are reduced. This down-regulation of PGHS-2 in pretibial fibroblasts may underlie the characteristic absence of inflammation in dermopathic skin.

Of potential importance to the accumulation of extracellular matrix components in dermopathic skin and in TAO is the demonstration of differential inducibility of plasminogen activator inhibitor type-1 (PAI-1) in fibroblasts from distinct anatomic regions (37). PAI-1 is a 50 kDa glyco-polypeptide that is a serine protease inhibitor. It can form complexes with both tissue and urinary forms of plasminogen activator. Its key function when accumulating in the extracellular matrix is to modulate the pericellular proteolytic environment and stabilize the matrix. In human fibroblasts, interferon-γ, leukoregulin and transforming growth factor-β regulate the expression of PAI-1 (37-40). In orbital fibroblasts, interferon-γ induces PAI-1 expression dramatically while it down-regulates expression or only modestly enhances PAI-1 synthesis in dermal fibroblast strains (37). Similar inductions in orbital cultures were noted after treatment with leukoregulin. This profound increase in PAI-1 mass elicited by pro-inflammatory cytokines might represent the basis for at least a portion of the extracellular protein accumulation in dermopathy and in orbital disease.

Mechanisms for the activation of fibroblasts in Graves' disease

The identity of the proximate signals that activate fibroblasts in Graves' disease remain uncertain. These are thought to emanate from bone marrow derived cells which are trafficked to the lesions. Lymphocytes and mast cells can be found in the affected tissue of the orbit and it is presumed that some factor(s) emanating from these and other bone marrow derived cells are acting locally to up-regulate the expression of fibroblast genes and their products that participate in tissue remodeling. A number of candidate molecules, including IL-1α and TGF-β have been identified and localized to affected orbital tissue with immunostaining (41). The techniques used may not have been specific, are certainly not quantitative and thus may have inaccurately portrayed the cytokine environment in the disease. Moreover, the limited access to tissue early in TAO, when such measurements might faithfully reflect those factors initiating the disease, has confounded efforts to identify the proximate causes of the orbital and dermopathic changes. With regard to dermopathic skin, very little is known about the cytokine environment in those lesions. The potential role of the antibodies associated with Graves' disease in directly activating fibroblasts has been suggested, but no consistent action of these immunoglobulins has thus far been convincingly demonstrated. Clearly, such an interaction would be possible, either through the thyrotropin receptor or utilizing another surface-displayed determinate.

It was shown recently that certain types of human fibroblasts, including those from the orbit, express the surface receptor CD40 (42). This member of the tumor necrosis factor-α (TNF-α) receptor family was originally found to be expressed on B lymphocytes and represents an important B cell activational molecule. Its natural ligand, CD154, also known as CD40 ligand, is a member of the TNF-α family and is expressed by T lymphocytes and mast cells. When CD40 displayed on the surfaces of fibroblasts is ligated with CD154 in cell culture, a number of inflammatory genes are activated, perhaps through an activation of NF-κB. These include the pro-inflammatory cytokines IL-6 and IL-8 (42). The expression of PGHS-2 is also up-regulated and this is mediated through an intermediate induction of IL-1α. This inductive process involves the mitogen-activated protein kinase pathway and results in substantial increases in PGE$_2$ production (43). Hyaluronan synthesis is up-regulated substantially in orbital fibroblasts by CD40 ligation in orbital fibroblasts but may not involve an increase in hyaluronan synthase expression. The increase in PGHS-2 expression and hyaluronan synthesis can be attenuated by glucocorticoids (43). Thus, the CD40/CD40 ligand bridge represents a novel pathway for fibroblast/lymphocyte crosstalk that could help explain how immunocompetent cells activate fibroblasts. Moreover, the findings define a novel pathway the disruption of which represents a potential therapeutic target for TAO and Graves' dermopathy.

TREATMENT OF DERMOPATHY

The uncertainty surrounding the pathogenesis of dermopathy has undermined development of rational and effective therapeutic strategies. Many approaches to treatment have been attempted with inconsistent results. Fortunately, most cases of dermopathy are relatively mild and do not require specific therapy. When the disease leads to concerns over the cosmetic appearance, tissue breakdown or infection, a number of strategies have been used. Compressive bandages, including Jobst stockings, have been very helpful in disease where there is some superficial lymphatic obstruction, such as is the case in the elephantiasic form of dermopathy.

Glucocorticoid steroids

In their review of glucocorticoid therapy in dermopathy, published 30 years ago, Benoit and Greenspan noted that most reports of clinical experiences with glucocorticoids contained single cases and that both the methods and the results varied widely (44). Thus, the lack of standardization in the early studies precluded meaningful comparisons between them. Kriss and co-workers reported a well-controlled series of 11 patients to whom fluocinolone acetonide as a 0.02% cream was applied directly on affected tissue over which occlusive plastic film was placed (45). The treatment was repeated 3-7 times per week and was followed by a maintenance regimen of 2-4 applications each month. The daily dosage never exceeded 2g per day. This strategy yielded improvement in all patients so treated. The use of systemic glucocorticoids for dermopathy is rarely indicated because of the morbidity associated with it. When aggressive orbital disease requiring such intervention is accompanied by dermopathy, improvement of the skin disease has been noted in many cases. In their series of dermopathic patients, Fatourechi *et al* found that of the 76 patients receiving topical steroids, 29 (38%) experienced a partial remission (4). This compared to an 18% rate in the control group.

Glucocorticoids probably exert most of their benefit on the extra-thyroidal lesions of Graves' disease through a down-regulation of inflammatory mediators. Because many of the lesions of dermopathy are not predominately inflammatory but appear to be largely a consequence of the disordered accumulation of hyaluronan, it should not be entirely surprising that this class of drug is not uniformly effective. The mechanism through which steroids might promote therapeutic action is uncertain. Lymphocytes and mast cells are present in TAO but appear to be absent or not abundant in dermopathic skin and could represent important targets for glucocorticoid action. On the other hand, fibroblasts have been shown to express the glucocorticoid receptor. The up-regulation of hyaluronan synthesis in cultured fibroblasts, provoked by pro-inflammatory cytokines such as leukoregulin, CD40 ligation and IL-1ß, can be partially attenuated by glucocorticoids (23). In addition, basal hyaluronan synthesis in dermal fibroblasts can be inhibited by these steroids (24). But the accumulation of hyaluronan in dermopathy probably occurs slowly, over relatively long time intervals and acute treatment with corticosteroids might not provide the sustained inhibition to meaningfully influence such an accumulation.

Alternative therapies

Beside glucocorticoid steroids, other agents have been evaluated in very limited studies, including the somatostatin analogue, octreotide (46). Plasmapheresis has also been attempted (47). These therapies have yielded positive results in some patients but the studies are too preliminary to conclude whether the modalities should be pursued.

CONCLUSIONS

Current understanding of the pathogenesis of myxedema and ophthalmopathy is very limited. The link between orbital, dermal and thyroidal tissues is uncertain as is the identity of the factor activating connective tissue in Graves' disease. Current treatment of both extrathyroidal components of the disease is inadequate. The most rewarding efforts directed toward therapy development are likely to be those which will yield fundamental insights into the anatomic site-selective signaling of connective tissue by the immune system.

REFERENCES

1.   **von Basedow KA** 1840 Exophthalmos durch hypertrophie des zellgewebes in der Augenhöhle. Wochenschr Ges Heilk Berl. 6:197
2.   **Smith TJ, Bahn RS, Gorman CA.** 1989 Connective tissue, glycosaminoglycans, and diseases of the thyroid. Endocrine Rev. 10:366-391.
3.   **Trotter WR, Eden KC.** 1942 Localized pretibial myxoedema in association with toxic goiter. Q J Med 11:229-240.
4.   **Fatourechi V, Pajouhi M, Fransway AF.** 1994 Dermopathy of Graves disease (pretibial myxedema): Review of 150 cases. Medicine. 73:1-7.
5.   **Truhan AP, Roenigk Jr HH.** 1986 The cutaneous mucinoses. J Am Acad Dermatol. 14:1-18.

6.   **Mullin GE, Eastern JS.** 1986 Cutaneous consequences of accelerated thyroid function. Cutis. 37:109-114.

7.   **Pegum JS, Grice K.** 1973 unusual skin eruption with eosinophilia associated with hyperthyroidism. Br J Dermatol. 88:295-301.

8.   **Matsuoka LY, Wortsman J, Uitto J, Hashimoto K, Kupchella CE, Eng AM, Dietrich JE.** 1985 Altered skin elastic fibers in hypothyroid myxedema and pretibial myxedema. Arch Intern Med. 145:117-121.

9.   **De Carli M, D'Elios MM, Mariotti S, Marocci C, Pinchera A, Ricci M, Romagnani S, Del Prete G.** 1993 Cytolitic T cells with Th1-like cytokine profile predominate in retroorbital lymphocyte infiltrates of Graves' ophthalmopathy. J Clin Endocrinol Metab. 77:1120-1124.

10. **Grubec-Loebenstein B, Trieb K, Sztankay A, Holter W, Anderi H, Wick G.** 1994 Retrobulbar T cells from patients with Graves' ophthalmopathy are CD8[+] and specifically recognize autologous fibroblasts. J Clin Invest. 93:2738-2743.

11. **Hufnagel TJ, Hickey WF, Cobbs WH, Jakobiec FA, Iwamoto T, Eagle RC.** 1984 Immunohistochemical and ultrastructural studies on the exenterated orbital tissues from a patient with Graves' disease. Ophthalmology 91:1411-1419.

12. **Smith RS, Smith TJ, Blieden TM, Phipps RP.** 1997 Fibroblasts as sentinel cells: synthesis of chemokines and regulation of inflammation. Am J Pathol. 151:317-322.

13. **Young DA, Evans CH, Smith TJ.** 1998 Leukoregulin induction of protein expression in human orbital fibroblasts: evidence for anatomical site-restricted cytokine-target cell interactions. Proc Natl Acad Sci USA. 95:8904-8909.

14. **Heufelder AE, Dutton CM, Sarkar G, Donovan KA, Bahn RS.** 1993 Detection of TSH receptor mRNA incultured fibroblasts from patients with Graves' ophthalmopathy and pretibial dermopathy. Thyroid. 3:297-300.

15. **Mengistu M, Lukes YG, Nagy EV,** 1994 TSH receptor expression in retroocular fibroblasts. J Endocrinol Invest. 17:437-441.

16. **Feliciello A, Porcellini A, Ciullo , Bonavolonta G, Avvedimento EV, Fenzi G.** 1993 Expression of thyrotropin-receptor mRNA in healthy and Graves' retroorbital tissue. Lancet. 342:337-338.

17. **Bell Andrea, Grunder L, Gagnon A, Parikh SJ, Smith TJ, Sorisky A.** 1999 Expression of functional TSH protein in human abdominal preadipocytes and orbital fibroblasts in primary culture. (Submitted for publication)

18. **Watson EM, Pearce RH.** 1947 The mucopolysaccharide content of the skin in localized (pretibial) myxedema. Am J Clin Pathol. 17:507-512.

19. **Sisson JC.** 1968 Hyaluronic acid in localized myxedema. J Clin Endocrinol Metab. 28:433-436.

20. **Shishiba Y, Tanaka T, Ozawa Y, Shimizu T, Kadowaki N.** 1986 Chemical characterization of high buoyant density proteoglycan accumulation in the affected skin of pretibial myxedema of Graves' disease. Endocrinol Jpn. 33:395-403.

21. **Horton MR, Burdick MD, Strieter RM, Bao C, Noble PW.** 1998 Regulation of hyaluronan-induced chemokine gene expression by IL-10 and IFN-gamma in mouse macrophages. J Immunol. 160:3023-3030.

22. **McKee CM, Penno MB, Cowman M, Burdick MD, Strieter RM, Bao C, Noble PW.** 1996 Hyaluronan (HA) fragments induce chemokine gene expression in alveolar macrophages. The role of HA size and CD44. J Clin Invest. 98:2403-2413.

23. **Smith TJ, Wang H-S, Evans CH.** 1995 Leukoregulin is a potent inducer of hyaluronan synthesis in cultured human orbital fibroblasts. Am J Physiol. 268:C382-C388.

24. **Smith TJ.** 1984 Dexamethasone regulation of glycosaminoglycan synthesis in cultured human skin fibroblasts: similar effects of glucocorticoid and thyroid hormones. J Clin Invest. 74:2157-2163.

25. **Smith TJ, Bahn RS, Gorman CA, Cheavens M.** 1991 Stimulation of glycosaminoglycan accumulation by interferon gamma in cultured human retroocular fibroblasts. J Clin Endocrinol Metab. 72:1169-1171.
26. **Cheung HS, Nicoloff JT, Kamiel MB, Spolter L, Nimni ME.** 1978 Stimulation of fibroblast biosynthetic activity by serum of patients with pretibial myxedema. J Invest Dermatol. 71:12-17.
27. **Shishiba Y, Imai Y, Odajima R, Ozawa Y, Shimizu T.** 1992 Immunoglobulin G of patients with circumscribed pretibial myxedema of Graves' disease stimulates proteoglycan synthesis in human skin fibroblasts in culture. Acta Endocrinol. 127:44-51.
28. **Kriss JP, Pleshakov V, Chien JR.** 1964 Isolation and identification of the long-acting thyroid stimulator and its relation to hyperthyroidism and circumscribed pretibial myxedema. J Clin Endocrinol Metab. 24:1005-1028.
29. **Shyjan AM, Heldin P, Butcher EC, Yoshino T, Briskin MJ.** Functional cloning of the cDNA for a human hyaluronan synthase. J Biol Chem. 271:23395-23399.
30. **Spicer AP, Olson JS, McDonald JA.** 1997 Molecular cloning and characterization of a cDNA encoding the third putative mammalian hyaluronan synthase. J Biol Chem. 272:8957-8961.
31. **Watanabe K, Yamaguchi Y.** 1996 Molecular identification of a putative human hyaluronan synthase. J Biol Chem. 271:22945-22948.
32. **Spicer AP, Kaback LA, Smith TJ, Seldin MF.** 1998 Molecular cloning and characterization of the human and mouse UDP-glucoase dehydrogenase genes. J Biol Chem. 273:25117-25124.
33. **Kaback LA, Smith TJ.** 1999 Expression of hyaluronan synthase mRNAs and their induction by IL-1ß in human orbital fibroblasts: potential insight into the molecular pathogenesis of thyroid-associated ophthalmopathy. J Clin Endocrinol Metab (in press).
34. **Smith WL, Garavito RM, DeWitt DL.** 1996 Prostaglandin endoperoxide H synthases (cyclooxygenases)-1 and -2. J Biol Chem. 271:33157-33160.
35. **Smith TJ, Jennings TA, Sciaky D, Cao HJ.** 1999 Prostaglandin-endoperoxide H synthase-2 expression in human thyroid epithelium: evidence for constitutive expression *in vivo* and in cultured KAT-50 cells. J Biol Chem. 274:15622-15632.
36. **Wang H-S, Cao HJ, Winn VD, Rezanka LJ, Frobert LJ, Evans CH, Sciaky DS, Young DA, Smith TJ.** 1996 Leukoregulin induction of prostaglandin-endoperoxide H synthase-2 in human orbital fibroblasts: an *in vitro* model for connective tissue inflammation. J Biol Chem. 271:22718-22728.
37. **Smith TJ, Ahmed A, Hogg MG, Higgins PJ.** 1992 Interferon-γ is an inducer of plasminogen activator inhibitor type 1 in human orbital fibroblasts. Am J Physiol. 263:C24-C29.
38. **Smith TJ, Higgins PJ.** 1993 Interferon gamma regulation of *de novo* protein synthesis in human dermal fibroblasts in culture is anatomic-site dependent. J Invest Derm. 100:288-292.
39. **Cao HJ, Hogg MG, Martino LJ, Smith TJ.** 1995 Transforming growth factor-ß induces plasminogena activator inhibitor type-1 in cultured human orbital fibroblasts. Invest Ophthalmol Vis Sci. 36:1411-1419.
40. **Hogg MG, Evans CH, Smith TJ.** 1995 Leukoregulin induces plasminogen activator inhibitor type-1 in human orbital fibroblasts. Am J Physiol. 269:C359-C366.
41. **Heufelder AE, Bahn RS.** 1993 Detection and localization of cytokine immunoreactivity in retro-ocular connective tissue in Graves' ophthalmopathy. Eur J Clin Invest. 23:10-17.
42. **Sempowski GD, Rozenblit J, Smith TJ, Phipps RP.** 1998 Human orbital fibroblasts are activated through CD40 to induce proinflammatory cytokine production. Am J Physiol. 274:C707-C714.
43. **Cao HJ, Wang H-S, Zhang Y, Lin H-Y, Phipps RP, Smith TJ.** 1998 Activation of

human orbital fibroblasts through CD40 engagement results in a dramatic induction of hyaluronan synthesis and prostaglandin endoperoxide H synthase-2 expression. J Biol Chem. 273:29615-29625.

44. **Benoit FL, Greenspan FS.** 1967 Corticoid therapy for pretibial myxedema: observations on the long-acting thyroid stimulator. Ann Int Med. 66:711-720.

45. **Kriss JP, Pleshakov V, Rosenblum A, Sharp G.** 1967 Therapy with occlusive dressings of pretibial myxedema with fluocinolone acetonide. J Clin Endocrinol Metab. 27:595-604.

46. **Chang TC, Kao SCS, Huang KM.** 1992 Octreotide and Graves' ophthalmopathy and pretibial myxoedema. Brit Med J. 304:158.

47. **Noppen M, Velkeniers B, Steenssens L, Vanhaelst L.** 1988 Beneficial effects of plasmapheresis followed by immunosuppressive therapy in pretibial myxedema. Acta Clin Belg. 43:381-383.

INDEX

Note: Page numbers in *italics* refer to illustrations; page numbers followed by *t* refer to tables.